Anti-Aging Therapeutics
Volume X
2007 Conference Year

Editors
Dr. Ronald Klatz
and
Dr. Robert Goldman

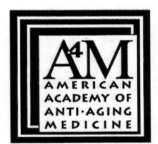 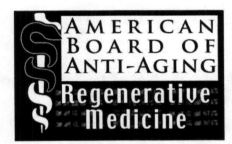 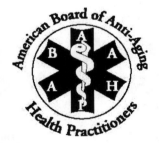

An official educational work published by A4M Publications
1510 West Montana Street
Chicago, IL 60614 USA
TEL: (773) 528-4333; FAX: (773) 528-5390; E-MAIL: a4m@worldhealth.net
WEBSITE: www.worldhealth.net

Visit
The World Health Network, at www.**worldhealth.net**, the Internet's leading anti-aging portal;
And
The A4M's Special Information Center, at **www.a4minfo.net**, the A4M's Publishing and Media Showcase

IMPORTANT – PLEASE READ

The content presented in the *Anti-Aging Therapeutics, volume 10* is for educational purposes only and is specifically designed for those with a health, medical, or biotechnological education or professional experience. *Anti-Aging Therapeutics, volume 10* does not prevent, diagnose, treat or cure disease or illness.

While potentially therapeutic pharmaceuticals, nutraceuticals (dietary supplementation) and interventive therapies are described in the A4M's *Anti-Aging Therapeutics, volume 10*, this work serves the sole purpose of functioning as an informational resource. Under no circumstances is the reader to construe endorsement by A4M of any specific companies or products. Quite to the contrary, *Caveat Emptor*. It is the reader's responsibility to investigate the product, the vendor, and the product information.

Dosing of nutraceuticals can be highly variable. Proper dosing is based on parameters including sex, age, and whether the patient is well or ill (and, if ill, whether it is a chronic or acute situation). Additionally, efficiency of absorption of a particular type of product and the quality of its individual ingredients are two major considerations for choosing appropriate specific agents for an individual's medical situation.

Furthermore, anyone with malignancy should consult their physician or oncologist prior to beginning, or continuing, any hormone therapy program.

Finally, please be mindful that just because a product is natural doesn't mean it's safe for everyone. A small portion of the general population may react adversely to components in nutraceuticals (especially herbal products). A complete inventory of interventions utilized by a patient should be maintained by physicians and health practitioners dispensing anti-aging medical care.

Anti-Aging Therapeutics, volume 10 is, again, designed for those with a health, medical, or biotechnological education or professional experience. It is not intended to provide medical advice, and is not to be used as a substitute for advice from a physician or health practitioner. If you are a consumer interested in any of the approaches discussed in these chapters, it is absolutely essential that you have a thorough discussion with your physician to understand all benefits and risks.

For those individuals interested in the diagnostics and/or therapies described by chapter authors of *Anti-Aging Therapeutics, volume 10*, A4M urges that you consult a knowledgeable physician or health practitioner, preferably one who has been Board Certified in Anti-Aging Medicine. You may find one by utilizing the Online Physician/Practitioner Locator at the A4M's educational website, www.worldhealth.net, or you may call our international headquarters in Chicago, IL USA at (773) 528-4333.

Table of Contents

* Denotes speaker at Spring 2007 Session of the Annual International Congress on Anti-Aging Medicine & Regenerative Biomedical Technologies;
** Denotes speaker at Summer 2007 Session;
*** Denotes speaker at Winter 2007 Session.

Chapter 1
Creating a Healthy Weight: The Foundation of Longevity

Wayne Scott Andersen, D.O. B.C.CCM, B.C. Anest*; Tom Lycan, Jr.
* Executive Director, The Health Institute; Medical Director,
Medifast and Take Shape for Life

ABSTRACT

The vast majority of Americans have become overweight and obese, an unsettling trend that has increased the rates of obesity-related disease, including but not limited to, diabetes, metabolic syndrome, and cardiovascular disease. Aside from a number of cultural factors, one problem may be the reactive approach to weight loss that many Americans take after having already become obese, an attitude that may lead to increased chances of regaining any weight that is lost. A weight loss protocol that focuses on achieving and maintaining an optimal weight through calorie restriction diet plans that incorporate meal replacements may aid in long-term weight control. This protocol recommends the consumption of low-calorie, low glycemic index (GI), portion-controlled meals in conjunction with the establishment of daily habits of health and regular exercise. If this protocol were to be successfully implemented on a large scale among both obese and non-obese Americans, it could have the potential to prevent cases of obesity and obesity-related illness.

Keywords: obesity, nutrition, longevity, dieting, exercise

OBESITY IN AMERICA
Epidemiology

The United States has seen its obesity rate reach epidemic levels as around two-thirds of the American adult population is now considered to be either overweight or obese (NHLBI *Obes Res.*, 1998). This trend has been seen nationwide to varying degrees, as currently, all states have at least 15% of their population considered to be obese (body-mass index [BMI, kg/m^2] greater than 30). Even worse, most longitudinal projections indicate that this trend will continue well into the 21st century. One Baylor University study found that by the year 2030, all 50 states will have at least 25% of their population considered to be obese (Foreyt and Poston, 2002; Hellmich and Manning; 2002).

Complications

In terms of health problems, it has been shown that obese individuals, on average, suffer from a wider range of ailments and to a greater degree of severity than do lean individuals. For example, a person's risk of developing Type II diabetes increases by twelve times if they are considered to be extremely obese (BMI greater than 35) as compared to a person within the normal BMI range (18.5 to 25). Not surprisingly, the incidence of Type II diabetes in the United States has increased along with the levels of obesity. In 2000, the Centers for Disease Control and Prevention (CDC) estimated that the lifetime risk of developing Type II diabetes for an American newborn was 1 in 3. In Hispanic-Americans and African-American newborns the estimated lifetime risk was increased to 2 in 5, and a female Hispanic-American newborn was further increased to 1 in 2. Currently, there are 21 million Americans suffering from diabetes and the CDC estimates that another 54 million Americans are at elevated risk of developing it (prediabetes) (CDC, 2007).

However, an even wider phenomenon than diabetes is metabolic syndrome, a cluster of related medical disorders whose principal cause is obesity (Zieve, 2004). As a result, metabolic syndrome has become increasingly common in the American population with an increase that is thought to have paralleled the rise in obesity (Weiss *et al*, 2004). First described by Reaven in 1988, metabolic syndrome typically entails obesity, central adiposity, insulin resistance, inflammation, hypertension, hypercholesterolemia, increased circulation of triglycerides and low-density lipoproteins (LDL), and decreased circulation of high-density lipoproteins (HDL). Now estimated to affect approximately 70 million Americans, metabolic syndrome carries an increased risk of premature aging, disability, diabetes, heart disease, cancer, stroke, infections, sleep disorders, and death (Must *et al*, 1992; Berenson *et al*, 1998; Steinberger *et al*, 2002).

Associated Costs

From an economic perspective, there are significant effects of these obesity-related disease burdens upon the American health system. There are great costs associated with the countless medications, surgeries, and other interventions recommended to obese patients by health professionals in order to improve their functionality, quality of life, and overall health. The result has been an emphasis by the entire healthcare economic system upon the sicker portion of the population. It has been estimated that the sicker 50% of the population has required a full 97% of total healthcare expenditures; and further, the sickest 5% of the population has required around 50% of total healthcare expenditures (Zuvekas and Cohen, 2007). Clearly, there is relatively little money being spent by the United States healthcare system to prevent healthy people from becoming sick. This oversight therefore misses an opportunity to prevent large numbers of Americans from developing disease in the first place and thus spares the economy from significantly larger health bills once they become sick.

WEIGHT LOSS
Preventive Treatment

This focus on the prevention of disease would work especially well with the treatment of obesity. The increased risk of illness that is associated with obesity is not permanent and can be reversed to a certain extent following weight loss. Williamson *et al* (1995) found that intentional weight loss reduced risk of death from a variety of illnesses and led to an overall increase in life expectancy. Therefore, if obesity is successfully treated by health professionals before it can cause significantly damaging health effects in a patient, obesity-related diseases may be prevented for that patient altogether.

Weight loss is a realistic goal for almost all patients. An editorial in the *Journal of the American Medical Association* proposed that if psychological and logistical barriers were removed then most patients could attain a healthy weight within a matter of months (Dansinger and Schaefer, 2004). However, the methods by which sustainable weight loss can be successfully attained has been the subject of countless debates, with new techniques and fads periodically emerging and being championed by doctors, nutritionists, and pharmaceutical companies. The only certainty seems to be that there is no silver bullet; none of the diets, medications, or dietary supplements are sufficiently effective by themselves.

Hindrances to Dieting
Culture

One major obstacle facing Americans are the tempting messages being received from society with regards to unhealthy meals in terms of their taste and convenience. Food chains compete to offer the largest portions and the tastiest quantities of sugars and fat in meals; macronutrients which appeal most to the basal instincts of hunger but are extremely unhealthy. This nutritional pollution started to become prevalent in the 1970's and by today has completely permeated American society. Marketplace portions are now 2-8 times as large as standard serving sizes and they are sold nearly instantaneously at fast food locations, while sugary soft drinks of no nutritional value are offered in massive 64 ounce containers to wash it down. This phenomenon has been relatively unique to the United States. A study conducted at Pennsylvania State University found that fast food locations from the same chain sold portions that were 25% larger in Philadelphia as compared to Paris, France. Similarly, the average time spent eating at the same chain was 22.2 minutes in Paris and just 14.4 minutes in Philadelphia (Rozin *et al*, 2003). At home, the most popular American cookbook describes dishes with an average of 25% larger portion sizes, 53% larger meat portions, and 24% smaller vegetable portions as compared to its equivalent French cookbook (Rozin *et al*, 2003). All of these factors most likely contribute to the difference in obesity between these two locations, as around 12% of the French population is considered to be obese (Marques-Vidal *et al*, 2002) as compared to 32% of the American population (Wang and Beydoun, 2007).

Macronutrient Composition

In terms of the macronutrients that are featured in the average American meal as compared to other countries, the most striking aspect is the focus on components which are not only unhealthy but also poor at satisfying hunger. Protein and complex carbohydrates provide a greater degree of satiety and are eaten disproportionately less in the United States. On the other hand, simple carbohydrates and fat provide less satiety and are eaten disproportionately more by Americans. The worst offender, dietary fat, has a strong epidemiological relationship with obesity largely because it of its high energy density, extremely efficient storage in the body, and high palatability. It is clear that a person whose daily intake features a large number of calories derived from fat, which is common in the United States, has a much greater risk of developing obesity. In the United States the average person's daily diet had 34% of the calories derived from fats (Kennedy *et al*, 1999).

A diet that features an excess of simple carbohydrates can also lead to obesity but for slightly different reasons. Similar to fat, simple carbohydrates offer high palatability and little cost but provide little satiety as compared to complex carbohydrates or proteins. However, simple carbohydrates create an additional problem because of their rapid degradation into sugars which are subsequently absorbed into the bloodstream. Generally within a half hour of consuming simple carbohydrates the blood sugar level rises sharply, with a spike in insulin levels following soon after until all of the circulating sugar is absorbed. The amplitude of that rise in blood sugar (with its accompanying insulin spike) is a measurement of the glycemic index (GI) for that food (Jenkins *et al*, 1981). Simple carbohydrates generally have the highest GI measurements as compared to other macronutrients, a distinction which can lead to adverse eating behavior. A number of studies (De Rougemont *et al*, 2007; Ebbeling *et al*, 2007; Bahadori *et al*, 2005) reported that participants who were administered lower GI meals tended to lose more weight than those who were administered higher GI meals or were *ad libitum* controls. This phenomenon seems to occur via the following mechanism. After consuming a snack with a high GI the resultant insulin spike tends to lower the blood sugar level at a much more drastic rate than for lower GI foods, leading to renewed hunger within a shorter period of time. This cycle repeats if the person continues to eat foods with high GI as their insulin levels remain consistently high but their feelings of hunger and satiety rapidly alternate. The net result is that even though simple carbohydrates do not store energy as efficiently as fat, their high GI index leads to high rates of consumption within short periods of time.

Exercise

Apart from diet, there are other common aspects of the American lifestyle that impede weight loss. In 2005, the National Academies' Institute of Medicine recommended 60 minutes of exercise for weight maintenance and 90 minutes for weight loss. However, it is clear that a large portion of the United States population does not engage in that adequate level of exercise. According to Macera *et al* (2005), the majority of US adults do not engage in moderate or vigorous-intensity physical activities to levels that are correlated with good health. Another measurement of exercise is the number of steps taken per day by a person, data that can be readily collected by an inexpensive pedometer. Tudor-Locke and Bassett (2004) proposed the widely-publicized guideline of 10,000 steps per day as being the threshold for the classification of an "active" lifestyle. However, a study of 1,000 American adults by Wyatt *et al* (2005) found that the average adult took 6,804 steps per day, well below the "active" cut-off.

PROTOCOL

It is of little surprise that in the face of these numerous challenges, even among those Americans who are able to lose weight, an estimated 85% of them gain it all back within two years, which mostly negates benefits upon longevity. Nevertheless, there are four general guidelines to weight loss that are effective if followed sufficiently: a decrease in caloric intake, an increase in caloric expenditure, a healthier selection of food, and an orientation towards overall health. Most importantly with regard to longevity, these four guidelines must be established and sustained over time. These methods can be successfully enacted with the help and guidance of the healthcare provider, thus increasing the length and quality of their patients' lives.

In order to help patients achieve the four general guidelines to weight control, healthcare providers play an important role in positively motivating patients toward behavior changes that will help them attain optimal health. This can be achieved through the following four actions on the part of the healthcare provider: (1) understanding the patient's mindset, (2) engaging the patient in long-term health planning, (3) maintaining an appropriate calorie restricted diet plan; and (4) helping the patient to develop his or her own habits of optimal health. Each of these four actions, their rationale, and how they might best be implemented is described below.

Patient's Mindset

The first aspect of the weight loss paradigm is the patient's attitude towards weight loss. Many patients regard being overweight as a temporary problem that needs to be solved only in the face of overwhelming pressure. This type of attitude can actually be detrimental to the weight loss process because it ignores the overall goal of weight loss, improving quality of life and longevity. In doing so, the patient does not even consider weight loss as necessary unless there is enough social pressure, even if they are nowhere near their optimal healthy weight. Once there is enough social motivation, the patient may drop enough weight to remove that pressure but does not focus on maintenance of that loss, often regaining that weight within a relatively short period of time. The net result is a conflict manipulation cycle of temporary weight gain, pressure, and then temporary weight loss.

Instead, the emphasis needs to be on the true goal of weight loss; optimal health and longevity. By taking in the big picture, the patient works consistently to maintain their ideal weight, and in the process he or she is less susceptible to the rising and ebbing motivation of social pressure. This attitude is also the proper mindset that is needed to face the constant health choices confronted by Americans on a daily basis. By constantly working to eat healthy foods and to exercise regularly while avoiding junk foods, a patient establishes their own habits of health as those choices become automatic. In contrast, a patient caught in a conflict manipulation cycle only makes healthy choices when they are under pressure to do so, reverting back to unhealthy choices the rest of the time. And while it may not matter whether a patient chooses to eat a meal of greasy fast food one time, if they choose to eat that meal every day for six months out of the year then all of those negative health effects quickly accumulate to significance.

Long-Term Planning

Once the correct attitude has been developed in the patient the long-term plan must be put into place. The long-term plan should be one that is broken up into four phases. Each phase is increasingly longer-term and wider in scope than the one before it, and all are tangible steps that can be followed as a guide. The first, immediate phase is weight loss with caloric restriction until the patient reaches their optimal weight. Insulin levels are stabilized and fat reserves are consumed as the patient sharply decreases their energy intake in relation to their energy expenditure. The second phase is maintenance, as the patient creates the habits of health that are needed to fully bring about improvements in longevity. The energy intake is increased to form an equilibrium with energy expenditure, with the emphasis upon proper nutrition and healthy foods. The third phase is adjusting the habits of health over time in accordance with the patient's age to maximize their anti-inflammatory benefits. This involves an increase in energy expenditure with exercise while continuing to match it to the energy intake from healthy foods. Finally, the fourth phase is the overarching emphasis upon longevity, wherein every diet and exercise decision is either consciously or unconsciously geared towards the improvement of lifetime health quality. This is primarily followed by avoiding excessive caloric intake while consuming adequate quantities of all necessary vitamins and nutrients on a daily basis.

One of the most distinctive aspects of this system is the emphasis that is placed upon lowering caloric intake as opposed to increasing caloric expenditure. The reason for this is two-fold; the difficulty of weight loss via exercise alone, and the idea that caloric restriction can lead to improvements in longevity. In terms of the former reason, while there is clearly a need for exercise to be an integral part of the weight loss process, few patients are capable of utilizing it alone for significant, lasting weight loss. The time constraints placed upon the average patient limit how much exercise can be completed, rarely allowing enough time to burn significantly more energy than is provided by the typical calorie-laden American diet. For example, a 180-pound person who does high-impact aerobics for 60 minutes is able to burn about as many calories as the 540 calories provided by a McDonald's Big Mac® (Nutristrategy, 2005; McDonalds, 2007). Even running a marathon (26.2 miles) burns around 2600 calories, roughly equivalent to just two-thirds of a pound of fat. As for the latter reason, data collected primarily from animal studies have indicated that mice fed caloric-restricted diets are more likely to live longer than mice with non-restricted diets. Therefore, while it is important to maintain the proper intake of nutrients and calories to avoid malnutrition, it could be beneficial in terms of longevity to eat fewer calories than what is consumed on average in the United States.

Calorie Restricted Diet Plans

This chapter will discuss two generalized methods for successfully implementing a caloric restriction diet as part of the first phase. Both have been clinically proven to be effective and are safe if utilized properly under the direction of qualified health-care providers. Both are designed to reduce excess visceral fat and decrease inflammation and both call for light meals to be eaten every three hours during the day. The first method is a low glycemic, moderate caloric restricted diet of meals that have been prepared using basic nutritional knowledge. The goal is to have an intake of around 1,200 calories per day and to maintain lean body mass by replacing dietary fat with complex carbohydrates as described in *Diabetes, Obesity, and Metabolism* (2005) and the *Journal of the American Medical Association* (2007). The second method consists of portion-controlled meal replacements that have balanced protein levels, low fat, and a low glycemic index. The goal is to have an intake between 800 and 1,000 calories per day while taking advantage of the pre-packaged meals that require little preparation or nutritional knowledge. A 2001 study in *Obesity Research* found that these type of diets can be very effective in terms of long-term weight loss if they are implemented correctly, as did a study in *Nutrition* (2000). The low glycemic index of the meals featured in both methods allow for the levels of blood sugar and insulin to remain in the normal range throughout the day, minimizing the feelings of hunger as much as possible. As for the frequent number of light meals, a study of school children found that children who ate 3 meals per day gained weight as compared to kids who ate 5-7 light meals per day. Another study of 379 men who ate 1-2 meals per day found that they were heavier and had higher cholesterol than men who ate more frequently.

Habits of Health

Once the first phase has been successfully completed the patient begins the second phase, engraining the habits of health while maintaining an equilibrium between caloric intake and expenditure. Many habits of health have been discovered by studying the National Weight Control Registry (2007), which is composed of men and women who have lost over 60 pounds and kept it off for at least 5 years. One example is the consumption of breakfast, a practice that is not followed by just 4% of the registry as compared to 25% within the general population. Over the course of the day the reported energy intake was the same between people who did or did not consume breakfast, indicating that if that first meal is skipped the person will fully compensate for those absent calories later in the day (Wyatt *et al*, 2002). Another example of a habit of health is regular exercise, a practice that was followed by 80% of the registry and by just 20% of people who were not able to maintain their weight loss (Kayman *et al*, 1990). On average, people from the registry who exercised burned 400 calories per day, roughly equivalent to an hour of jogging.

CONCLUDING REMARKS

Obesity in the United States has reached epidemic proportions with the potential for an extremely large negative impact upon the healthcare system. By implementing a proactive protocol that focuses on the long-term goal of optimal health, longevity has the potential to be improved in a large number of Americans at very low cost.

REFERENCES

1. Bahadori B, Yazdani-Biuki B, Krippl, P, Brath H, Uitz E, Wascher TC. Low-fat, high-carbohydrate (low-glycemic index) diet induces weight loss and preserves lean body mass in obese healthy subjects: results of a 24-week study. *Diabetes, Obesity and Metabolism*. 2005;7:290-293.
2. Berenson GS, Srinivasan SR, Bao W, Newman WP III, Tracy RE, Wattigney WA. Association between multiple cardiovascular risk factors and atherosclerosis in children and young adults. *N Engl J Med*. 1998;338:1650-1656.
3. Centers for Disease Control and Prevention (CDC). (2007). "Diabetes Disabling Disease to Double by 2050." Accessed on Sept 12, 2007, at: http://www.cdc.gov/nccdphp/publications/aag/ddt.htm
4. Dansinger ML, Schaefer EJ. Low-fat diets and weight change. *JAMA*. 2006;295:94-95.
5. De Rougemont A, Normand S, Nazare JA, Skilton MR, Sothier M, Vinoy S, Laville M. Beneficial effects of a 5-week low-glycaemic index regimen on weight control and cardiovascular risk factors in overweight non-diabetic subjects. *Br J Nutr*. 2007;6:1-11.
6. Ditschuneit HH, Flechtner-Mors M. Value of structured meals for weight management: risk factors and long-term weight maintenance. *Obes Res*. 2001;9 Suppl 4:284S-289S.
7. Ebbeling CB, Leidig MM, Feldman HA, Lovesky MM, Ludwig DS. Effects of a low–glycemic load vs low-fat diet in obese young adults: a randomized trial. *JAMA*. 2007;297:2092-2102.

8. Foreyt JP, Poston WS. Consensus view on the role of dietary fat and obesity. *Am J Med.* 2002;113 Suppl 9B:60S-62S.

9. Hellmich N, Manning A. (2002). "Health and Behavior; Scales tipping toward diabetes." USA Today. Accessed on 9/16/07 at: http://www.usatoday.com/news/health/2002-10-23-stopgain_x.htm

10. Jenkins DJ, Wolever TM, Taylor RH, Barker H, Fielden H, Baldwin JM, Bowling AC, Newman HC, Jenkins AL, Goff DV. Glycemic index of foods: a physiological basis for carbohydrate exchange. *Am J Clin Nutr.* 1981;34:362-366.

11. Kayman S, Bruvold W, Stern JS. Maintenance and relapse after weight loss in women: behavioral aspects. *Am J Clin Nutr.* 1990;52:800-807.

12. Kennedy ET, Bowman SA, Powell R. Dietary-Fat Intake in the US Population. *Journal of the American College of Nutrition.* 1999;18:207-212.

13. National Institutes of Health, National Heart, Lung, and Blood Institute. Clinical guidelines on the identification, evaluation, and treatment of overweight and obesity in adults--the evidence report. *Obes Res.* 1998;6 (suppl 2):51S-209S. [Published erratum appears in *Obes Res.* 1998:6:464].

14. Macera CA, Ham SA, Yore MM, Jones DA, Ainsworth BE, Kimsey CD, Kohl HW 3rd. Prevalence of physical activity in the United States: Behavioral Risk Factor Surveillance System. *Prev Chronic Dis.* 2005;2:A17. Epub 2005 Mar 15.

15. Marques-Vidal P, Ruidavets RB, Cambou JP, Ferrières J. Trends in overweight and obesity in middle-aged subjects from southwestern France, 1985-1997. *International Journal of Obesity.* 2002;26:732-734.

16. McDonald's. (2007). McDonald's USA nutrition facts for popular menu items. Accessed on Sept 21, 2007, at: http://www.mcdonalds.com/app_controller.nutrition.index1.html

17. Must A, Jacques PF, Dallal GE, Bajema CJ, Dietz WH. Long-term morbidity and mortality of overweight adolescents: a follow-up of the Harvard Growth Study of 1922 to 1935. N Engl J Med 1992;327:1350-1355.

18. National Weight Control Registry. (2007). Accessed on Sept 21, 2007, at: http://www.nwcr.ws/

19. Nutristrategy. (2005). Calories burned during exercise. Nutristrategy nutrition and fitness software. Accessed on Sept 21, 2007, at: http://www.nutristrategy.com/activitylist.htm

20. Reaven GM. Banting Lecture 1988: role of insulin resistance in human disease. *Diabetes.* 1988;37:1595-1607.

21. Rothacker QD. Five-year self-management of weight using meal replacements: comparison with matched controls in rural Wisconsin. *Nutrition.* 2000;16:344-348.

22. Rozin P, Kabnick K, Pete E, Fischler C, Shields. The ecology of eating: smaller portion sizes in France Than in the United States help explain the French paradox. *C Psychol Sci.* 2003;14:450-454.

23. Steinberger J, Daniels SR. Obesity, insulin resistance, diabetes, and cardiovascular risk in children: an American Heart Association scientific statement from the Atherosclerosis, Hypertension, and Obesity in the Young Committee (Council on Cardiovascular Disease in the Young) and the Diabetes Committee (Council on Nutrition, Physical Activity, and Metabolism). *Circulation.* 2003;107:1448-1453.

24. Tudor-Locke C, Bassett DR Jr. How many steps/day are enough? Preliminary pedometer indices for public health. *Sports Med.* 2004;34:1-8.

25. Wang Y, Beydoun MA. The obesity epidemic in the United States--gender, age, socioeconomic, racial/ethnic, and geographic characteristics: a systematic review and meta-regression analysis. Epidemiol Rev. 2007;29:6-28.

26. Weiss R, Dziura J, Burgert TS, *et al.* Obesity and the metabolic syndrome in children and adolescents. *N Engl J Med.* 2004;350:2362-2374.

27. Wyatt HR, Grunwald GK, Mosca CL, Klem ML, Wing RR, Hill JO. Long-term weight loss and breakfast in subjects in the National Weight Control Registry. *Obes Res.* 2002;10:78-82.

28. Wyatt HR, Peters JC, Reed GW, Barry M, Hill JO. A Colorado statewide survey of walking and its relation to excessive weight. *Med Sci Sports Exerc.* 2005;37:724-730.

29. Zieve FJ. The metabolic syndrome: diagnosis and treatment. *Clin Cornerstone.* 2004;6 Suppl 3:S5-13.

30. Zuvekas SH, Cohen JW. Prescription drugs and the changing concentration of health care expenditures. *Health Aff* (Millwood). 2007;26:249-257.

ABOUT THE AUTHOR

Dr. Wayne Scott Andersen is a board certified Anesthesiologist and Critical Care Specialist. A graduate of the University for the Health Sciences, Kansas City, Missouri, his post doctoral training included a residency training at Cleveland Clinic in Cardiovascular Anesthesiology and fellowship training at the University of Miami in Surgical Critical Care Medicine. As the tenth board certified physician in the nation in Critical Care, Dr. Andersen helped pioneer the emerging subspecialty of intensive care medicine. Observing the pivotal role nutrition plays in recovery from illness inspired Dr. Andersen to redirect his focus into the preventative arena of nutritional intervention. He is convinced that education, tools and support are required to create long-term solutions to creating optimal health. Dr. Andersen observes that: "Significant results fuel and motivate the individual to pursue a healthier lifestyle."

Chapter 2
Medical Marijuana: Scientific Mechanisms and Clinical Indications

David Bearman, M.D.
Substance Use and Abuse Expert;
Medical Consultant to Zona Seca Drug Treatment Program

ABSTRACT

Finally in the early 21st century, medicinal cannabis is being rediscovered by physicians and patients alike. This paper discusses the current state of medicinal marijuana in the United States. The contemporary medicinal use of cannabis in the context of the 5000-year history of the therapeutic use of cannabis will be examined. This includes cannabis use in ancient times, the use of cannabis in patent medicines, and its use in the early 20th century. The modern medicinal cannabis research that started in 1949 will also be discussed. The paper will cover the current legal status of medicinal cannabis, recent research, the role of the FDA, physician practice standards, medical indications, and mechanisms of action.

INTRODUCTION

We stand at the dawn of a new era for medicinal cannabis. Since 1964, when Dr. Raphael Mechulam, of Jerusalem University, isolated tetrahydrocannabinol (THC) we have learned more about the marvels of the brain's neurochemistry. There has developed a greater understanding of the role of serotonin in depression and we have had the discovery of endorphins, the naturally-occurring opiates, and the endocannabinoid system. In 1992, Professor Mechulam described the endocannabinoid system. He characterized the endogenous cannabinoid receptors and the endogenous cannabinoids that bind to these receptors.

We have crossed the threshold into exciting cannabis-related treatments for many conditions and symptoms. Cannabis gives relief from chronic pain which arises from a myriad of pain-producing illnesses; cannabis provides both analgesia and anti-inflammatory relief for autoimmune diseases such as rheumatoid arthritis, fibromyalgia, complex sympathetic dystrophy, and restless leg syndrome; and assists many with mental health problems, including attention deficit disorder (ADD), post-traumatic stress disorder (PTSD), depression, and obsessive compulsive disorder (OCD) – to name but a few conditions which have been shown to benefit from cannabis and cannabinoids.

THE HISTORY OF MEDICINAL MARIJUANA
The Current Situation

All surveys conducted over the past 10 to 15 years concerning the medicinal use of cannabis have revealed that more than 70% of the American public believe that the medicinal use of cannabis should be legal if a physician recommends it. The results of the most recent survey reveals that approximately 80% of adult Americans now share this view. Given these findings it is of no surprise that 12 states in the U.S. have legalized the medicinal use of cannabis. Bill Richardson, Governor of New Mexico, signed the latest state medicinal cannabis legislation into law in April 2007.

The State of Oregon has a mandatory patient identification program; therefore state officials know exactly how many physicians in Oregon have recommended cannabis to at least one of their patients. 2340 physicians in Oregon have recommended the use of cannabis to one or more of their patients. Over in California, there is a voluntary patient identification card program. Because the program is voluntary we can only estimate the number of doctors in the State of California that have recommended cannabis to their patients. Typical estimates range between 3000 and 5000 physicians.

Many healthcare organizations recognize the medical utility of cannabis. Well over a 100 health-related entities including the American Public Health Association, the American Academy of Family Physicians, the American Pain Management Association, the Institute of Medicine and the American Nurses Association, have officially come out in favor of the medicinal use of cannabis.

A Brief History of the Medicinal Use of Marijuana

It is not clear how far back the medicinal use of cannabis goes. The first official recognition of marijuana's medical usefulness is usually attributed to Shen Nung, the second emperor of China and also their God of Agriculture and Pharmacy. Shen Nung is credited with identifying 300-400 medical herbs by personally testing their properties, and is recognized as being responsible for the *Pen Tsao Ching*, which is considered the first *Materia Medica*. Chinese oral history states that this written in 2637 B.C.

Unfortunately, we do not have a copy of that first *Materia Medica*. The oldest *Materia Medica* we do have is from India. It is thought to have been written somewhere between 1100 and 1700 BC. Like all major *Materia Medica* ever written, including ones from Egypt, Greece, and Rome, it contains references to the medicinal use of cannabis.

When the 1937 Marijuana Tax Act hearings were held, the American Medical Association (AMA) testified against the proposed legislation. Dr. William Woodward, the AMA's chief lobbyist and both a doctor and a lawyer, testified before the House Ways and Means Committee that "The AMA knows of no dangers from the use of cannabis." At that time cannabis had been in the USP for over 75 years and was found in 28 patent medicines then still on the market.

The AMA not only made it clear that it thought the act should not be passed, but they also strongly urged that if the legislation passed, it should not be called the Marijuana Tax Act. This was because in those days no one in the medical profession used the term medical marijuana – it was always referred to as cannabis. The AMA pointed out that marijuana was a slang term which was unfamiliar to most people, including those in the medical field and the industries (e.g. paint and varnish, and bird seed) that relied on hemp. It was confusing not to use conventional terminology.

Today the government has purposely created untrue and unnecessary confusion between hemp and what was known as cannabis (which we now have come to call marijuana). There is a big difference between industrial hemp and cannabis, or marijuana. Hemp is what industrial cannabis is called. Hemp is tall and spindly and is used to make paper and fiber. It contains approximately 0.3% THC, the most pharmacologically active chemical of the 483 chemicals in cannabis. Medicinal cannabis is shorter, much bushier and more densely flowered than hemp. Cannabis (aka marijuana, weed, grass) contains somewhere between 4% and 10% or 11% THC and, in rare instances, as much as 20% THC.

Some supporters for the legalization of marijuana suggest that George Washington grew cannabis for medicinal or recreational purposes because he separated the male and the female plants. The male plant produces hemp with its long strong fibers for rope, cloth and paper. The female plant produces cannabis, as the female has an abundance of flowering tops and a higher concentration of THC. However, Washington was probably separating the males from the females to improve the production of hemp. Until 1883, hemp had been the number one agricultural commodity in the world for 1000 years.

Dr. William B. O'Shaughnessy reintroduced cannabis to Western medicine in 1839. O'Shaughnessy had spent several years in India. While there he heard of cannabis' medicinal use, and he conducted several years of animal and human research on cannabis. However, medically he is probably best known as the physician who discovered that the best way to treat cholera is to replace all the fluids that have been lost. Cannabis remained a popular medicine during the 19th century. In the 1890s, Sir Joshua Reynolds prescribed tincture of cannabis to Queen Victoria for the treatment of premenstrual syndrome. Cannabis is still used for that indication today.

Sir William Osler, M.D., considered the founder of modern medicine, wrote the first textbook of internal medicine in the late 1890s. In his textbook, Osler wrote that cannabis was the most effective treatment for migraine headaches. That opinion was held for many years by numerous prominent physicians. As late as 1942, Dr. Morris Fishbein, long-time editor of the *Journal of the American Medical Association,* wrote an article stating that cannabis was the most effective treatment available for migraine headaches. And as cannabis is reemerging as a therapeutic agent, physicians are once again recommending cannabis to relieve the symptoms of migraines.

Cannabis was in the United States Pharmacopeia (USP) from 1854 until 1941. During that time it was the third or fourth most common ingredient in patent medicines. Prominent drug companies, such as Sqibb, Eli Lilly, Merck, and Parke-Davis all had products that contained cannabis. People consumed these medicants with benefit and without reporting significant adverse side effects.

In the 1920s and 1930s, as medicine evolved into the modern medicine of today, manufactured pharmaceuticals began to appear. The increasing numbers and presumed specificity of these manufactured pharmaceuticals caused many to discount herbal medicine. Many of the modern physicians of the 30s, 40s, and 50s did not believe that plants which grew naturally and were used by primitives could be as effective as manufactured pharmaceuticals produced by chemists and pharmacologists.

Federal control over medicinal cannabis in the United States began in the late 1930s. First came the 1937 Marijuana Tax Act. This law did not make cannabis illegal. Instead it added bureaucratic impediments which made it more cumbersome for drug companies to use cannabis in medications. It became necessary for pharmaceutical companies to keep records on cannabis and to pay a tax on its use. Therefore many drug companies began to omit cannabis from their medications.

Then, the Federal Food, Drug, and Cosmetics Act (1938) came about. This act was passed as a result of a sulfa drug produced by Massengill, which sadly contained a compound similar to antifreeze. This led to the death of 100 people. It was this act that gave the Food and Drug Administration (FDA) the power to decide whether or not a drug was safe. As a result of this, all future pharmaceuticals required the FDA to certify their safety.

This 1938 law grandfathered in the medications, including cannabis, that were on the market at that time. Soon in 1942, cannabis fell out of the United States Pharmacopeia. This was largely because drug companies were not using it anymore. Later cannabis was bureaucratically and arbitrarily categorized as a "new" drug and therefore was required to be covered by the 1938 Act. A legal challenge is currently in the courts that cannabis does not require FDA approval because it is covered by the grandfather clause.

In 1969, the Marijuana Tax Act was declared unconstitutional in a case involving the famed 60's guru and former Harvard professor, Timothy Leary, Ph.D. whose mantra was *Turn on, tune in, drop out.* However, we are now constrained by the Controlled Substances Act, which was passed in 1970. Cannabis is placed in Schedule I, which is reserved for drugs that have no known medical use in the U.S. This law is thought by many conservative Republicans to abuse the 9th and 10th amendments to the Constitution, which limit the powers of the federal government and protect state's rights.

Between 1978 and 1992, a program called the Compassionate Investigational New Drug (IND) Program, existed in the U.S. The purpose of this government program was to provide cannabis to patients who the government deemed received medicinal value from it. It required going through a cumbersome bureaucracy to get approval. At its height the IND had 15 patients enrolled in the program and 25 more approved (some texts say the numbers were 12 on the program and 28 or 35 approved). Each one on the program, be it twelve or fifteen, received 300 hand-rolled 0.9 gram cannabis cigarettes per month from the federal government.

The program was closed to new entrants in 1991 because too many people were applying. In the words of Dr. Mason, head of the United States Public Health Service at the time, the first Bush administration was concerned that if too many patients were on the program, the public might get the idea that marijuana was actually good for you. In fact if hundreds of patients were on the program it would have made it difficult for the federal government to continue to contend that marijuana has no medical value. There are still five surviving patients who remain in the program, four who receive their 300 marijuana cigarettes each month in the mail; the fifth gets his 300 every three weeks.

Modern Day Research into the Medicinal Use of Marijuana

The United States government has largely stood in the way of constructive research regarding the medicinal use of cannabis. One of the leading medicinal cannabis practitioners in California, and in the United States, was the late Dr. Todd Mikuriya, who was in charge of marijuana research for the federal government at the National Institute of Mental Health (NIMH) for a short period of time in the late 1960s. Mikuriya was very familiar with the India Hemp Commission Report (1894), produced by the British in India, having read all 3340 pages of it. He was very excited about scientifically exploring the possibilities surrounding the medicinal use of cannabis. However, Mikuriya soon found that the government was more excited about finding out about anything that was wrong with cannabis. The government made clear their aversion to understanding how cannabis worked and why it had been used medicinally for at least 3000 years, and the NIMH and Mikuriya soon parted company.

Current federal drug czar John Walter, has said that there is no research that shows that cannabis is useful from a medicinal point of view. Former drug czar General McCaffrey has said that cannabis was Cheech and Chong medicine. Both of these bureaucrats have evidently done limited literature searches into the subject. If they had, they would have found that there has been quite a lot of research into the medicinal use of cannabis both here and abroad. Much of this research has produced positive findings about cannabis' medicinal efficacy.

The first modern study of the medicinal use of cannabis was conducted in 1949. The results of that study suggested that cannabis may be useful in dealing with seizures. Not surprisingly, I have a number of patients today, who get a great deal of relief from seizures by using cannabis. In the 1970s and 1980s studies were conducted in eight different states, including Georgia, Tennessee, New York, California, and New Mexico, which demonstrated that cannabis was useful in treating nausea and as an appetite stimulant.

The next breakthrough for the modern day medicinal use of cannabis occurred in 1985. In response to increasing medicinal use of cannabis by AIDS patients and cancer victims, the U.S. government encouraged the development and approval of synthetic delta-9 THC. This product is marketed under the trade name Marinol®. It does have therapeutic benefits. The FDA has approved it for treatment of nausea in cancer patients and/or treatment for appetite stimulation in AIDS patients. Off label, it has been used to treat pain, ADD/ADHD and other conditions. I am the largest prescriber of Marinol® in the Santa Barbara County. However, I find that it has more side effects, costs more, does not work as well as cannabis, and may cause dysphoria. Nevertheless for many, it is effective with few side effects.

In 1992, Mechulam characterized the endocannabinoid system, the system of receptor sites and neurotransmitters that explain why cannabis affects us as it does. Even though we know less about the enocannabinoid system than other neurotransmitter systems, the endocannabinoid system is the largest neurotransmitter system in the brain.

Another great leap forward in the modern day medicinal cannabis research came about in 1999, when GW Pharmaceuticals, a British phytochemical company, started to conduct research on six different strains of cannabis and combinations of these strains. They developed different tinctures of cannabis delivered under the tongue via a metered sprayer.

GW's research effort was in response to the 1997 report of the House of Lord's Science and Technology Committee and a growing need to address the medical needs of British Multiple Sclerosis (MS) patients who were being arrested for possession of marijuana in embarrassing numbers. The MS patients were using marijuana because it was providing relief from muscle spasm and pain with few side effects.

In 2000, the California Marijuana Research Center (CMRC) was set up at the University of California at San Diego School of Medicine. The CMRC has administered more than eighteen FDA-approved smoked cannabis medical studies done at four UC Medical Schools, including a study by Dr. Daniel Abrams *et al* published in the February 2007 issue of the *Journal of Neurology*. Abrams' study was designed to determine the effect of smoked cannabis on the neuropathic pain of HIV-associated sensory neuropathy. The results showed that even the government's low-grade cannabis was capable of reducing daily pain by 34%. These results led the authors to conclude: *"Smoked cannabis was well tolerated and effectively relieved chronic neuropathic pain from HIV-associated sensory neuropathy. The findings are comparable to oral drugs used for chronic neuropathic pain."*

Research conducted by Dr. Donald Tashkin, a noted pulmonologist at UCLA, has found revealing and possible counter-intuitive findings about the pulmonary effects of cannabis. Some of Tashkin's research (Tashkin *et al*) clearly shows that cannabis is a bronchodilator and is useful in treating asthma. This is consistent with the historical fact that in the 1920's Australia and France had cannabis containing smokables for treatment of asthma.

Another of Tashkin's studies, reported at the 2006 International Cannabinoid Research Society (ICRS), demonstrated that cannabis smokers actually have a reduced risk of lung cancer over non-smokers. Tashkin states that more research is needed to confirm or refute this finding. But when paired with the Kaiser-Permanente survey of 65,000 patient charts, which found no difference in cancers of the mouth, throat and lungs in people who smoked nothing and those who smoked cannabis, it strongly suggests that smoking cannabis either lowers cancers of the respiratory tree or has no effect on respiratory cancer rates.

The Medicinal Marijuana Movement

The arrest of Robert Randall in 1972 triggered the medicinal marijuana movement. Randall was going blind. He was also a recreational user of cannabis. One night he noticed that it alleviated some of his symptoms. After that he started using marijuana therapeutically and growing it. After he was arrested for cultivating a few plants, Randall sued the government. He contended that he would go blind if he did not continue to use cannabis.

The government had Randall evaluated both at UCLA and at John Hopkins, who both found that cannabis was the only treatment that lowered Randall's intraocular pressure. They concurred that without cannabis he would go blind. Subsequently, as part of a legal settlement, the government agreed to begin sending him cannabis. The Compassionate Investigational New Drug (IND) Program emanated from the court settlement to Randall's lawsuit.

At the time the IND program was terminated in 1991, there were 15 people in the program. A further 28 had been approved and were waiting to get their cannabis from the government. But the program was terminated because too many people had applied – hundreds, possibly up to two thousand people had submitted the paperwork to get on the program and were waiting to have their requests for medicinal marijuana processed by the government. The sheer number of people waiting to see if they could be accepted on the program, and the government's commitment to total prohibition of cannabis, was more than enough to make the government concerned, and the IND program was axed.

No more people were approved for the program. Those who were newly approved but had not yet received any cannabis from the government never got it. Only the 15 IND patients receiving government marijuana in 1992 were grandfathered in and continued to receive it. Dr. Mason, head of the USPHS at the time, is quoted as saying, *"If there are too many people on this program people will get the wrong idea that there is something good about marijuana."*

MEDICAL MARIJUANA TODAY
Who Might Benefit From Medical Marijuana?

Cannabis is of great benefit to a vast number of people with a wide range of conditions. Tens of millions more would benefit if it were obtainable through conventional distribution. Pain is the number one condition treated with cannabis by doctors in California, Oregon, and Colorado – three of the 12 the states in which it is legal to use cannabis under state law if it is approved or recommended by a physician. Migraine is another condition for which cannabis can be extremely effective. Some of my patients have told me that if they take cannabis with the onset of their migraine prodrome it prevents the migraine from developing. Other migraine sufferers say that while cannabis does not prevent the migraine from occurring, it makes them less severe, and does help to control the symptoms.

Cannabis can also provide great relief from nausea, is an appetite stimulant, and helps with depression. All of which are of great benefit to AIDS and cancer patients. Cannabis seems to be particularly good at dealing with pain issues associated with arthritic or autoimmune conditions. This is likely because of its analgesic and anti-inflammatory properties. Of course, it is well known that cannabis is useful for helping people with sleeping difficulties.

Other conditions that cannabis may benefit include: seizures, glaucoma – cannabis decreases intraocular pressure by approximately 25% – peripheral neuropathy, asthma, and irritable bowel syndrome. Research by Professor Daniel Piomelli, a pharmacologist at the University of California, Irvine, demonstrates that cannabis may also be of benefit to people with bipolar disorder, Tourette's syndrome, ADD, and panic attacks. Clinical experience supports Professor Piomelli's contention.

One of the most exciting uses for cannabis is for treatment of PTSD. This is very important for servicemen returning from the war in Iraq. In California, unlike other states where the medicinal use of cannabis is legal, we do not only have a discrete list of conditions that physicians are allowed to recommend cannabis for. California has a list of specific conditions, but physicians also have the legal right to use their discretion to recommend cannabis for "any other medical condition" for which we feel cannabis will be medically useful. This has allowed cannabis to be used for the psychological problems noted above.

The Great Debate

The medical marijuana movement has had its fair share of critics. The majority of them do not have a medical background. The critics tend to be of the belief that the medicinal use of cannabis is a hoax, and has more to do with legalizing cannabis for recreational purposes than to relieve the symptoms of people who are ill. If something (say Valium or morphine) has medicinal value and people want to utilize it therapeutically, that does not mean that society is also sanctioning its recreational use. These are two different issues and this effort to confuse the two is unfortunate because cannabis has significant medicinal value.

Fortunately, many leading figures and organizations have publicly supported the medicinal cannabis movement. The former Surgeon General of the United States, Dr. Joycelyn Elders, said that there is an overwhelming amount of evidence to show that cannabis can relieve certain types of pain. An 1997 editorial published in the *New England Journal of Medicine*, said that they thought that the federal policy of preventing physicians from prescribing marijuana for ill patients was "*misguided, heavy-handed, and inhumane.*" Furthermore, the government-funded Institute of Medicine report into the medicinal use of marijuana concluded that cannabis does indeed have medicinal properties.

Dr. Andrea Barthwell, who served as Deputy Director for Demand Reduction in the Office of National Drug Control Policy (ONDCP), between 2002 and 2005 has had an interesting changing of position. During her time at the ONDCP she was highly critical of medical marijuana. However, she is now is a paid lobbyist for GW pharmaceuticals, the company that makes Sativex®, which is tincture of cannabis.

Another person who seems to have dramatically changed his opinion on medical marijuana is Bob Barr, a former member of the United States House of Representatives. Barr was a vigorous opponent of marijuana and a strong supporter of the War on Drugs. However, since joining the Libertarian Party, Barr has seemingly reversed his previous opinions. He is now a paid lobbyist for the Marijuana Policy Project, whose goal is to legalize the recreational use of marijuana. He bases this change on solid Libertarian philosophy – that after 9/11 the federal government accrued too much power to itself at the expense of the states.

Is Medical Marijuana Safe?

There is no question that cannabis is safe. Every governmental study ever done by the U.S., Canadian, Australian, British, and European countries has recommended the legalization of the recreational use of cannabis, never mind its medicinal use. Of course, the FDA has already approved Marinol®, which is a synthetic version of delta-9 THC. Delta-9 THC is the most pharmacologically active ingredient in cannabis, but it is also the most euphoric, and so Marinol® causes more euphoria and therefore more dysphoria than cannabis, and it is perfectly legal. Sativex®, a whole plant alcohol extract (tincture of cannabis), is made from two strains of cannabis; one high in THC and the other in CBD. Sativex® was approved for sale in Canada and has been marketed there by Bayer AG for several years.

In 1988 after a two-year rescheduling hearing FDA Chief Administrative Law Judge wrote that cannabis was one of the safest therapeutic agents known to man. This was after over 5000 pates of testimony. He concluded that American doctors should be able to prescribe marijuana.

Administering Medical Marijuana

The most well known method of taking cannabis is smoking it. However, in recent years vaporization has become more and more popular. Vaporization involves heating up the cannabis to a temperature which releases the volatile cannabinoid-containing oils that are in the plant into the air. At present, there are a couple of hundred different kinds of vaporizers on the market. The vaporization point for the various chemicals in cannabis is 190 to 340 degrees Fahrenheit and the combustion point is 451 degrees Fahrenheit. The smoke produced by vaporization is both cooler and contains about 70% fewer irritants than smoking marijuana cigarettes (aka joints).

Cannabis can also be consumed sublingually. That is the way that Sativex®, an under the tongue metered spray, is administered. It can also be ingested orally, which is how Marinol® is administered. It is also possible to use cannabis topically. Topical application of tincture of cannabis is an effective route of administration for people with arthritis of the hands, wrists, and feet. This tincture can provide pain relief and diminish swelling in the small joints of the fingers, wrists, and even ankles and toes of a patient whose small joints are afflicted by arthritis.

The respiratory route of administration is generally the best because the therapeutic effects of cannabis are almost instantaneous when taken in via the lungs. The respiratory route also allows for easy dose titration. The respiratory route can be via smoking or vaporizing. Vaporizing provides about 70% less irritants than smoking.

The problem with taking cannabis orally is that absorption rates vary, depending on the motility and contents of the gastrointestinal tract. Unless you are using Marinol® the dose may vary. If it is too much it can cause dysphoria, which can last for a couple of hours.

How Does Marijuana Exert its Medicinal Effects?

Cannabis is a 21-carbon molecule that contains 483 chemicals, of which 66 are cannabinoids. Many of the 483 compounds have medicinal value. Research continues to gain more knowledge about these molecules. Recently a hearing was held before the DEA Chief administrative law judge, Mary Ellen Bittner. The DEA was ordered to give a license to Dr. Albert Craker at the University of Massachusetts, who is an expert in medicinal plants, so that he could grow cannabis. His research goal is investigation of the ingredients in various strains of cannabis to determine which of the chemicals are most effective at treating the wide variety of medical conditions that respond to the medicinal use of cannabis.

How does cannabis exert its medicinal effects? The medicinal effects of cannabis are mediated by the endocannabinoid system. An increase in cannabinoids either endogenous or exogenous, increases the amount of the neurotransmitter dopamine in the brain. We know that dopamine acts in a different way to any other neurotransmitter. Instead of stimulating the next neuron on the pathway up the CNS, dopamine actually doubles back on itself and de-polarizes the neuron that just released it by reversing the concentration of sodium and potassium inside and outside the cell. The effect of this is that it slows down neurotransmission.

So, if a person is having migraines caused by an overload of the electrical circuits in a certain part of the brain, slowing down the speed of neurotransmission, leads to fewer neural impulses, which in turn, decreases the likelihood or severity of a migraine. The same thing is true of people that have panic attacks, if you have negative thoughts that are moving at warp speed to the midbrain, you are overwhelming the emotional control center of the brain, the limbic system. Cannabis slows down the speed of neurotransmission exposing the cerebral cortex to fewer slower moving neural stimuli. This allows the higher centers of the brain to have time to more rationally assess the relative danger or the negativity and put a more rationale point of view on that sensory input.

One suggestion is that cannabis and cannabinoids increase the amount of free dopamine in the brain by freeing dopamine from binding to another neurochemical, dopamine transporter. The dopamine transporter and dopamine bond form an electrochemical bond. This ties up the dopamine so the dopamine is not free to act as one of the brain's "off switches". We were all taught in medical school that 70% of the brain is there to turn off the other 30% – dopamine is one of the "off switches" that helps modulate sensory input. Therefore, if there is not enough dopamine present in the brain, certain parts of it become overloaded, and the illness you have depends upon the part or parts of the mid-brain that is being overloaded.

Cannabinoids compete with dopamine for the binding sites on the dopamine transporter, and in sufficient quantity it wins, thus freeing up more dopamine to help slowdown the speed of neurotransmissions. This, in my opinion and many others, is responsible for much of the therapeutic value of cannabis. Although it has effects on certain receptor sites in the brain that contribute to its therapeutic value. It probably directly affects the appetite and sleep centers in the brain, decreases the perception of pain, and centrally decreases nausea. Peripherally, cannabinoids stimulate CB2 receptors in the GI tract, which is what makes cannabis valuable in treating Crohn's Disease and IBS.

The Law Surrounding the Medical Use of Marijuana

The use of medical marijuana in California is governed by the Compassionate Use Act of 1996, or Proposition 215. In January 1997, Dr Marcus Conant and five other physicians filed a class action lawsuit against the federal government in response to threats made by government officials that the DEA would revoke the BNDD license for writing prescriptions and Medicare participation, and possibly prosecute, any doctor who recommended marijuana to a patient. They felt that this infringed on the right of any American's free speech and specifically that the federal government was trying to unconstitutionally limit physician advice.

A preliminary injunction prohibiting federal officials from threatening or punishing physicians for recommending medical marijuana was issued by the 9th Circuit in April 1997, and a permanent injunction was issued in September 2000. However, in June 2001, the Bush administration filed an appeal challenging the permanent injunction. Finally, in October 2002, after a long and protracted legal battle, the Ninth Circuit Court of Appeals unanimously upheld the right for doctors to recommend marijuana to their patients. The Justices emphasized that it is the role of the states, not the federal government, to regulate the practice of medicine. This decision was then appealed to the U.S. Supreme Court who declined to hear it.

The outcome of this legal battle is that physicians now have protection from the federal government to use their First Amendment free speech right to answer their patients' questions regarding marijuana. So, if a patient asks you if you think cannabis might be helpful for their arthritis, you now have the federal court certified freedom to answer them without fear of the federal government harassing you.

The Medical Board of California has been the principal impediment to the smooth implementation of Proposition 215. As past Medical Director of the oldest County-organized Medi-Cal Managed Care Program in the Country, and former Director of a California State University (CSU) student health center, I have over 20 years experience in quality assurance .As such I am greatly disappointed at the quality of the quality assurance provided by the California Medical Board. Their guidelines are vague, their process frequently opaque. They have intimidated physicians to the point that there has been a reluctance on the part of many Californian physicians to do anything that might bring them to the attention of the medical board, because any sort of disagreement with them is aggravating, time consuming, and expensive – and that is when you win.

As I said, the MBC guidelines are vague, not necessarily bad. What is bad is that their very vagueness allows wide latitude for interpretation by the MBC. This has created a barrier. The courts have ruled that the MBC has illegally attempted to investigate doctors for approving cannabis even when the MBC has received no quality of care complaint. This has been intimidating to many physicians.

The MBC guidelines state that there needs to be a *bona fide* doctor-patient relationship, a good-faith patient's history and physical examination must be performed and you need to review relevant medical records. The guidelines also state that you have to have a plan with objectives and demonstrate that the patient has a condition that will benefit from the use of cannabis.

If a physician is making medicinal cannabis recommendations, it is imperative to keep good records, preferably typed so that other people can read them. You also need to follow-up the patient as is appropriate. The MBC says you need to see them at least once a year. If the patient's primary treating physicians were not so intimidated by the MBC, these criteria would be very easy to accomplish.

The problem is that different physicians have different ideas about just about everything. The same is true with physicians who make frequent recommendations for medicinal cannabis. Some physicians who operate HMO style practices have given the medicinal marijuana movement a bad name. These doctors may see the patient only briefly before granting their approval for medicinal cannabis. The position they have taken seems to go something like this: if a patient tells them that they have a particular medical problem and that cannabis is useful to them, these doctors will recommend cannabis. They say that they have no reason not to approve its use when it provides medical benefit, because they see cannabis as being extremely safe, and because they can.

I take a more conservative point of view. First, we pre-screen the prospective patient at the time a person desires to make a 215 appointment. We do not make an appointment for just anyone. Unless we have pretty good idea that they are likely to qualify, we do not make a prospective patient an appointment. Before the office even issues an appointment to see me we want to know what the patient's diagnosis is, whether other healthcare practitioners have seen them, and if their problem adversely affects their ability to work or to do activities of daily living. If their responses sound reasonable, we will give them an appointment. We try to see their medical records before their appointment, or if not, we have them bring them in with them.

If a patient arrives without their records and decides to proceed with their appointment, they are advised that the most they can expect is an "in process" letter which states I will approve with receipt of confirming records. In a few instances, where a physical exam documents a serious problem (e.g., missing limb, S/P lumbar or cervical fusion, multiple knee surgeries), a recommendation may be made without records in hand. Just because a patient has got an appointment to come in and see a doctor for a medical marijuana approval does not mean they are going to get one. At present, most cannabinologists believe that the patient should have a documented and/or demonstrable medical problem.

I tell all my patients about the voluntary patient identification program that exists in California – remember in Oregon the patient participation program is mandatory. Therefore, in California, a patient does not need to participate in the program to be within the law, but it gives the patient something to show the police to prove that they did not write up the letter themselves. In total, the appointment takes 45 to 60 minutes.

CONCLUDING REMARKS

Where do we go from here? The question is whether or not we are going to let people take responsibility for their own health. Why should people suffer unnecessarily? Cannabis has provided millions world-wide with relief from chronic pain caused by a myriad of pain-producing illnesses. Cannabis has significantly improved the quality of life of people with cancer, Aids, arthritis, and the list goes on. The medical marijuana movement is not concerned with decriminalizing or legalizing cannabis for recreational use. It is concerned with helping people with serious illnesses and disabilities to get on with their lives.

The real issue is whether or not the pharmaceutical companies will take control over the medical use of this plant through patenting strains and creating synthetic cannabinoids while being protected by the government, or whether people will be able to grow a safe, cheap, effective medication for themselves.

REFERENCES

Abrams DI, Jay CA, Shade SB, Vizoso H, Reda H, Press S, Kelly ME, Rowbotham MC, Petersen KL. Cannabis in painful HIV-associated sensory neuropathy: a randomized placebo-controlled trial. *Neurology*. 2007;68:515-521.

Fishbein M. Migraine Associated with Menstruation. *J Amer Med Assoc.* 1942; 237:326.

Tashkin DP, Shapiro BJ, Lee YE, Harper CE. Effects of smoked marijuana in experimentally induced asthma. *Am Rev Respir Dis.* 1975;112:377-386.

Angle, Nichol, et al. *Scientific American*. December 8, 2004.

Hergenrather, Mikuriya and Bearman. *Crohn's Disease and Cannabis* at ICRS, 2006.

Grottenherman, Russo, Ethan. *Cannabis and Cannabinoids*.

1988 Recommendation of FDA Chief Administrative Law Judge Francis Young.

Emerging Issues for the 21st Century. ABC-Clio. Medical Marijuana

ABOUT THE AUTHOR

Dr. David Bearman received his M.D. from the University of Washington School of Medicine. He graduated with honors from the University of Wisconsin with an undergraduate degree in Psychology. He was the Director of Medical Services for the Santa Barbara Regional Health Authority (SBRHA) since its inception in 1983 through June 1997, and was then promoted to Senior Health Care Advisor/Grants Development Director. In 1999 as a result of Dr. Bearman's efforts, the California Healthcare Foundation allocated $10 million to several health entities located in Santa Barbara County for a county-wide medical data exchange system. SBRHA is the oldest County Organized Health System (COHS) in California and the U.S. As Medical Director for SBRHA's first 14 years he developed and implemented Quality Assurance (QA) Utilization Review (UR) system and on-site review; created Peer Review and Quality Improvement Committee and developed Targeted Case Management Program. He has a long and illustrative background in the field of drug abuse treatment and prevention, been prominent in the community clinic movement having started in Seattle the 3rd Free Clinic in the Country, directed the Haight Ashbury Drug Treatment Program, and founded the Isla Vista Medical Clinic in 1970. He has been Medical Director of Santa Barbara County Methadone Maintenance Clinic and Ventura County Opiate Detox Program, taught courses on substance abuse at UCSF, UCSB, and SDSU, been a consultant to Hoffman LaRoche, NIDA, and the National PTA, directed several conferences, delivered numerous professional talks, consulted widely, and been an expert witness in over 100 civil, criminal, and family court cases and currently is Medical Director of Zona Seca.

Chapter 3

Methyltetrahydrofolate: Metabolic and Clinical Significance in Aging

Teodoro Bottiglieri, Ph.D.
Professor, Baylor University Medical Center Institute of Metabolic Disease

ABSTRACT

Folate and folic acid are forms of a water-soluble B vitamin. Folate occurs naturally in food whereas folic acid is the synthetic form of this vitamin that is found in supplements and fortified foods. Genetic, drug, and dietary interactions may predispose certain groups in the population to an increased risk of folate deficiency that can lead to marcocytic anemia, fatigue, irritability, peripheral neuropathy, restless leg syndrome, diarrhea, weight loss, insomnia, depression, dementia, cognitive disturbances, and psychiatric disorders.

The aging population is particularly susceptible to folate deficiency. More recent studies suggest that folate deficiency may contribute to depressive symptoms and cognitive impairment of the aging brain, and may also accelerate the progression of Alzheimer's disease.

Clinical studies have shown that folate supplementation may be beneficial in the treatment of depression and age-related cognitive decline. Most treatment studies have used the synthetic form of folic acid, which is converted to other forms of folate in the body. However, 5-methyltetrahydrofolate (5-MTHF) is the biological form that is absorbed at the gut level, and transported across the blood brain barrier, which may offer more beneficial effects.

The aim of this paper is to review the role of folate in age-related disorders, mechanisms of toxicity, diagnostic techniques, and treatment strategies.

INTRODUCTION

Folate and folic acid are forms of a water-soluble B vitamin. Folate occurs naturally in food whereas folic acid is the synthetic form of this vitamin that is found in supplements and fortified foods. Genetic, drug, and dietary interactions may predispose certain groups in the population to an increased risk of folate deficiency that can lead to marcocytic anemia, fatigue, irritability, peripheral neuropathy, restless leg syndrome, diarrhea, weight loss, insomnia, depression, dementia, cognitive disturbances, and psychiatric disorders.

The aging population is particularly susceptible to folate deficiency. More recent studies suggest that folate deficiency may contribute to depressive symptoms and cognitive impairment of the aging brain, and may also accelerate the progression of Alzheimer's disease.

This paper will explain the role of folate metabolism in cell function, identify factors that can lead to folate deficiency, define the impact that folate deficiency can have on the aging brain, and consider relevant treatment strategies.

THE IMPORTANCE OF THE FOLATE AND METHYLATION CYCLES

Most people have heard of folic acid, however many people are not aware of the reduced forms of folate that are present in cells. These include dihydrofolate (DHF), tetrahydrofolate (THF), formyl-tetrahydrofolate (CHO-THF), 5,-10-methylene-tetrahydrofolate (CH_2-THF), and 5-methyl-tetrahydrofolate (CH_3-THF or 5-MTHF). All of these forms of folate are intermediates of the folate cycle that originate from folic acid, which is present in food and dietary supplements, and each has specific biological functions, including:

- The synthesis of purines, the building blocks of DNA
- The synthesis of methionine, which is important for methylation reactions
- The metabolism of homocysteine

Folic acid is absorbed by the gut and is converted to THF and then onto CH_2-THF. As can be seen in Figure 1, purine synthesis takes place during this reaction. CH_2-THF is then converted to 5-MTHF, which is a cofactor for the synthesis of biopterin and neurotransmitters. 5-MTHF is the form of folate that is taken up into the cells and is also used to methylate homocysteine and thus keep homocysteine levels down as low as possible. The methylation of homocysteine by 5-MTHF results in the production of THF and methionine. The methionine that is formed is utilized for the synthesis of S-adenosylmethionine (SAM), which is a critical metabolic intermediate in the pathway because it is one of the only molecules that can methylate macromolecules and small molecules such as DNA, proteins, phospholipids, and neurotransmitters. More than 100 different methylation reactions use SAM and the synthesis of SMA is dependent upon the folate cycle and the folate methylation cycle being functional. A byproduct of that reaction is S-adenosylhomocysteine (SAH), which is converted to homocysteine.

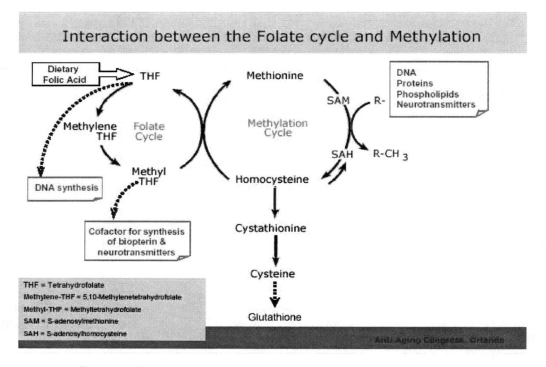

Figure 1. The interaction between the folate cycle and methylation

The correct functioning of the folate cycle and the folate methylation cycle is dependent upon a number of key enzymes, including: 5, 10 methylenetetrahydrofolate reductase (MTHFR), methionine synthase (MS), cystathionine β-synthase (CBS), methionine adenosyltransferase (MAT), and S-adenosyl-homocytsteine hydrolase (SAHase). (Fig.2)

There is a common polymorphism that is prevalent in the general population known as C677T, and people who are homozygous for this polymorphism have what is know as a TT genotype. The effect of this polymorphism is that it reduces the activity of MTHFR by approximately 60%, and that will actually predispose these people to hyperhomocystinemia if they have a low folate status. This is because the folate cycle is not working as efficiently as it should because of the drop in activity of MTHFR. This polymorphism is unheard of in African-Americans; however it affects approximately 10% of Caucasians and 20% of Latin and Mediterranean people.

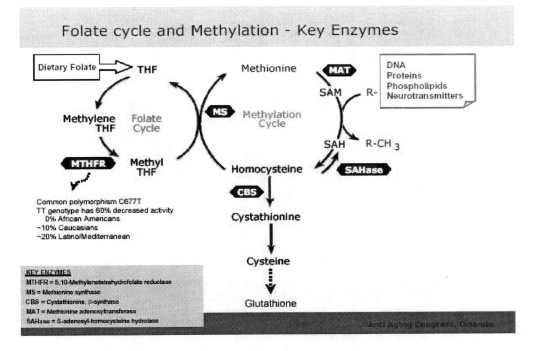

*Figure 2. The presence of a number of key enzymes is vital
if the folate cycle and methylation cycle are to function correctly.*

It is not just enzymes that are vital for the correct functioning of the folate and methylation cycles, the presence of sufficient amounts of the B-vitamins, vitamin B6, B12, and B2 is also essential (Fig. 3). These B-vitamins function along with the enzymes as cofactors to drive the reactions and keep the pathway running efficiently.

A deficiency in vitamin B2, B6, or B12 will lead to an increase in homocysteine levels and an increase in SAH levels. This is because the reaction that converts SAH to homocysteine is bi-directional, and the cells actually prefer to make SAH from homocysteine rather than SAH being generated from methylation reactions. If you induce hyperhomocystinemia, and this has been shown in many models in animal studies and transgenic models, you get elevations of SAH. The ratio of SAM to SAH is critical for determining the rate of methylation reactions, and the imbalance in the SAM/SAH ratio caused by increased homocysteine levels has been shown to inhibit the methylation cycle in both *in vitro* and animal models.

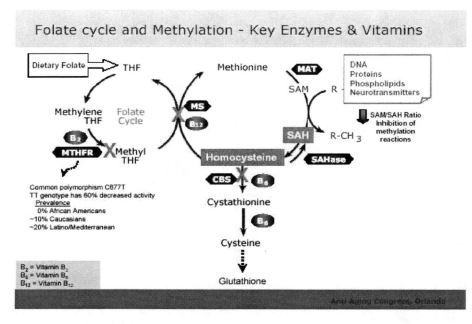

Figure 3. A number of B-vitamins are vital for the correct functioning of the folate and methylation cycles.

A vast amount of literature has been published on the relationship between homocysteine and vascular disease. A landmark study by Nygard *et al* was published in the *New England Journal of Medicine* back in 1997. The results of this study showed that elevated plasma homocysteine levels were associated with an increased risk of mortality (Fig. 4). Results of that study showed that it is necessary to keep plasma homocysteine below 9 µmol/l in order to reduce the risk of mortality from cardiovascular disease.

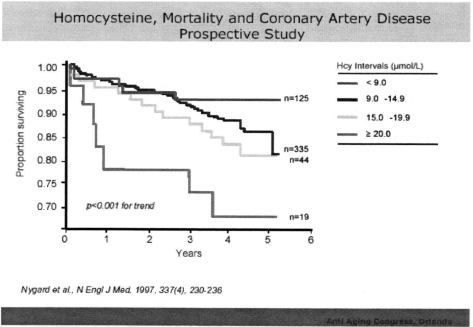

Figure 4. The relationship between plasma homocysteine level, mortality, and coronary artery disease.

Another important study was The Hordaland Homocysteine Studies by Ueland *et al*, a population-based study of more than 18,000 men and women. The results of this study showed that homocysteine is not just an independent risk factor for vascular disease, but also for mortality. Study results also showed that elevated homocysteine levels interacted with traditional physiologic and life-style risk factors of mortality. For example, people with diabetes and homocysteine level of 15 µmol/l or more were found to have nearly a 20-fold increased risk of relative mortality.

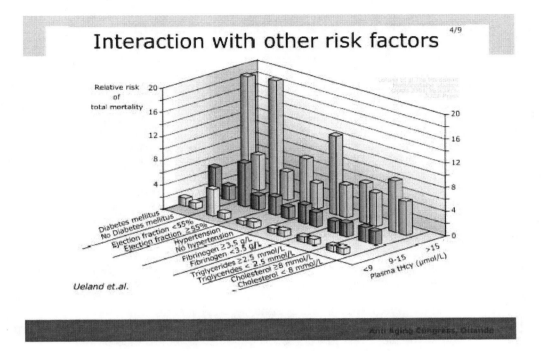

Figure 5. The results of The Hordaland Homocysteine Studies revealed that homocysteine was not just an independent risk factor for vascular disease, but also for mortality. Study results also showed that elevated homocysteine levels interacted with physiologic and life-style risk factors of mortality.

FOLATE DEFICIENCY

There are numerous causes of folate deficiency, the most obvious of which is nutritional. Other causes include:

- Defects in utilization – alcohol, pregnancy and lactation
- Malabsorption
- Disease states – cancer, liver disease, hemodialysis
- Drug-induced deficiencies – methotrexate, nitrous oxide, anticonvulsants
- Inherited disorders – severe MTHFR deficiency, MTHFR C677T polymorphism, methionine synthetase deficiency
- Auto-antibodies to folate receptor (FR) – cerebral folate deficiency

Of course, it is possible for a person to have dietary, genetic, and drug interactions and these can all compound to produce an even lower level of folate in the body, or even push somebody even into a state of negative folate balance, which will increase their homocysteine levels.

Clinical symptoms of folate deficiency include:
- Megaloblastic anemia
- Mental retardation
- Ataxia
- Peripheral neuropathy
- Cognitive dysfunction (dementia)

- Psychiatric disorders (depression)
- Endothelial dysfunction (vascular disease)
- Restless leg syndrome
- Fatigue
- Irritability
- Insomnia

FOLATE DEFICIENCY AND NEUROPSYCHIATRIC DISEASE

Back in the 1980s, Shorvon *et al* conducted a study to investigate the incidence of neurological and psychiatric complications in patients with megaloblastic anemia due to vitamin B12 or folate deficiency. Their results showed that roughly a third of participants were suffering from cognitive dysfunction, a staggering 56% of patients with folate deficiency had affective disorder, and 40% of those with B12 deficiency had peripheral neuropathy. Approximately a third of participants had no symptoms whatsoever, but we now know that if these patients had been left untreated for long enough every one of them would have gone on to develop some form of neurological or psychiatric complication.

In 1993 Crellin *et al* reviewed a number of studies conducted between 1967 and 1990 investigating the incidence of folate deficiency in psychiatric populations. The results of this review revealed that the incidence of folate deficiency in patients with depression and schizophrenia was 25-35% and 12-36% in psychogeriatric patients. Severe B12 deficiency is quite rare these days as is severe folate deficiency; however, it is important to remember that these deficiencies still exist.

The Relationship between Folate Deficiency and Depression

Numerous studies have linked folate deficiency with depression. However a particularly interesting study was conducted by Morris *et al* in 2003. This study was particularly interesting simply because food has been fortified with folate in the US since 1998. Folate status has improved somewhat since the fortification program began, however the results of this study showed that depression is linked to a low folate status, and that there are still US citizens with a low folate status.

Prior to the folate fortification program, Fava *et al* published a paper investigating the relationship between folate and homocysteine levels in depressed patients. The incidence of folate deficiency in that study was approximately 26%, which is higher than it is in the US today. Study results showed that patients that were folate deficient responded less well to antidepressant treatment than depressed patients with normal serum folate. This finding has been supported by those of other studies.

Such findings spurred Coppen and Bailey to study whether treating depressed patients with folic acid in addition to their standard antidepressant treatment would improve their clinical outcome. The results of their study showed that adding folic acid to fluoxetine did indeed improve the clinical outcome, but only in women. Folic acid appeared to have no effect on the men in this study, however when the researchers analyzed the blood and looked at serum folate and homocysteine levels in the male group, they found that serum folate did not go up significantly and homocysteine levels did not drop significantly, whereas they did in the female group. The authors concluded that this was due to poor compliance by the men.

So, there are numerous studies that support the link between folate deficiency and depression, but what could be the reason for this? Research suggests that the key to the link between folate deficiency and depression is likely to be found at the neurotransmitter level, and it seems probable that folate deficiency has deleterious effects upon neurotransmitter metabolism. There are studies that have shown that folate deficiency effects methylation reactions in the brain, of course we can speculate as to which methylation reaction is altered, but it is probably a multifactorial effect. Animal studies have shown that folate deficiency lowers serotonin levels, and human studies have shown that depressed folate deficient patients have lower levels of cerebrospinal fluid 5-hydroxyindoleacetic acid (CSF 5-HIAA), the marker for serotonin (Bottiglieri *et al*). Low levels of CSF 5-HIAA have also been found in folate deficient adults with epilepsy (Botez *et al*) and children with severe metabolic defects affecting the folate pathway (Hyland *et al*).

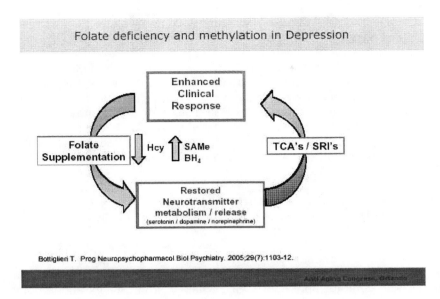

Figure 6. The relationship between folate deficiency and methylation in depression.

These findings led to the development of a hypothesis suggesting that patients who have depression and who respond poorly to antidepressants are in a state of negative folate balance, thus meaning that they are folate deficient. If you give supplementary folate to these patients, you will lower their homocysteine levels and normalize both their SAM levels and their BH4 (tetrahydrobiopterin) levels. That will result in a restored neurotransmitter metabolism, and if your patients are also taking their antidepressant medication, that will enhance their clinical response.

Hyperhomocystinemia and Dementia – Is There a Link?

There is a growing body of evidence to support the association between hyperhomocystinemia and dementia. In fact, evidence suggests that vascular dysfunction may well be a major component in the pathology of Alzheimer's disease.

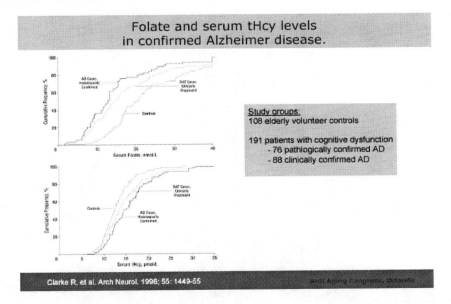

Figure 7. The link between low serum folate and elevated homocysteine levels in confirmed Alzheimer's disease.

Clarke *et al* measured serum folate and homocysteine levels in people that had been clinically diagnosed or histopathologically confirmed as having Alzheimer's disease. The results of this study showed that low blood levels of folate and elevated homocysteine levels were indeed associated with Alzheimer's disease. As can be seen in Figure 7, there is a shift to the left in the cumulative frequency curve in the top graph for folate, indicating low serum folate levels, and a shift to the right in the bottom graph, indicating increased homocysteine levels among patients diagnosed with Alzheimer's disease.

A number of other studies have supported this effect, and they all suggest that elevated homocysteine is a risk factor for dementia of approximately two-fold. In the study by Clarke *et al*, that was as high as 4.5 fold in the participants with histopathologically confirmed Alzheimer's disease. However, Anello *et al* found that having both hyperhomocystinemia and the MTHFRT **C**677T genotype increases the risk of dementia by 6.28-fold.

We studied the relationship between plasma homocysteine, folate, vitamin B12 levels, and the MTHFR C677T genotype in an Italian population of patients with dementia (Bottiglieri *et al*, 2001). Our results showed that people with a low serum folate and the TT genotype are at greater risk for hyperhomocystinemia than people who eat a poor diet with a negative folate balance and the CC (normal) genotype. This suggests that it may be prudent to screen people for the TT genotype, because if their homocysteine levels are not coming down they may well need a higher dose of folate.

Another interesting study which we conducted a number of years back (Bottiglieri *et al*, 2000) examined folate levels in cerebrospinal fluid (CSF) obtained from patients undergoing elective surgery. The people in this study were cognitively intact. They had no dementia and no other illnesses; they were having hip replacements and so forth. The results of this study showed a definite age-related decline in CSF folate levels. Our findings were confirmed in another study published several years later.

Therefore, there is a natural age-related decline in folate levels, which may be associated with the age-related cognitive decline that we also see in the population. Another study, which we published (Serot *et al*), found that homocysteine levels increase with age. So, it appears that low folate and high homocysteine levels are really a problem of aging. However, the good news is that these are problems we can address and remedy simply by giving people supplementary folate.

Folate Deficiency – Neurotoxic Mechanisms

All of these findings have enabled us to theorize the apparent neurotoxic mechanisms triggered by folate and/or vitamin B12 deficiency (Bottiglieri, 2005). These mechanisms are summarized in Figure 8.

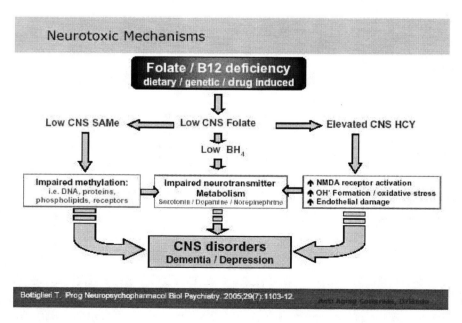

Figure 8. Neurotoxic mechanisms associated with folate deficiency.

Folate and/or B12 deficiency can lead to low folate levels in the central nervous system (CNS). This can affect a number of pathways, and lead to low SAM levels in the CNS and elevated homocysteine levels. Low SAM levels leads to high SAH levels, which inhibit or impair methylation reactions. This has a major effect on the methylation of DNA and proteins and phospholipids and receptors. Low folate levels also affect tetrahydrobiopterin (BH4) levels, which in turn affects the neurotransmitter system.

Elevated homocysteine levels are problematic in the sense that there is a lot of literature showing that increased homocysteine can give rise to the activation of NMDA receptors. Overactivation of NMDA receptors can allow calcium to get into the cells, which can trigger a cascade of processes that result in cell death. Overactivation of NMDA receptors also results in increased oxidation and hydroxyl radical formation, which gives rise to oxidative stress, and can also cause endothelial damage. These different mechanisms may converge to produce various affects in the CNS that may lead to dementia and depression.

Treating Folate Deficiency

What can be done to treat folate deficiency? The most obvious thing to do is give the patient supplementary folate and other B vitamins. There are many different forms of folate and other B vitamins available, either in combination or alone. D, L-folic acid is probably the cheapest. However L-methyl-tetrahydrofolate (MTHF) is the form of folate taken up by cells and is also the form of folate with the greatest bioavailability, thus leading to higher plasma levels of MTHF (Fig. 9).

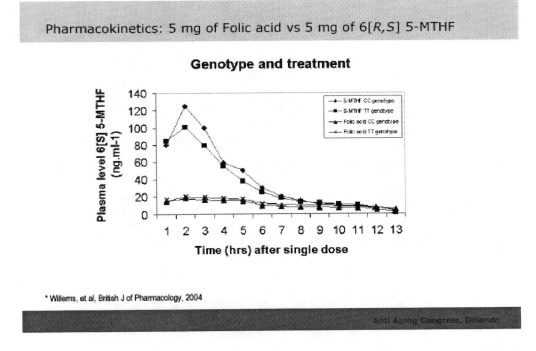

Figure 9. Plasma levels of 5-MTHF after taking 5 mg of folic acid versus 5 mg 5-MTHF.

What about restoring vitamin B12 levels? Cyanocobalamin or methylcobalamin can be used to restore vitamin B12 levels. Methylcobalamin is preferable as it directly targets the methylation pathway because it is utilized by the enzyme that converts methylfolate to tetrahydrofolate.

CONCLUDING REMARKS

In conclusion, we now know that folate is required for the synthesis of DNA, critical methylation reactions, and to maintain low levels of homocysteine. Deficiency of folate is common in the aging population and is associated with neuropsychiatric complications including depression and dementia. These deficient states can be effectively treated with folate supplementation. Research suggests that folate supplementation may also augment the efficacy of antidepressants. Various forms of folate are available in combination with other B vitamins that can enhance folate-dependent pathways. 5-MTHF is the form of folate which is transported across cells and the blood brain barrier and provides a greater bioavailability, and is thus the treatment of choice for folate deficiency.

REFERENCES

Anello G, Gueant-Rodriguez RM, Bosco P, Gueant JL, Romano A, Namour B, Spada R, Caraci F, Pourie G, Daval JL, Ferri R. Homocysteine and methylenetetrahydrofolate reductase polymorphism in Alzheimer's disease. *Neuroreport*. 2004;15:859-861.

Botez MI, Young SN. Effects of anticonvulsant treatment and low levels of folate and thiamine on amine metabolites in cerebrospinal fluid. *Brain*. 1991;114:333-348.

Bottiglieri T. Homocysteine and folate metabolism in depression. *Prog Neuropsychopharmacol Biol Psychiatry*. 2005;29:1103-1112.

Bottiglieri T, Parnetti L, Arning E, Ortiz T, Amici S, Lanari A, Gallai V. Plasma total homocysteine levels and the C677T mutation in the methylenetetrahydrofolate reductase (MTHFR) gene: a study in an Italian population with dementia. *Mech Ageing Dev*. 2001;122:2013-2023.

Bottiglieri T, Reynolds EH, Laundy M. Folate in CSF and age. *J Neurol Neurosurg Psychiatry*. 2000;69:562.

Clarke R, Smith AD, Jobst KA, Refsum H, Sutton L, Ueland PM. Folate, vitamin B12, and serum total homocysteine levels in confirmed Alzheimer disease. *Arch Neurol*. 1998;55:1449-1455.

Coppen A, Bailey J. Enhancement of the antidepressant action of fluoxetine by folic acid: a randomised, placebo controlled trial. *J Affect Disord*. 2000;60:121-130.

Crellin R, Bottiglieri T, Reynolds EH. Folates and psychiatric disorders. Clinical potential. *Drugs*. 1993;45:623-636.

Fava M, Borus JS, Alpert JE, Nierenberg AA, Rosenbaum JF, Bottiglieri T. Folate, vitamin B12, and homocysteine in major depressive disorder. *Am J Psychiatry*. 1997;154:426-428.

Hyland K, Smith I, Bottiglieri T, Perry J, Wendel U, Clayton PT, Leonard JV. Demyelination and decreased S-adenosylmethionine in 5,10-methylenetetrahydrofolate reductase deficiency. *Neurology*. 1988;38:459-462

Morris MS, Fava M, Jacques PF, Selhub J, Rosenberg IH. Depression and folate status in the US Population. *Psychother Psychosom*. 2003;72:80-87.

Nygard O, Nordrehaug JE, Refsum H, Ueland PM, Farstad M, Vollset SE. Plasma homocysteine levels and mortality in patients with coronary artery disease. *N Engl J Med*. 1997;337:230-236.

Serot JM, Barbé F, Arning E, Bottiglieri T, Franck P, Montagne P, Nicolas JP. Homocysteine and methylmalonic acid concentrations in cerebrospinal fluid: relation with age and Alzheimer's disease. *J Neurol Neurosurg Psychiatry*. 2005;76:1585-1587.

Shorvon SD, Carney MW, Chanarin I, Reynolds EH.The neuropsychiatry of megaloblastic anaemia. *Br Med J*. 1980;281:1036-1038.

Ueland PM, Nygård O, Vollset SE, Refsum H. The Hordaland Homocysteine Studies. *Lipids*. 2001;36:S33-39.

Willems FF, Boers GH, Blom HJ, Aengevaeren WR, Verheugt FW. Pharmacokinetic study on the utilisation of 5-methyltetrahydrofolate and folic acid in patients with coronary artery disease. *Br J Pharmacol*. 2004;141:825-830.

ABOUT THE AUTHOR

Dr. Teodoro Bottiglieri's research focuses on understanding the role of homocysteine, B vitamins, and methylation in the central nervous system. The research conducted in his laboratory has application to many disease states, including diagnosis of in-born errors of metabolism, and age-related disease including vascular dysfunction, depression, Parkinson's disease, and dementia.

Chapter 4
21ST Century Ultrasound: The New Physical Examination

Eric R. Braverman, M.D.
Director, PATH Research Foundation;
Director, Integrative Medicine Program, Cabrini Medical Center

ABSTRACT
A head-to-toe ultrasound should be an option to all patients, whose financial situation allows, as an important supplement to the routine physical exam for the reasons described in the paper.

INTRODUCTION
The superiority of an ultrasound physical exam to a routine physical exam done with one's hands is considerable. Today's physical is simply inadequate and inferior. Just as we have evolved from using a rolled up piece of paper applied to a woman's chest to a classic tube stethoscope device, we must make the transition from this outdated examination to an ultrasound exam. The ultrasound exam makes fingers in the rectum and hands in the vagina and listening to the neck obsolete. The ultrasound exam allows us to see every organ. We can see nodules, pre-cancers, damage, changes in shape and size due to disease or dysfunction of the organ, inflammation, and calcifications. Ultrasound can even detect dehydration in a patient. Ultrasound is superior in every way to a physical exam.

Physicians who conduct manual examinations of the human body miss things on a regular basis. Modalities such as the MRI, CAT, and PET scans are useful in identifying disease. For example, the MRI can recognize multiple sclerosis and specific cancers, the CAT scan is useful in finding bleeds in the brain and lung tumors, and the PET scan may find spot cancers. Although important, these imaging techniques cannot compare to ultrasound in terms of its global general review. Thus, a head-to-toe ultrasound should be an option to all patients, whose financial situation allows, as an important supplement to the routine physical exam.

HEAD-TO-TOE ULTRASOUND
Transcranial Ultrasound
Measures blood flow in the eye blood vessels and middle cerebral arteries (the main arteries into the brain).
Benefits: Can detect aneurysms and damaged blood vessels; can provide information regarding migraines and dementia; most brain diseases are acquired. Can also detect increased velocity of the blood flow due to vascular spasm or blockage.
Recommended Nutritional Supplements: Vitamins C, E, and K, flavonoids, Coleus Forskholii, and omega-3 fatty acids

Carotid Ultrasound
Measures blood flow through main artery in the neck to brain
Benefits: Can show early changes in blood flow, thickening of the intima, and advanced atherosclerotic disease – blockages.
Recommended Nutritional Supplements: Vitamins C and E, carnitine, flavonoids, Co-enzyme Q10, and omega-3 fatty acids

Thyroid Ultrasound
Shows goiterous changes, enlarged thyroid, cancer masses, nodules, calcifications, cysts, and atrophy even in patients with normal physical exam.
Benefits: Early diagnosis of disease is possible with this ultrasound.
Recommended Nutritional Supplements: low cruciferous diet and iodine and tyrosine if hormone level is low

Echocardiogram

Shows heart size (all four chambers), ejection fraction, changes in wall motion as a sign of previous or current heart attack and heart failure; early changes in heart appearance due to increased alcohol intake or increased blood pressure. Can detect damaged heart valves such as: mitral, tricuspid, pulmonic, and aortic. Can also detect changes/enlargements in left/right ventricle left/right atrium.
Benefits: Can predict early atrial fibrillation and heart failure, and can suggest coronary artery disease.

Breast Ultrasound

This is the best test to find breast cysts. Also shows nodules, masses, and calcifications at times in patients with negative breast exam.
Benefits: Can detect cancers and pre-cancers.
Recommended Nutritional Supplements: Vitamins B6 and E, Co-enzyme, and omega 6 fatty acids

Abdominal Ultrasound

Shows enlarged liver, and spleen at times, in patients with normal physical exams or in obese patients; allows the detection of early changes of alcoholic hepatitis, fatty liver, gall stones, gall bladder wall thickening, liver cyst, hemangiomas, other benign tumors and cancer, calcifications, cysts/calcifications of pancreas, and atherosclerotic changes in the abdominal aorta.
Benefits: Can identify damage caused by drugs and infections. Can detect pancreatic cancer or previously benign cysts, sarcomas, abdominal aortic aneurysms, and spleen calcification.
Recommended Nutritional Supplements: Lipoic acid, N-Acetyl Cysteine, milk thistle, and S-adenosyl methionine

Renal Ultrasound

Shows kidney stones, cysts, and tumors – often as an accidental finding in patients without complaints. Can also show fluid collection in kidneys (hydronephrosis), enlargement, or kidney atrophy.
Benefits: Early diagnosis of disease is possible with this ultrasound.
Recommended Nutritional Supplements: Magnesium and vitamin B6

Pelvic Ultrasound

Can detect uterine enlargement, fibroids, changes in ovaries (increased size, cysts, tumors), prominent endometrium, endometrical cancers, cervical cysts, sarcomas, myosarcomas, and fluid collection due to advancing ovarian cancer. Also can determine bladder size and identify bladder stones.
Benefits: Early diagnosis of disease is possible with this ultrasound.
Recommended Nutritional Supplements: Vitamin C

Prostate Ultrasound

Shows size of prostate, its nodules, calcifications, masses, bladder size and function, enlarged prostate, abnormal growth in prostate/bladder, presence of residual urine in patient with enlarged prostate at times in patient with normal DRE.
Benefits: Early diagnosis of disease is possible with this ultrasound.

Scrotal Ultrasound

Size of testicles and epididymus, presence of varicocele, spermatocele, water in testicles, information regarding infertility, cancer, overuse of testosterone-shrunken testicles, smaller testicles as a result of aging and hormonal change, calcifications, tumors at times not found on physical exam.
Benefits: Early diagnosis of disease is possible with this ultrasound.
Recommended Nutritional Supplements: Vitamin E, selenium, zinc, saw palmetto, pygeum africanus, and stinging nettle.

CONCLUDING REMARKS

The superiority of an ultrasound physical exam to a routine physical exam done with one's hands is considerable. Today's physical is simply inadequate and inferior. All patients, whose financial situation allows, should be offered a head-to-toe ultrasound examination as an important supplement to the routine physical exam.

ABOUT THE AUTHOR

Dr. Eric Braverman is the Director of The Place for Achieving Total Health (PATH Medical), with locations in New York, NY, Penndel, PA (metro-Philadelphia), and a national network of affiliated medical professionals. Dr. Braverman received his B.A. Summa Cum Laude from Brandeis University and his M.D. with honors from New York University Medical School, after which he performed post-graduate work in internal Medicine with Yale Medical School affiliate. Dr. Braverman is the author of five medical books, including the *PATH Wellness Manual*, which is a user's guide to alternative treatment. He has appeared on CNN (Larry King Live), PBS, AHN, MSNBC, Fox News Channel and local TV stations. Dr. Braverman has been quoted in the *New York Post, New York Times* and the *Wall Street Journal*.

Chapter 5
Electrotherapy

Eric R. Braverman, M.D.*; Kenneth Blum, Ph.D.; Ray Smith, Ph.D.;
Manpreet Kalra, BSc; Mallory Kerner
* Director, PATH Research Foundation; Director, Integrative Medicine Program, Cabrini Medical Center

ABSTRACT

In an increasingly technological age, electricity may become the norm for treating and preventing a range of disorders from PMS to anxiety. The benefits of such treatment have been proven time and again, and have been recognized for hundreds of years. The following will outline many of these benefits, and will introduce a specific and promising development in electrotherapy: Cranial Electrotherapy Stimulation (CES). After outlining some important studies and hypotheses about CES, new directions for further research and discoveries of the effects of CES on the brain will be discussed.

INTRODUCTION

Electrotherapy has long been used for regulating heart rhythms and healing bone fractures. Vagus nerve stimulation, which involves implanting a lead under the skin and using a stimulator to send electric impulses to the left vagus nerve, has been shown to influence both sympathetic and parasympathetic cardiovascular modulation in patients with epilepsy.[1] A 3M Transcutaneous Electrical Nerve Stimulation (TENS) device, which is a small, portable, battery-operated device that sends mild electrical impulses to the body, is used for chronic back or neck strains and sprains, joint injuries, degenerative diseases, osteoarthritis and bursitis, and postoperative recovery. TENS can help in the regaining of strength and endurance, and provides proven pain relief without drugs. TENS can also help to alleviate symptoms of reflex sympathetic dystrophy, multiple sclerosis, and other medical conditions of the nervous system.

When used on the head, TENS is called Cranial Electrotherapy Stimulation (CES). CES has been used for healing muscles, and as a Fine Electrical Stimulator (FES) it enables stroke patients to perform fine motor tasks such as opening the hands. CES has caused an average improvement of over 50% in test scoring of hospitalized psychiatric patients and inpatient alcoholics with measured anxiety.[2] It has reduced stress measure related to withdrawal syndrome, by at least 40%, in every studied instance for inpatient substance abusers. It has caused an average reduction of 50% in the depression score of: long-term psychiatric patients, university counseling center clients, post-withdrawal alcoholic patients, and hospitalized para- and quadriplegics.[3] It has caused significant improvement in sleep onset time, sleep efficiency, percentage of bed-time sleep, percent sleep time in stages 1 and 4, and percent sleep time for delta-wave sleep in insomniacs.[4] Because symptoms of depression, anxiety, substance abuse, withdrawal syndrome, and insomnia are so widespread in a variety of psychiatric diagnoses, CES is a useful adjunct in treating a broad range of disorders including schizophrenia, learning disabilities, and hyperactivity.

CES – A BRIEF HISTORY AND OVERVIEW

CES has a long history. The idea that electricity heals is not a new one. The use of electricity in therapeutic disorders dates back in scientific history to Mesmer, who in the eighteenth century tried to use magnetism for a variety of medical problems. Allen Childs, MD, Assistant Professor of Pharmacy at the University of Texas at Austin, suggests that electrical therapies actually date back to ancient Egypt.

CES began in the Soviet Union in 1953 under the rubric, "Electrosleep," as its primary focus was the treatment of sleep disorders. East Block nations soon picked it up as a treatment modality and its use had spread worldwide by the late 1960s when animal studies on CES began in the United States at the University of Tennessee and at what is now the University of Wisconsin Medical School. These were soon followed by human clinical trials at the University of Texas Medical School in San Antonio, the University of Mississippi Student Counseling Center, and the University of Wisconsin Medical School. As of April 1990, there were over 100 published CES studies appearing in the American literature. Currently, many researchers around the United States are actively studying the device and therapy, and I am sure our ability to use it effectively will continue to grow.

Open marketing of the CES device began in the early 1970s in the United States for the clinical conditions of anxiety, depression, and insomnia. Under the 1976 Medical Devices Amendment, the FDA grandfathered CES devices, which are currently marketed as previously, but limited to the earlier treatment claims (depression, anxiety and insomnia) until such time as a Premarket Approval Application is submitted to FDA for new treatment claims.

In summary, CES is the FDA's term for any application of 4 milliamps or less of electricity across the head for medical purposes. Its use requires a prescription. Currently, all approved devices give biphasic, 100 Hz, 0.5 - 4.0 milliamps, on a 20% duty cycle. Having followed recommendations of the National Research Council and after over 20 years of medical experience with CES in America, the FDA now considers the side effects of CES to be nonsignificant. For that reason their policy is not to require an Investigational Device Exemption prior to experimental studies of CES. Pacemakers are a contraindication for use of the device.

To date, more than eleven thousand persons own CES devices, which have been prescribed for their home use. In this technological age when we are surrounded by electromagnetic fields and currents, CES treatment may be necessary as an antidote and for maintenance of fully optimum health. Electromagnetic "pollution" from video screens, televisions, stereophonic equipment, microwaves, hairdryers, and phone lines may be destroying our health and may require a device of this type, using similar forces but directed differently. It is likely that CES incorporates some of the benefits of electroconvulsive shock therapy (ECT), without the damaging effects of high amounts of current. CES may provide natural levels of supplementary current to keep the brain healthy in the electrical age. Although technological progress has brought with it a host of new challenges for our Earth and our health, we have also discovered the antidote for many of these problems. However, more research is to be done in order to grasp the full nature of the damage from electromagnetic fields, and also what can be gained from using electrotherapy as a treatment modality.

We now know that CES devices impact brain chemistry. CES devices are thought to raise alpha waves, raise blood levels of endorphins, and increase the efficiency of conversion of amino acids into the brain's neurotransmitters, and together they are more effective than amino acid augmentation alone. Modulating the neurotransmitters in the brain helps to rebalance the immune system and help with aspects of all depression and anxiety type symptoms. Therefore, there is hope that this new brain bioelectrical approach can be extremely successful and may actually become a first line therapy for psychiatric disorders because of its noninvasiveness and low level of side effects. Other possible applications of CES are menstrual cramping, stiff neck, headache, and other pain; allergic reactions, temporal lobe disorders, withdrawal syndrome, and restoration of cognitive function. CES may be a very useful alternative to drug treatments in individuals who have treatment resistant anxiety and/or depression.

The usual treatment is 15, 30, or 60 minutes twice daily for stress; often individuals wear it overnight with a timer that turns it off after 1 hour. The device possesses an automatic shut-off valve. The intensity of current should be set at a comfortable level. The best placement of electrodes will be near the left hand over the wrist and on the third eye.

Patients who first use the CES device can often experience benefit in the first 30-minute session. Often a good marker of its benefits is that it will induce relaxation and/or improve sleep. It should be noted that individuals using this device may initially feel a tingling sensation. This is a good and normal reaction. For other individuals an appropriate trial may be concurrent use with amino acids or antidepressants, which require at least three weeks to reach their full effect, and sometimes as much as two months.

CES and Substance Abuse

Smith[5] was one of the first to study the relationship between substance abuse and depression. He notes that codeine (an opiate) stimulates the production of norepinephrine and will produce a high in the presence of endorphins. As a result of codeine abuse an excess of norepinephrine accumulates in the nerve synapse thus causing the brain to temporarily cease production of this neurotransmitter. With this decrease in norepinephrine levels a severe depressive state is produced as the neurochemical levels in the brain are no longer homeostatically balanced (Budzynski, 1990).

According to Smith and Ostrander, [6] alcohol and valium bind to the endorphin receptor sites. This results in the brain shutting down its manufacture of the natural endorphin due to a surplus endorphin accumulation in the synapse. Since the natural endorphins inhibit the overproduction of norepinephrine, the lack of a normal true endorphin level allows the norepinephrine to range out of control, causing severe anxiety reaction and panic states. Along with this reaction there are all the other symptoms of the classic withdrawal syndrome or delirium tremors. This situation progressively worsens, in that after several days, a severe chemical depression results from an overproduction of norepinephrine causing a rebound shutdown of its production. CES can stop this cycle.[7, 8, 9]

CES and Depression

Smith (1985) reported on 5 studies that involved depression. Overall, the analysis indicated that there was an average reduction of 50% in the depression scores of alcoholic patients as a result of CES treatment.

CES and Cognitive Brain Dysfunction

Very often the serious addictive state is accompanied by an insidious and progressive condition known as Korsakoff's psychosis. This is an advanced condition that manifests itself as a destruction of normal brain functioning, particularly in the area of recent or short-term memory losses[10] and in the ability to process information dealing with abstract symbols.

Statistics have shown that CES treatment halts and significantly reverses brain dysfunction in patients as measured on seven different psychological scales of cognitive function, bringing many such functions back to the level of the preaddiction state in the majority of patients studied.[7] Research findings indicate that CES stimulated the production of acetylcholine in the memory channels of the hippocampal gyrus that, in turn, improved cognitive functioning in alcoholics.[11]

CES for Treatment of Anxiety and Withdrawal

CES is used to stimulate brain tissue to produce neurochemicals up to a level of prestress homeostasis. Research findings state that CES appears to stimulate the production of the beta endorphins (supporting the hypothesis that a mild effect is produced at the hypothalamic area of the brain) that in turn, tend to "inhibit the increased levels of norepinephrine from unduly stimulated neuroreceptors on the locus ceruleus so that anxiety and associated panic states are effectively blocked."[12]

The locus ceruleus is a cluster of neurons located in the dorsal brain stem, adjacent to the fourth ventricle. More than half of the noradrenergic neurons in the central nervous system are located within its boundaries. This relatively small collection of neurons has numerous and important projections to the cortex, the limbic system, the medullary and spinal centers affecting cardiovascular sympathetic activity, hypothalamus, and other important brain neurotransmitter systems.[13]

A study by Gold[14] has indicated that endorphins and exogenous opiates inhibit the activity of the locus ceruleus. Drugs (or CES) that inhibit the function of the locus ceruleus and block elicited behaviors and visceral phenomena are hypothesized to be useful in the medical treatment of opiate withdrawal. This was Gold's hypothesis and he found that Clonidine (a drug which inhibits the locus ceruleus and locus ceruleus mediated noradrenergic activation) is an efficacious nonopiate treatment for opiate withdrawal. This finding supports the data found with CES since it also inhibits the locus ceruleus and produces the same effect as Clonidine in blocking anxiety, but without the rebound depression obtained when using Clonidine.

Another important finding resulting from CES studies is that CES is highly effective when used in conjunction with methadone withdrawal for heroin addicts. (Methadone is often used with heroin addicts – substituting one addicting drug for another). A study by Gomez[15] shows a major decrease in withdrawal time coupled with a significant reduction in anxiety.

Transcutaneous Electrical Nerve Stimulation for the Treatment of Primary Dysmenorrhea and Pain Relief

Traditionally, we have been treating dysmenorrhea with nonsteroidal drugs such as Motrin or Ponstel. For some women pain is so severe that they need to be placed on natural progesterone or birth control pills. For the women who do not obtain complete relief from pills, who have contraindications or side effects from using the nonsteroidal anti-inflammatory drugs, or who do not wish to use a medication, TENS is a new, non-drug method for relieving the pain of dysmenorrhea. A study was done using TENS for dysmenorrhea at the Department of Obstetrics and Gynecology at the University of Illinois College of Medicine, showing that TENS, in addition to reducing the pain of dysmenorrhea in most of the study participants, also significantly reduced diarrhea, fatigue, menstrual flow, and clot formation, as compared with these conditions in women who were not using TENS.[16] The TENS was safe and did not affect the length or amount of menstrual flow. The TENS has 3 electrodes that are placed on each side of the umbilicus (belly button) and one right over the pubic area. The patient adjusts the amount of electricity to produce a comfortable tingling sensation or to achieve satisfactory pain relief.

The reason why TENS is postulated to reduce dysmenorrhea involves two theories: the gate control theory and the endorphin-mediated pain relief theory. The gate control theory is that one stimulates the sensory nerve fibers affecting the uterus, and this blocks the transmission of pain related impulses. The second theory is the release of our natural endogenous endorphins. These endorphins are natural potent analgesics, and it has been demonstrated that these endorphins can be released with low frequency electrical stimulation. Adding nutrients and/or medicine to potentiate endorphins, e.g. D-phenylalanine, Trexan, can strengthen this effect.

In summary, TENS is an effective method for some women in relieving dysmenorrhea. TENS also can be used with nonsteroidal, anti-inflammatory drugs like Motrin. The nutrients, borage oil, fish oil, B-6, and magnesium, can replace drugs. In fact, the two together (TENS and nutrients) are even more effective than over-the-counter pain medication. The TENS is a non-medication alternative that can be used for some women who want to avoid using medication altogether.

Pulsing Brain Hormones by CES?

A recent reference[17] showed once again that the brain electrically pulses its own hormones. Evidence will increasingly show that electromagnetic fields affect pulsing of the brain's hormones, and that this is affecting the mental health of America. One out of two Americans now are suffering from a mental disorder. So much of this is biochemical and we want people to know that their mood problems and depression are greatly a result of our environment. Hormones released by electrical pulse may be aided by the electrical pulses of the CES device.

CONCLUDING REMARKS

A significant amount of research has been conducted in the field of CES. There have been other successful studies concluded in the areas of stress, anxiety, and reduction of pain (Smith, 1985, 2007).

So far we have found that CES can be a valuable adjunct to existing therapy in the treatment of alcohol withdrawal. In substance abuse recovery programs, CES stimulates an increase in beta-endorphin levels and also acetylcholine levels that block anxiety and improve cognitive functioning in alcoholics. Also, when used in conjunction with other modalities, it results in quicker recovery in alcoholism, cocaine, heroin, and other drug abuse. New studies have shown CES benefits with opioid withdrawal.[18, 19]

CES has several advantages over many treatments of alcoholism: it does not require the ingestion of another potentially addictive substance, and once shown how to use the device it is easy to treat oneself. It appears to be effective in cases of chronic tension states, depression, and sleep disturbance. It reduces stress, and turning a switch on a CES device is much easier than learning a method of relaxation (e.g. Zen). Drug addiction appears to occur commonly in people with significant depression, anxiety, and insomnia. Thus, CES may be both a treatment and prophylactic device. Finally, there are no side effects when it is used properly. As stated by Ostrander, there is no other treatment modality designed to help the brain bring its neurochemistry back to pretrauma levels of homeostasis; or to allow cognitive functioning to return to normal patterns within weeks instead of the usual months or, in some cases, years, which is often the case with substance abuse situations. Stress reduction and relaxation seem to be important benefits of CES even in people without mental disorders or substance abuse problems.

We are currently researching the effect that different frequencies and milliamps have on results. Most drug users can tolerate and enjoy higher milliamps than patients with anxiety, depression, and insomnia alone. Already, different frequencies have FDA acceptance for use in treating chronic pain and PMS. The age of electromedicine seems to be dawning.

Braverman *et al* have shown through brain mapping that many serious disorders of the brain are associated electrical rhythm disturbances.[20] CES may normalize a variety of these rhythm disturbances in diverse psychiatric conditions. The brain wave, P300 is significantly improved by CES. This wave is associated with drug craving and is probably a marker for decreased attention span. Braverman *et al* have provided other data for the mechanism by which CES corrects abnormal electrophysiology of the brain.

REFERENCES

1. Stemper B, Devinsky O, Haendl T, Welsch G, Hilz MJ. Effects of vagus nerve stimulation on cardiovascular regulation in patients with epilepsy. *Acta Neurol Scand*. 2007 Nov 13; [Epub ahead of print]
2. Krupitsky EM, Burakov AM, Karandashova GF, Katsnelson JaS , Lebedev VP, Grinenko AJa , Borodkin JuS. The administration of transcranial electric treatment for affective disturbances therapy in alcoholic patients. *Drug Alcohol Depend*. 1991;27:1-6.
3. Smith R. *Cranial Electrotherapy Stimulation - its first fifty years, plus three: a monograph*. Mustang, OK: Tate Publishing; 2007.
4. Bobblit WE. Electrosleep as a Sleep Induction Method. *Psycho Forum* 1969.
5. Smith R. Cranial Electrotherapy Stimulation. In: Joel Myklebust (ed). *Neural Stimulation*. Florida: A Uniscience Publication, CRC Press, Inc.; 1985:15;1-45.
6. Ostrander DR. *CES: An Overview of the Effectiveness as a Treatment Modality.* 1989.
7. Schmitt R, Capo T, Frazier H, Boren D. Cranial electrotherapy stimulation treatment of cognitive brain dysfunction in chemical dependence. *J Clin Psychiatry*. 1984;45:60-1, 62-63.
8. Grinenko A, Drupitskiy EM, Lebedev VP. Metabolism of biogenic amines during treatment of alcohol withdrawal syndrome by transcranial electric treatment. *Biogenic Amines*. 1988;5:527-536.
9. Braverman E, Blum K, Smayda R. A commentary on brain mapping in 60 substance abusers: can the potential for drug abuse be predicted and prevented by treatment? *Current Therapeutic Research*. 1990;48:569-585.
10. Smith R. The Effects of Cerebral Electrotherapy on Short Term Memory Impairment in Alcoholic Patients. *The Intern J of Addictions*. 1977:575-582.
11. Smith RB. Confirming evidence of an effective treatment for brain dysfunction in alcoholic patients. *J Nerv Ment Dis*. 1982;170:275-278.
12. Budzynski T. Cranial Electric Stimulation and the Practitioner. *CES Labs*. 1989:1-51.
13. Foote S. Locus Ceruleus. In: George Adleman (ed). *Encyclopedia of Neuroscience*.   Boston, Birkhouser Inc: 1987; 596-597.
14. Gold MS, Byck R, Sweeney DR, Kleber HD. Endorphin-locus coeruleus connection mediates opiate action and withdrawal. *Biomedicine*. 1979;30:1-4.
15. Gomez E, Mikhail AR. Treatment of methadone withdrawal with cerebral electrotherapy (electrosleep). *Br J Psychiatry*. 1979;134:111-113.
16. Dawood MY, Ramos J. Transcutaneous electrical nerve stimulation (TENS) for the treatment of primary dysmenorrhea: a randomized crossover comparison with placebo TENS and ibuprofen. *Obstet Gynecol*. 1990;75:656-660.
17. O'Byrne KT, Knobil E. Electrophysiological approaches to gonadotrophin releasing hormone pulse generator activity in the rhesus monkey. *Hum Reprod*. 1993;8 Suppl 2:37-40.
18. Westermeyer J. Rapid opioid detoxification with electrosleep and naloxone. *Am J Psychiatry*. 1990;147:952-953. Comment on: *Am J Psychiatry*. 1989;146:1349.
19. Vining E, Kosten TR, Kleber HD. Clinical utility of rapid clonidine-naltrexone detoxification for opioid abusers. *Br J Addict*. 1988;83:567-575.
20. Braverman E, Smith R, Smayda R, Blum K. Modification of P300 amplitude and other electrophysiological parameters of drug abuse by cranial electrical stimulation. *Current Therapeutic Research*. 1988;48:586-596.
21. Koch M. *Electromagnetic fields: a guide to understanding what they are and how to reduce your exposure to them*. Alachua, FL: Teslatronics, Inc.; 1991.
22. US Congress, Office of Technology Assessment, *Biological effects of power frequency electric and magnetic fields – background paper*, OTA-BPE-53 (Washington, DC: U.S. Government Printing Office, May 1989)
23. Brodeur P. *Currents of death: power lines, computer terminals and the attempts to cover up their threat to your health*. Simon and Shuster; 1989.
24. Dodge CH. *High voltage in extremely low frequency communications systems: Health and Safety concerns*. Congressional Research Service, The Library of Congress, Washington, DC, 1984.

25. Sheppard AR, Eisenbud M. *Biological effects of electric and magnetic fields of extremely low frequency.* New York, New York University Press; 1977.
26. Becker RO, Marino AA. *Electromagnetism and life.* New York: State University of New York, New York Press; 1985.
27. Aldrich TE, Easterly CE. Electromagnetic fields and public health. *Environ Health Perspect.* 1987;75:159-171. Review.

ABOUT THE AUTHOR

Primary author Dr. Eric Braverman is the Director of The Place for Achieving Total Health (PATH Medical), with locations in New York, NY, Penndel, PA (metro-Philadelphia), and a national network of affiliated medical professionals. Dr. Braverman received his B.A. Summa Cum Laude from Brandeis University and his M.D. with honors from New York University Medical School, after which he performed post-graduate work in internal Medicine with Yale Medical School affiliate. Dr. Braverman is the author of five medical books, including the *PATH Wellness Manual*, which is a user's guide to alternative treatment. He has appeared on CNN (Larry King Live), PBS, AHN, MSNBC, Fox News Channel and local TV stations. Dr. Braverman has been quoted in the *New York Post, New York Times* and the *Wall Street Journal*.

Chapter 6
Genomic Approach to Cancer Treatment
Stanislaw R. Burzynski, M.D., Ph.D.
President, The Burzynski Clinic (Houston, Texas USA)

ABSTRACT

Medical practices over the past century have reflected powerful philosophical doctrines. The human being as an individual has been neglected and the ideology of a "melting pot" in the United States and the "human masses" in communist countries has occupied a prominent place. Failure of this same approach has also been visible in oncology. Identical chemotherapeutic agents prescribed to all patients with the same type of cancer helped some of them, but produced serious toxicity in the vast majority. The understanding that all cancers are associated with changes in gene expression influenced dramatic changes in the diagnosis and therapy of cancer and the creation of personalized treatment. This approach consists of identification of genes involved in cancer in individual patients, and treatment with targeted pharmaceuticals that selectively kill cancer cells containing these abnormal genes. The Burzynski Clinic (BC) in Houston routinely performs analyses of the most important oncogenes in the blood samples of new patients. A personalized treatment plan, which consists of the newest agents selected from a group of over 20 cutting-edge medications, is then designed based on these results. Antineoplastons A10I and AS2-1I are pharmaceuticals introduced by our team that affect multiple genes and are used in phase II and for proposed phase III clinical trials. The prodrug of antineoplaston AS2-1I, phenylbutyrate, is also commonly administered in our medical oncology practice. Using this individualized principle, BC treats patients diagnosed with over 50 different types of malignancies including breast, prostate, colon, lung, head and neck, ovarian, pancreatic, esophageal, liver, renal, bladder, brain, malignant melanoma, and lymphoma. Japanese, European, and our teams published results have all reported remarkable objective responses in breast, colon, pulmonary, liver, prostate, bladder cancers, and different types of brain tumors. In a group of 1100 evaluable patients with difficult-to-control cancers treated in our medical oncology practice at BC, 45% obtained objective responses, 37% stabilization and 18% failed to respond and developed progressive disease. It is expected that the introduction of new methods of gene expression analysis and new gene targeting therapies will lead to better and a more durable control of cancer.

Keywords: antineoplastons treatment, cancer treatment, genetic testing, genomics in cancer, personalized treatment, targeted therapy

INTRODUCTION

The beginning of the 21st century coincided with the 100th anniversary of radiation therapy as well as the introduction of new exciting molecular-targeted therapies for cancer treatment. The realization that all cancers are associated with changes in gene expression has influenced dramatic changes in the diagnosis and therapy of cancer and the creation of personalized treatment. This approach consists of identification of genes involved in an individual patient's cancer and treatment with targeted pharmaceuticals that selectively kill cancer cells containing these abnormal genes. The aim of this paper is to try to answer the question: Does a personalized treatment approach improve the results of cancer therapy? The most important strategies used in The Burzynski Clinic will also be reviewed.

GENOME, EPIGENOME, AND CANCER

After determining a sequence of the human genome, it was discovered that only 10% of genes are active in adult life; therefore, approximately 90% of our genes are silenced.[1] The system of biochemical factors called the epigenome consists of molecular switches that silence and activate genes throughout our lifetime.[2] Silencing of tumor suppressor genes triggers higher oncogene activity leading to mutations and an increased risk of cancer. Decreased activity of tumor suppressors and increased activity of oncogenes lead to cancer, but the inverse controls cancer (Fig. 1). Since epigenomes are systems of molecular switches which target gene expression, normalization of gene expression based on epigenetic mechanisms is a very attractive approach to control cancer.

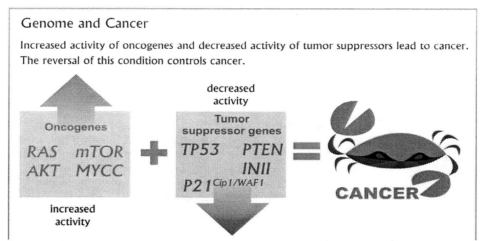

Figure 1. Altered activity of oncogenes and tumor suppressor genes in cancer.

GENE-TARGETED THERAPY AND ANTINEOPLASTONS

Drugs that were initially approved for oncological indications which were directed against single specific targets raised tremendous hopes and excitement as well as disappointment. Currently, the emphasis of research is centered around drugs affecting multiple targets. In summary, there are over 20 targeted therapeutics approved by the FDA and the number is growing rapidly[3] (Fig. 2). Currently available targeted medications are either monoclonal antibodies injected intravenously or "small molecules" administered orally.

In some cases, treatment with new drugs has resulted in spectacular responses, but unfortunately they have been short lived.[4] The hope that these new drugs would provide long term control of cancerous cells is unrealistic. Pharmaceuticals affecting multiple targets may show higher clinical activity, but their application may lead to unacceptable toxicity. Ultimate success in controlling malignant processes would require elimination of cancerous stem cells and the introduction of medications that not only affect multiple targets, but also multiple pathways[5,6] (Fig. 3). Such formulations have been introduced by our group under the name of antineoplastons, which consists of a class of 12 anti-tumor agents.[3] Chemically, antineoplastons are peptides, amino acid derivatives and organic acids introduced by our team for Phase II clinical trials in 1994 (Fig 4).

Antineoplastons are multi-targeted medications affecting the hubs of the gene expression network, multiple signaling pathways, the cell cycle, cell death, and cellular and nuclear transports, thereby resulting in a better chance for durable results. For over 30 years, we have been developing multi-targeted therapies with antineoplastons and we were among the first researchers in the world to work on cancer epigenetics.[1,3]

- ● The most important inhibitors of growth factor signaling:
  Imatinib, Erlotinib, Trastuzumab, Cetuximab, Bevacizumab, Panitumumab and Gefitinib
- ● Inhibitors of signal transduction pathway intermediates:
  Lonafarnib-interrupts RAS pathway
  Temsirolimus-interrupts AKT/mTOR pathway
  Enzastaurin-interrupts PKC pathway
- ● Monoclonal antibodies targeting CD antigens:
  Rituximab targeting CD20
  Alemtuzumab targeting CD52
- ● The most important agents affecting multiple targets:
  Sunitinib, Sorafenib, Lapatinib and Dasatinib - they interact with multiple kinases involved in angiogenesis and signal transduction

Figure 2. The most important gene-targeted medications.

How to Effectively Control Cancer?

● The ultimate success in controlling cancer would require elimination of neoplastic stem cells

● Introduction of medications that not only affect multiple targets

● But also multiple pathways.

Figure 3. The most important directions in effective control of cancer.

Antineoplastons, 12 Anti-tumor Agents

● Chemistry

Peptides, amino acid derivatives, carboxylic acids

● Discovery

Described first in 1968 as peptide fractions in plasma - Ph.D. thesis of Stanislaw R. Burzynski, M.D.

● Synthetic Antineoplastons

Antineoplaston A10, Antineoplaston AS2-1, Antineoplaston A10 I, Antineoplaston AS2-1 I and Phenylbutyrate - Prodrug of AS2-1

Figure 4. Antineoplastons currently used in cancer treatment.

PERSONALIZED CANCER TREATMENT

In our clinic, an individualized treatment plan is developed for each patient based on the results of oncogene testing of the blood samples or pathology specimens.[7] Patients with a number of over-expressed oncogenes have a better chance to respond positively to treatment than patients who do not. Due to strict FDA admission criteria, only a small percentage of patients can be enrolled into the clinical trials with antineoplastons. The majority of patients are treated with a combination of targeted pharmaceuticals based on the identification of oncogenes and the type and stage of their cancer (Fig. 5).

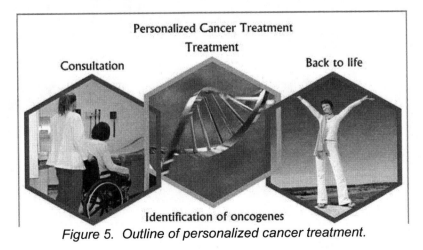

Figure 5. Outline of personalized cancer treatment.

39

Antineoplastons are not available to such patients due to FDA restrictions, but FDA-approved phenylbutyrate, which is metabolized into antineoplaston AS2-1I, is prescribed to these patients. Treatment of a typical patient consists of phenylbutyrate, several targeted agents, supplements, and a proper diet. Determination of a response is based on standard National Cancer Institute (NCI) criteria and requires a decrease of tumor measurements after the treatment. Using this individualized treatment principle, the Burzynski Clinic treats patients diagnosed with over 50 different types of malignancies including breast, colon, lung, prostate, head and neck, ovarian, pancreatic, esophageal, liver, kidney, bladder, brain, malignant melanoma, and lymphoma. In a group of 1100 evaluable patients with difficult-to-control cancers treated in our medical oncology practice, 45% of patients obtained objective responses, 37% had stabilization, and 18% failed to respond and developed progressive disease. This treatment is much better tolerated than standard chemotherapy and radiation, with either no side effects or minimal adverse reactions noted. The best responses are documented in breast, prostate, colon, ovarian, and head and neck cancers, and non-Hodgkin's lymphoma with the highest objective response rates of 60% (Fig. 6, 7, 8).

Personalized Treatment at Burzynski Clinic
Comparison of Responses in Common Cancers (as of Jan 1, 2008)

Diagnosis	Number of patients	Objective response (%)	Stable disease (%)	Progressive disease (%)
Breast cancer	194	60	25	15
Non-Hodgkin's lymphoma	77	55	34	11
Carcinoma of unknown primary	28	54	39	7
Prostate cancer	210	51	40	9
Head and neck cancer	40	50	33	17
Colon cancer	110	47	31	22
Ovarian cancer	34	47	29	24
Uterine and vulvar cancer	22	45	23	32
Lung cancer	92	34	45	21
Malignant melanoma	33	31	24	45

Figure 6. Responses to personalized treatment at Burzynski Clinic.

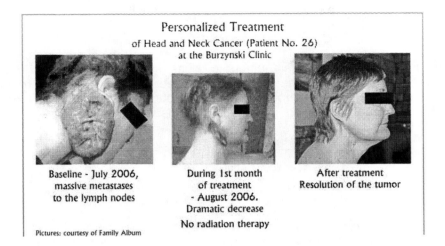

Baseline - July 2006,
massive metastases
to the lymph nodes

During 1st month
of treatment
- August 2006.
Dramatic decrease
No radiation therapy

After treatment
Resolution of the tumor

Pictures: courtesy of Family Album

Figure 7. Complete response of squamous cell carcinoma of the oropharynx metastatic to the cervical lymph nodes. A 49-year-old female diagnosed on November 15, 2004, initially treated with combination chemotherapy with 5-fluorouracil, cisplatin, and docetaxel which was discontinued due to high toxicity. She refused radiation therapy. She began a personalized treatment plan (phenylbutyrate, erlotinib, bevacizumab, and low-dose chemotherapy) at Burzynski Clinic on July 18, 2006. Treatment was discontinued on January 12, 2007. She is currently tumor-free.

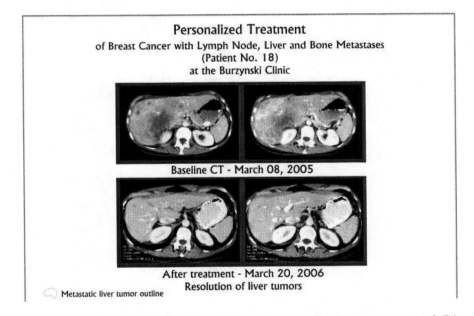

Baseline CT - March 08, 2005

After treatment - March 20, 2006
Resolution of liver tumors

Metastatic liver tumor outline

Figure 8. Partial response of metastatic breast cancer after personalized treatment. A 51-year-old female diagnosed on March 18, 2005, with infiltrating ductal carcinoma of the breast with lymph node, liver, and bone metastases. She refused standard treatment. She began a personalized treatment plan (phenylbutyrate, trastuzumab, bevacizumab, sunitunib, and low-dose chemotherapy) on March 30, 2005. She is currently in remission.

CLINICAL TRIALS WITH ANTINEOPLASTONS

Patients who are not good candidates for treatment with targeted therapies are enrolled into our clinical trials with antineoplastons. Twelve FDA-supervised phase II trials confirmed antitumor activity in advanced cases of different types of brain tumors in adults and children (Fig. 9). In addition to clinical trials conducted at our clinic, Japanese and European teams have confirmed remarkable objective responses using antineoplastons in the treatment of colon, lung, breast, and liver cancers, and malignant brain tumors. The deadliest brain tumors, inoperable brainstem gliomas were selected for Phase III trial, which is scheduled to start soon.

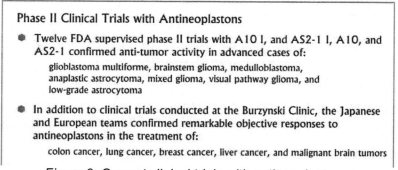

Phase II Clinical Trials with Antineoplastons

● Twelve FDA supervised phase II trials with A10 I, and AS2-1 I, A10, and AS2-1 confirmed anti-tumor activity in advanced cases of:

glioblastoma multiforme, brainstem glioma, medulloblastoma, anaplastic astrocytoma, mixed glioma, visual pathway glioma, and low-grade astrocytoma

● In addition to clinical trials conducted at the Burzynski Clinic, the Japanese and European teams confirmed remarkable objective responses to antineoplastons in the treatment of:

colon cancer, lung cancer, breast cancer, liver cancer, and malignant brain tumors

Figure 9. Current clinical trials with antineoplastons.

Inoperable low-grade astrocytomas are the most common brain tumors in children. In evaluable children diagnosed with this type of brain tumor treated in our phase II trials, 63% obtained complete disappearance or more than 50% decrease of their tumor size, 30% had stabilization, (less than 50% decrease of tumor size and no progression), and only 7% developed progressive disease (Fig. 10). Five year survival in this group exceeded 70% of patients.[8]

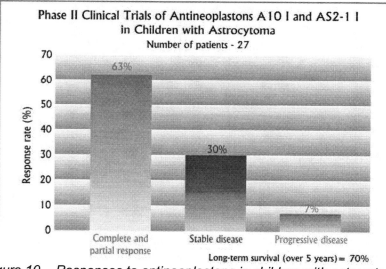

Figure 10.   Responses to antineoplastons in children with astrocytoma.

The results of standard treatments are disappointing in glioblastoma multiforme (GBM), the most common malignant brain tumor of adult patients. In a large series of patients with GBM, less than 2% survived 3 years after diagnosis in North America and approximately 3% survived 2 years after diagnosis in Western Europe (Fig. 11). In a group of 88 evaluable patients with GBM treated in phase II trials with antineoplastons, 25% were long-term survivors (over 2 years) and the maximum survival now exceeds 13 years[9] (Fig 12).

A Japanese group from the University of Kurume Medical School presented encouraging results in the treatment of patients with colon cancer with liver metastases with antineoplastons in conjunction with chemotherapy. The study compared the results of treatment of patients who received antineoplastons with chemotherapy and patients who received chemotherapy alone. The addition of antineoplastons increased 5-year survival to 91% compared with 39% in the control group that received chemotherapy alone.[10]

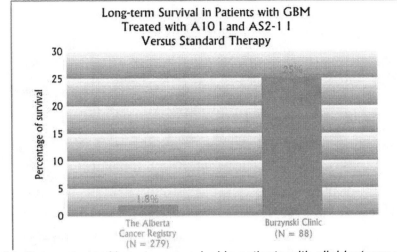

Figure 11. Comparison of long-term survival in patients with glioblastoma multiforme with standard therapy and antineoplastons.

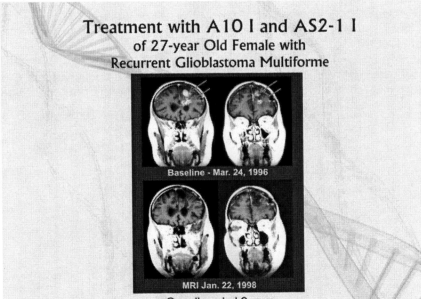

Figure 12. Complete response of glioblastoma multiforme (GBM) after treatment with antineoplastons. The patient was diagnosed with GBM on July 28, 1994, and initially treated with surgical resection, radiation therapy, and two types of chemotherapy. She started A10I and AS2-1I on April 2, 1996. Magnetic resonance imaging of the head with gadolinium indicates gradual decrease and disappearance of the tumor.

CONCLUDING REMARKS

Personalized treatment based on identification of oncogenes involved in cancer allows successful therapy of patients who have failed standard radiation and chemotherapy. Antineoplaston treatment results in objective responses and long-term survival in difficult-to-treat malignant brain tumors and colon cancer. Dynamic expansion of research on targeted therapies and identification of patients who are prospective responders promises much better results in cancer treatment in the near future.

REFERENCES

1. Burzynski SR. Age Management Treatments Which Target Silenced Genes. In: Redberry GW (ed.) *Gene Silencing: New Research.* New York, NY: Nova Sci Pub; 2006:33-80.
2. Jones PA, Martienssen R. A blueprint for a Human Epigenome Project: the AACR Human Epigenome Workshop. *Cancer Res.* 2005;65:11241-11246.
3. Burzynski, SR. Targeted Therapy for Brain Tumors. In: Yang AY (ed.) *Brain Cancer Therapy and Surgical Interventions.* New York, NY: Nova Sci Pub.; 2006;77-111.
4. Green MR. Targeting targeted therapy. *N Engl J Med.* 2004;350:2191-2193.
5. Kondo T, Setoguchi T, Taga T. Persistence of a small subpopulation of cancer stem-like cells in the C6 glioma cell line. *Proc Natl Acad Sci U S A.* 2004;101:781-786.
6. Kitano H. Cancer as a robust system: implications for anticancer therapy. *Nat Rev Can.* 2004;4:227-235.
7. Ross JS, Fletcher JA, Linette GP, Stec J, Clark E, Ayers M, Symmans WF, Pusztai L, Bloom KJ. The Her-2/neu gene and protein in breast cancer 2003: biomarker and target of therapy. *Oncologist.* 2003;8:307-325.
8. Burzynski SR. Treatments for Astrocytoma in Children: Current and Emerging Strategies. *Pediatr Drugs* 2006;8:167-178.
9. Weaver RA, Burzynski SR, Janicki TJ, Burzynski B, Jurida G, Szymkowski B. Long-term survival in patients with glioblastoma multiforme treated in phase II studies with ANP. *Neuro-Oncol.* 2005;7:299.
10. Ogata Y, Tsuda H, Matono K, Kumabe T, Saitsu H, Hara H, Akagi Y, Araki Y, Sata M, Shirouzu K. Long-term survival following treatment with antineoplastons for colon cancer with unresectable multiple liver metastases: report of a case. *Surg Today.* 2003;33:448-453.

ABOUT THE AUTHOR

Dr. Stanislaw Burzynski graduated with honors in 1967. From 1970 to 1977 he was a faculty member at Baylor College of Medicine in Houston. In 1977 he established the Burzynski Research Institute. Dr. Burzynski is the discoverer of antineoplastons, holder of more than 220 patents, and author of the new theory of aging and more than 220 publications.

Chapter 7
The Ironic Life-Saving Potential of Diabetic Sugar Diets
Nick Delgado Ph.D.
President, Ultimate Medical Research

ABSTRACT

Diabetic sugar diets that you believe can kill you ironically can save your life. Fat is the real culprit, because it desensitizes insulin; causing all blood sugar levels to rise to diabetic levels.

Keywords: diabetes, diet, Kempner, rice and fruit, insulin, heart disease

INTRODUCTION

Diabetic sugar diets that you believe can kill you ironically can save your life! Fat is the real culprit, because it desensitizes insulin; causing all blood sugar levels to rise to diabetic levels. Blood sugar will usually rise in the presence of too many fats. It is important to remember that the majority of clients are not saints, and they sometimes like to overeat when dinning out.

Dr Kelly M West once stated that as fat increases in the diet and in the blood, insulin and sugar in the blood will rise also. This is not an effect of sugar but of fat intake. Dr James Anderson, a world authority on endocrinology from the University of Kentucky, states that eating a diet containing high levels of complex carbohydrates and very low levels of fat enables insulin to work properly and control blood sugar, and that following such a diet may even reduce the need for insulin.

There are two general types of diabetes: insulin-dependent type 1 and dietary-induced type 2. Both improve on a Delgado-type of diet, with type 1 diabetics having less complications and type 2 diabetics, in many cases, reducing or eliminating their need for insulin, especially when one increases the intake of raw vegetables, fruit, beans, peas, and brown rice, along with an added daily blended drink of vegetables and fruit.

DIETARY THERAPY FOR DIABETES AND HEART DISEASE

In every experiment reported in the medical literature, from Dr Himsworth's studies on fat and insulin response that took place in the 1930's, to Dr Anderson's studies on the benefits of a diet containing high levels of complex carbohydrates in the 1970's and 1980's, dietary therapy has been shown over and over again to be of great benefits to people with diabetes, yet for some reason these studies have been ignored or forgotten!

Dr Walter Kempner of Duke University was interested in the effect of diet on diseases such as hypertension and diabetes. He had previously observed that such diseases were rare in nations were rice was a stable food. Kemper devised his own Rice Diet, which included rice, fruit, juices, and vitamins, and began to determine its efficacy by monitoring the effect it had upon diabetic patients. Because the patients involved in the study had fragile kidneys and could not tolerate even small amounts of protein in the diet the researchers added one pound of white sugar to their diet in order to ensure the patients got enough calories – patient with failing kidneys can survive and improve on a diet with less than 6% of calories from Protein, 10% fat, and at least 84% carbohydrates. Therefore, to save these patients kidneys, they had to design a diet that was completely the opposite of what one would believe would help a diabetic.

To everyone's shock and amazement these diabetic patients who were scheduled for kidney dialysis improved dramatically. Doctors monitored their daily blood sugar levels, lipids, and insulin response; since they believed that they would have to increase their dose of insulin, yet because the foods were low in fat (fat not sugar desensitizes insulin) all of the patients reduced their need for insulin or were able to stop taking insulin completely! Thus showing that, in the short-term at least, sugar does not worsen diabetes in the presence of a low-fat diet. An additional benefit of this very low fat diet was fat loss, simply because rice and fruit are low in calories and rich in fiber.

Be sure to understand that we are not suggesting adding sugar to your patients' diet. However, a high-fiber, high-complex carbohydrate diet will be well tolerated by most diabetics and heart patients.

CONCLUDING REMARKS

This paper does not say nor imply that sugar is good for you. Sugar contains empty calories, and if the diet of patients in Kempner's study was higher in calories or fats, over time this would cause a raise in triglyceride levels and would worsen the diabetic condition. Because their diet was low in total calories and fat (less than 10% of calories from fat), the blood sugar remained well controlled thus enabling many patients to come off insulin. This amazing discovery was all but lost in the literature, until Nathan Pritikin retold the story of Walter Kempner at a medical conference held back in 1979.

REFERENCES

1. Kempner W. Treatment of hypertensive vascular disease with rice diet. *Am J Med*. 1945;8:545-577.
2. Murphy RJF. The effect of `rice diet' on plasma volume and extracellular fluid space in hypertensive subjects. *J Clin Invest*. 1950;29:912-917.
3. Samaha FF. Low-Carbohydrate as Compared with a Low-Fat Diet in Severe Obesity. *N Engl J Med*. 2003 May 22; 348(21):2074-2081.
4. Foster GD. A Randomized Trial of a Low-Carbohydrate Diet for Obesity. N Engl J Med. 2003;348:2082-2090.
5. Swank RL, Nakamura H. Oxygen availability in Brain Tissues after Lipid Meals. *Am J Physiology*. 1960;198:217-220.
6. Scherer R. Morarescu A, Ruhenstroth-Bauer G. The significance of plasma lipoproteins on erythrocyte aggregation and sedimentation. *British J Hematology*. 1977;32:235.
7. Lissner L, Levitsky DA, Strupp BJ, Kalkwarf HJ, Roe DA. Dietary fat and the regulation of energy intake in human subjects. *Am J Clin Nutr*. 1987;46:886-892.
8. Fries ED. Salt, volume and the prevention of hypertension. *Circulation*. 1976;53:589-595.
9. Keys A, Mickelsen O. The Relation in Man between Cholesterol Levels in the Diet and in the Blood. *Science*. 1950:112:79-81.
10. Ginsberg HN, Karmally W, Siddiqui M, Holleran S, Tall AR, Blaner WS, Ramakrishnan R. Increases in dietary cholesterol are associated with modest increases in both LDL and HDL cholesterol in healthy young women. *Arterioscler Thromb Vasc Biol*. 1995;15:169-178.
11. Ginsberg HN, Karmally W, Siddiqui M, Holleran S, Tall AR, Rumsey SC, Deckelbaum RJ, Blaner WS, Ramakrishnan R. A dose-response study of the effects of dietary cholesterol on fasting and postprandial lipid and lipoprotein metabolism in healthy young men. *Arterioscler Thromb*. 1994;14:576-586.
12. Lichtenstein AH. Dietary fat, carbohydrate, and protein: effects on plasma lipoprotein patterns. *Journal of Lipid Research*. 2006;47:1661-1667.
13. Kolata G. *Science*. 1982;216:38-39.
14. West KM. Diabetes in American Indians and other native populations of the New World. *Diabetes*. 1974;23:841-855.
15. Wendorf M. Perspectives in Diabetes Archaeology of NIDDM. *Diabetes*. 1991;40:161-165.
16. Jenkins D, Barnard N, Anderson JW. Type 2 diabetes and the vegetarian diet. *Am J Clin Nutr*. 2003;78:610S-616s.

ABOUT THE AUTHOR

Dr. Nick Delgado serves as President of Stem Cell Genetic Research International, and President of Ultimate Medical Research. Nick directed Nathan Pritikin Longevity Health, presenter for Mastery University of Robbins Research International, and is the author of 10 books. Nick is considered to be one of the strongest men in the world in dumbbell lifts, placing first this year at the Arnold Classic. He is a Certified Hypnotherapist and TimeLine Therapist of Advanced NLP coaching, Diplomat for the American Academy of Anti-aging Medicine. At www.ultimatemedicalresearch.com, Nick shares the latest news on ways to improve quality of life, breakthroughs with cord blood adult stem cells, methods of restoring sexual function and energy, and how to become "Lean N Fit".

Chapter 8
Key Steps to Longevity:
Your Love Life, A High Fiber Diet, and Exercise
Nick Delgado Ph.D.
President, Ultimate Medical Research

ABSTRACT

One of the secrets of longevity is to eat a diet as close to nature as possible. It is vital to eat foods that have been produced with little or no processing, and raw food that is free of fats should be eaten as often as is possible. However, we now believe that anti-aging requires an integrated approach – diet is not the only secret to a long and healthy life, a positive attitude and connections with social networks that foster love are important to longevity. We believe that eating a proper diet, regular exercise, supplementation and various other alternative approaches can help to slow the inevitable decline of aging and extend life expectancy. The aim of this paper is to discuss these approaches and examine how they can be used to prolong life.

Keywords: longevity, centenarians, sex, fiber, T3, thyroid

INTRODUCTION

One of the secrets of longevity is to eat a diet as close to nature as possible. It is vital to eat foods that have been produced with little or no processing, and raw food that is free of fats should be eaten as often as is possible. However, we now believe that anti-aging requires an integrated approach – diet is not the only secret to a long and healthy life, a positive attitude and connections with social networks that foster love are important to longevity. We believe that eating a proper diet, regular exercise, supplementation and various other alternative approaches can help to slow the inevitable decline of aging and extend life expectancy.

STEPS TO LONGEVITY
The Importance of Hormones

Maintaining youthful levels of hormones is essential for a long and healthy life. Dr Alfred Wolf from Germany has spoken numerous times of the importance of restoring hormone levels with bioidentical hormones and balancing estrogen metabolism.

In *Estrogen Metabolism the Male Toxin*, reprinted in the Winter 2003 edition of *Anti-Aging Medical News* I described what Dr Wolf suspected, which was that certain harmful estrone-like metabolites are more toxic than originally expected, and that these metabolites may be contributing to the rise of breast cancer, prostate cancer, obesity, and heart disease. Indeed, in a study by Muller *et al* published in *Circulation*, it was found that elderly men with higher estrogen levels had faster progression of carotid atherosclerosis than men with higher bio-available testosterone levels.

Free T3 levels have been shown to be a strong predictor of death in cardiac patients. Iervasi *et al* found that having a low T3 concentration (or low-T3 syndrome) is a strong independent predictive marker of poor prognosis in cardiac patients. Results showed that there was a highly significant increase in the incidence of cardiac and cumulative deaths in patients with low T3 levels compared with patients with normal T3 levels. The authors also speculated that low-T3 syndrome may well be directly implicated in the evolution and prognosis of cardiac disease. The implications of this study are particularly important since free T3 is a thyroid test rarely requested by conventional endocrinologists.

Low testosterone levels have also been associated with an increased risk of certain cancers. In prospective studies Stattin *et al* discovered that the incidence of prostate cancer was lower in men with high testosterone levels and higher in men with elevated estrogen levels.

Today, we are able to carry out a full hormonal profile on patients by measuring hormone levels in urine, blood and saliva. Therefore it is easy for us to identify deficiencies and monitor treatment. We also have a better understanding of hormone metabolites, and we are aware that that elevated levels of certain metabolites can be harmful to life expectancy (risk of breast or prostate cancer). Of course, the goal with hormone replacement is to restore hormones to youthful levels. Hormones are like most things in life – too little or too much is usually a bad thing. According to Dr Thierry Hertoghe, a renowned expert on hormonal deficiency, extreme levels of hormones should be avoided at all costs; the balance needs to be right. It is important to note that only bioidentical hormones should be used for hormone replacement therapy.

Dietary Intervention

In my PhD thesis and the book *Grow Young and Slim* 3rd edition, I reported on my study of dietary intervention in 769 individuals. At the start of the study, each participant had their blood pressure checked, lipid tests, and carotid artery exams. These measurements were re-taken every six-months for the two-year study period. The participants followed a diet devised by myself and took regular exercise. They also took part in neuro-linguistic programming to ensure compliance. The results showed that triglyceride and so-called "bad" LDL cholesterol levels fell dramatically – by as much as 50% in some participants, insulin requirement was reduced, and glucose levels, blood pressure, and carotid artery measurements of the artery walls all improved.

The Japanese are renowned for their longevity, even though Japanese people smoke more than American citizens, this is because their diet is far superior to ours. The traditional Japanese diet is based upon complex carbohydrates and moderate amounts of starch, in the form of brown rice and vegetables. They eat little meat and no dairy products. In 2004, the average lifespan of Japanese women was 85.59 years and 78.64 years for men, which is four to five years longer than that of the average American.

Here in America, vegetarians live longer that the average US citizen, whilst vegans live even longer. Results of a study by Fraser and Shavlik showed that vegetarian Adventists do even better, with women living, on average, to 88.6 years and men to 85.3 years. In fact, a direct comparison with other white Californians found that vegetarian Adventists live, on average, 10 years longer. However, even vegetarian Adventists still eat too much dairy, eggs, soy protein, and vegetable oils in their diets to achieve the full potential of human longevity, thus leaving the opportunity to add a few more years to those people who are fully informed.

The November 2005 issue of National Geographic magazine carried an excellent article entitled *"The Secrets of Living Longer."* This article reported on three groups of long-lived people from Okinawa in Japan, Sardinia in Italy, and Loma Linda in California. The one thing that these three groups of people had in common was that they ate a plant-based diet.

I differ from those who think a high protein diet is healthy. It is wrong to believe that you must eat protein to have muscle density, and that you must eat high cholesterol foods in order to produce the sex hormones needed to build muscle. I also disagree with the belief that the best source of protein is lean meat, in my opinion, meats like chicken and fish contain too much protein and too much cholesterol.

Many old school bodybuilders believe that caveman was a hunter, or a meat eater, I believe they were gatherers. We maybe hunted occasionally, but we probably got most of our protein from a diet rich in tubers, vegetables and fruit.

Sex and Longevity

Anyone with an interest in longevity should read the book *Centenarians: People over 100: a Triumph of Will and Spirit* by Lynne Adler (Health Press, 1995). In writing this book, Adler found that these long-lived people had more than 20 key factors in common with each other. One of which was their optimistic approach to life while being highly adaptable to change. However, those that lived the longest maintained relationships with a significant other. It is thought that the facts that these people were usually highly sexually active when they were younger, and that some continued to enjoy sex into their advanced years, might have contributed to a higher production of certain hormones. Thus, suggesting that regular sexual activity may help to prolong life and increase levels of hormones that improve quality of life as we age.

Results of a study by Davey Smith *et al*, which tracked 1,000 middle-aged men for more than 10 years revealed that mortality risk was 50% lower in men who had sex twice a week than it was in men who had sex less often.

The Kinsey Institute in Indiana continues to do research on the healthy benefits of sex. In summary, medical discoveries by the American Heart Association and American Association of Urologists have confirmed that sex is good for your overall health. Benefits to be gained from regular sex include:

- Improved cardiovascular health
- Improved respiratory health
- Boosts the immune system
- Improves bladder control
- Reduces pain
- Burns calories
- Anti-depressant properties
- Mild sedative
- Reduces stress
- Promotes longevity

THE TRUTH ABOUT LONGEVITY

To live longer than 114 years is extremely uncommon. More than 99% of humans die long before their 114th birthday. Dr Alexander Leaf, a Professor of Medicine at Harvard Medical School exposed the lies about longevity made by people living in Hunza, Pakistan and in Vilcabamba, Ecuador. People living in these areas claimed to be living in excess of 120 years old; however these claims were proven untrue by Dr Leaf.

The best verified records of extreme longevity and true extension of quality of life are found in people living in Bama, China and Okinawa, Japan. Both of these communities eat a high complex carbohydrate and low fat diet, where rice is a staple food. What is interesting about these people living in rural areas of Japan and China is that they seem to have much higher testosterone, DHEA and estrogen levels than is normal for their age – centenarians living in these areas have the hormone levels of the average 70-year-old American.

CONCLUDING REMARKS

Proven methods of increasing longevity include: regular physical activity, maintaining intimate and social connections, and eating a diet rich in fiber, low in fat, and high in nutrient density. Hormone replacement with bioidentical hormones, where hormones are replaced to youthful levels (never supraphysiological levels) may also help people to live longer with an improved quality of life, thus enabling us to enjoy our golden years.

REFERENCES

1. Coles LS. Demography of human super centenarians. *J Gerontol A Biol Sci Med Sci.* 2004;59:B579-586.
2. Hayflick L. "Anti-aging" is an oxymoron. *J Gerontol A Biol Sci Med Sci.* 2004;59:B573-578.
3. History of Average Lifespan: http://www.cdc.gov/nchs/data/hus/hus04trend.pdf#027
4. Muller M, van den Beld AW, Bots ML, Grobbee DE, Lamberts SW, van der Schouw YT. Endogenous sex hormones and progression of carotid atherosclerosis in elderly men. *Circulation.* 2004;109:2074-2079. Epub 2004 Apr 19.
5. Iervasi G, Pingitore A, Landi P, Raciti M, Ripoli A, Scarlattini M, L'Abbate A, Donato L. Low-T3 syndrome: a strong prognostic predictor of death in patients with heart disease. *Circulation.* 2003;107:708-713.
6. Stattin P, Lumme S, Tenkanen L, Alfthan H, Jellum E, Hallmans G, Thoresen S, Hakulinen T, Luostarinen T, Lehtinen M, Dillner J, Stenman UH, Hakama M. High levels of circulating testosterone are not associated with increased prostate cancer risk: a pooled prospective study. *Int J Cancer.* 2004;108:418-424.
7. Davey Smith G, Frankel S, Yarnell J. Sex and death: are they related? Findings from the Caerphilly Cohort Study. *BMJ.* 1997;315:1641-1644.
8. Fraser GE, Shavlik DJ. Ten years of life: Is it a matter of choice? *Arch Intern Med.* 2001;161:1645-1652.
9. Meyer T, Kovács S, Ehsani A, Klein S, Holloszy J, Fontana L. Long-Term Caloric Restriction Ameliorates the Decline in Diastolic Function in Humans. *J Am Coll Cardiol.* 2006;47:398-402.
10. Rowe JW, Andres R, Tobin JD, Norris AH, Shock NW. The effect of age on creatinine clearance in men: a cross-sectional and longitudinal study. *J Gerontology.* 1976;31:155-163.
11. Average lifespan of the Japanese: http://search.japantimes.co.jp/print/news/nn07-2005/nn20050723b2.htm
12. Rush B. *PHILADELPHIA DOCTOR. Medical Inquires and Observations by Dr. Benjamin Rush.* 4th edition. Published in Philadelphia in 1815 and reissued in facsimile by Arno Press.
13. Younger hearts with calorie restriction: http://www.eurekalert.org/pub_releases/2006-01/wuso-cra011206.php

14. Luigi Cornaro: http://www.soilandhealth.org/02/0201hyglibcat/020105cornaro.html
15. Mair W, Piper MD, Partridge L. Calories do not explain extension of life span by dietary restriction in Drosophila. *PLoS Biol.* 2005; 3:e223. Epub 2005 May 31.
16. Lissner L, Levitsky DA, Strupp BJ, Kalkwarf HJ, Roe DA. Dietary fat and the regulation of energy intake in human subjects. *Am J Clin Nutr.* 1987;46:886-892.
17. Yu BP, Kang CM, Han JS, Kim DS. Can antioxidant supplementation slow the aging process? *Biofactors.* 1998;7:93-101.
18. Lichtenstein AH, Russell RM. Essential nutrients: food or supplements? Where should the emphasis be? *JAMA.* 2005; 294:351-358.
19. Bartke A, Chandrashekar V, Dominici F, Turyn D, Kinney B, Steger R, Kopchick JJ. Insulin-like growth factor 1 (IGF-1) and aging: controversies and new insights. *Biogerontology.* 2003;4:1-8.
20. Miller RA. Genetic approaches to the study of aging. *J Am Geriatric Soc.* 2005;53:S284-286.
21. Holzenberger M. The GH/IGF-I axis and longevity. *Eur J Endocrinol.* 2004;151:S23-27.
22. Life expectancy of dogs: http://www.pets.ca/pettips/tips-46.htm
23. Samaras TT, Elrick H, Storms LH. Is height related to longevity? *Life Sci.* 2003;72:1781-802.
24. Hoppe C, Molgaard C, Juul A, Michaelsen KF. High intakes of skimmed milk, but not meat, increase serum IGF-I and IGFBP-3 in eight-year-old boys. *Eur J Clin Nutr.* 2004;58:1211-1216.
25. Cadogan J. Milk intake and bone mineral acquisition in adolescent girls: randomized, controlled intervention trial. *BMJ.* 1997;315:1255-1260.
26. Heaney R. Dietary changes favorably affect bone remodeling in older adults. *J Am Diet Assoc.* 1999;99:1228-1233.
27. Arjmandi BH, Khalil DA, Smith BJ, Lucas EA, Juma S, Payton ME, Wild RA. Soy protein has a greater effect on bone in postmenopausal women not on hormone replacement therapy, as evidenced by reducing bone absorption and urinary calcium excretion. *J Clin Endocrinol Metab.* 2003;88:1048-1054.
28. Allen NE, Appleby PN, Davey GK, Kaaks R, Rinaldi S, Key TJ. The associations of diet with serum insulin-like growth factor I and its main binding proteins in 292 women meat-eaters, vegetarians, and vegans. *Cancer Epidemiol Biomarkers Prev.* 2002;11:1441-1448.
29. Allen NE, Appleby PN, Davey GK, Key TJ. Hormones and diet: low insulin-like growth factor-I but normal bioavailable androgens in vegan men. *Br J Cancer.* 2000;83:95-97.
30. Larsson SC, Wolk K, Brismar K, Wolk A. Association of diet with serum insulin-like growth factor I in middle-aged and elderly men. *Am J Clin Nutr.* 2005;81:1163-1167.
31. Giovannucci E, Pollak M, Liu Y, Platz EA, Majeed N, Rimm EB, Willett WC. Nutritional predictors of insulin-like growth factor I and their relationships to cancer in men. *Cancer Epidemiol Biomarkers Prev.* 2003;12:84-89.
32. Holmes MD, Pollak MN, Willett WC, Hankinson SE. Dietary correlates of plasma insulin-like growth factor I and insulin-like growth factor binding protein 3 concentrations. *Cancer Epidemiol Biomarkers Prev.* 2002;11:852-861.
33. Nemet D, Cooper DM. Exercise, diet, and childhood obesity: the GH-IGF-I connection. *J Pediatr Endocrinol Metab.* 2002;15 (Suppl 2):751-757.
34. Rattan SI. Aging intervention, prevention, and therapy through hormesis. *J Gerontol A Biol Sci Med Sci.* 2004;59:705-709.
35. Mehlman MJ, Binstock RH, Juengst ET, Ponsaran RS, Whitehouse PJ. Anti-aging medicine: can consumers be better protected? *Gerontologist.* 2004;44:304-310.

ABOUT THE AUTHOR

Dr. Nick Delgado serves as President of Stem Cell Genetic Research International, and President of Ultimate Medical Research. Nick directed Nathan Pritikin Longevity Health, presenter for Mastery University of Robbins Research International, and is the author of 10 books. Nick is considered to be one of the strongest men in the world in dumbbell lifts, placing first this year at the Arnold Classic. He is a Certified Hypnotherapist and TimeLine Therapist of Advanced NLP coaching, Diplomat for the American Academy of Anti-aging Medicine. At www.ultimatemedicalresearch.com, Nick shares the latest news on ways to improve quality of life, breakthroughs with cord blood adult stem cells, methods of restoring sexual function and energy, and how to become "Lean N Fit".

Chapter 8
The Right Stuff: Use of ALCAT Testing to Determine Dietary Factors Affecting Immune Balance, Health, and Longevity

Roger Davis Deutsch
CEO, Cell Sciences Systems (US) & ALCAT Europe

ABSTRACT

The aging processes, described by Denham Harmon in the 1950s, are manifesting at earlier ages. Metabolic syndrome, characterized by obesity, diabetes, and cardiovascular disease, has sharply increased in recent years. Many observational studies support the thesis that the deleterious effects exerted by free radicals, upon lipid membranes, DNA, and protein structures, forms the common underlying basis of the many diverse degenerative aging disorders. The inability to tolerate foods and environmental factors induces chronic activation of the innate immune system and gives rise to inflammatory processes, which includes excess production of reactive oxygen species and the release of preformed and newly synthesized mediators of inflammation. A simple blood test (the ALCAT test) can be used to identify food and other factors that induce innate immune system activation. This review article describes the relationships between inflammatory processes, degenerative disorders, and dietary factors.

Keywords: nutrigenomics, metabolic syndrome, innate immunity, specific immunity, allergy, food Intolerance, food sensitivity

INTRODUCTION

Since the introduction of the free radical theory of aging by Denham Harmon in 1956[1] numerous findings have supported the notion that random damage induced by reactive oxygen species (ROS) exerts deleterious effects on a wide range of cellular and tissue structures resulting in degeneration and aging. On the other hand, it has also been demonstrated that certain foods containing sirtuins, such as resveratrol (found in red wine) can switch on the same genes that are activated during times of calorie restriction thereby exerting a regenerating effect, or down regulation of the P53 gene.[2]

Whilst other foods induce hormonal secretions associated with the activation of proinflammatory genes, such as foods having a high glycemic index that induce insulin secretion. It is quite possible that food induced inflammatory bowel promotes sugar cravings as activated immune cells in the gut consume serotonin, thus possibly creating a deficit of this key neurotransmitter in the brain.[3] Yet, other foods exert anti-inflammatory effects, such as foods high in n-3 fatty acids (EPA, DHA), e.g. oily fish, which induce a decrease in inflammatory cytokine production from monocytes, notably, IL-1, IL-6, and TNF-alpha.[4]

Chronic inflammation is the primary cause of free radical generation and the common soil of most, if not all, of the diseases of aging. The most significant source of free radicals, as well as preformed and newly synthesized inflammatory mediators, is the activated innate immune system. Further, clinical observations suggest a link between genetic differences and how each individual reacts to food and other environmental exposures as a function of biochemical individuality. Adverse reactivity to foods and other environmental substances activates the innate branch of the immune system, generating release of toxic inflammatory mediators and reactive oxygen and nitrogen species.

Chronic activation of innate immunity appears to underlie and form a common basis for a wide range of generative diseases associated with the aging; including, diabetes, obesity, cardiovascular disease, arthritis, dementia, auto-immunity, and others.

In some instances an infectious agent is demonstrable. However, in many cases no specific antibody is demonstrable and the inciting environmental factor is presumed to be other than microbial.

Commonly eaten, but constitutionally incompatible foods and additives, as well as other environmental exposures, seem to be associated with chronic activation of innate immunity and therefore a major contributor to degenerative processes.

IMMUNITY

A basic review of salient features of the immune system, for the non-immunologist, is in order. Many authors have drawn military parallels describing the human immune system as being similar to a country's defenses. Like a military organization, the immune system must function under tight regulation. If it breaks down, the effects may be devastating. An enemy might attack without resistance; or, the army might grossly overreact to a harmless situation, dropping bombs or launching missiles on a pack of boy scouts or a Salvation Army parade. Simple as it sounds, the military needs to react when it should, and not react when it shouldn't. So too must the immune system. The damage to the organism resulting from immune dysfunction could be every bit as calamitous as that to the nation if its military organization failed.

Put differently, the immune system is a double edged sword. Under ideal circumstances it diligently discriminates between self and non-self; selectively protecting, through the aegis of powerful biological weaponry against a plethora of pathogenic micro-organisms and; like rooting out enemy infiltrators, it also guards against abnormal cell proliferation, eliminating malignant cells before they can multiply and corrupt the population.

Normally, the immune system performs efficiently and unnoticed by the host. However, in states of disarray, its effects are anything but unnoticed. Given the complexity of the system, as well as the fact that molecular similarities sometimes exist between self and foreign proteins, it is little wonder that on occasion it does fail. Failure might manifest in different ways. Over reaction to otherwise innocuous substances is termed allergy. The self destruction when the immune response is turned against the host, which is termed auto-immunity, can be devastating, as in multiple sclerosis, rheumatoid arthritis, myasthenia gravis, systemic lupus, and others. This would be similar to a military unit mistakenly attacking their own town folk.

A prominent feature of innate immunity is the phagocytic cells. The killing mechanisms of phagocytes are very effective. They have been compared with infantry soldiers. In some respects they are actually more like kamikaze pilots. Phagocytes will engulf foreign pathogens into vacuoles then, merging with cytoplasmic granules containing highly toxic preformed proteolytic enzymes, destroy the pathogen. Like a kamikaze, they are usually destroyed in the process. In addition to these enzymes an activated phagocyte will also generate free radicals and other toxic reactive oxygen and nitrogen species. These can be taken up by nearby cells causing peroxidation of lipids in cell and organelle membranes, deformation of protein structures and damage to both nuclear and mitochondrial DNA.

It is noteworthy that overloading the macrophage/monocyte system with the need to clear apoptotic neutrophils (i.e. dead kamikazes) allows some of them to undergo secondary necrosis, whereby uncleared cell fragments release their nucleosome fragments, which themselves may promote further inflammation and auto-immunity.[5] We often see that a commonly eaten food or food additive, will wipe out as much as 20% of the live neutrophils, in vitro, as determined by the ALCAT test method. This could well describe a model whereby food intolerance induces auto-immunity.

Interaction between the neutrophil and/or macrophage and the invader is facilitated by the cell surface receptors' ability to recognize molecular repeat structures on pathogen surfaces. Phagocytes also possess lectin receptors capable of recognizing mannose molecules on pathogens. However, many foods also contain lectin molecules and can easily be mistaken for pathogens, setting off a damaging response.

In some instances cells are assisted by the complement cascade of serum proteins, to effect binding of these markers on the pathogen surface, a process termed, opsonization. This occurs even on the very first exposure and is characteristic of innate immunity. Prior exposure is not necessary to initiate it and repeated exposure does not enhance it.

When bacteria with a polysaccharide capsule present, direct leukocyte contact is inhibited by the capsule. The 'solution' involves B-lymphocyte production of a specific antibody capable of recognizing a particular molecular structure, or epitope, associated with the micro-organism in order to facilitate binding. Phagocytes possess Fc γ receptors to facilitate this. Endocytosis and the further destructive sequence of events soon follow. This is characteristic of adaptive or, specific immunity as the antibody that is specific to the antigen (antibody generator) requires priming through prior exposure, and mounts a more efficient response upon re-exposure, as the formed antibodies increase their binding capacity as a result of affinity maturation.

When a virally infected or a cancerous cell, displaying altered surface markers presents, the altered cell will be destroyed by the direct killing action of a cytotoxic lymphocyte (CTL) or a natural killer (NK) cell.

If the host is attacked by a large pathogen, such as a parasite, other granulocytic cells (mast cells and basophils) release pre-formed histamine in a rather explosive fashion to attack the larger foe. This process is usually antibody mediated. Neutrophils may also react in this fashion toward a larger pathogen (or food macromolecule) in a process called frustrated phagocytosis.

Inappropriate activation, that is, reacting to a harmless substance such as a pollen grain as though it were a parasite, is termed allergy. Failure of the surveillance and neutralization of cancerous cells can result in neoplastic growth. Excessive generation of free radicals and reactive oxygen (and nitrogen species) and proteolytic enzymes, let's call this intolerance, results in chronic inflammation, tissue and DNA damage, and leads to premature aging and possibly cancer. Inappropriate activation of CTL, and other defense mechanisms, aimed at self proteins, induces auto-immunity.

These imbalances, as well as simple nutritional strategies to redress them, will be examined in this review. As these responses are organism specific and involve cellular and molecular mechanisms, a practical cellular laboratory technique for determination of offending dietary factors to be avoided, the ALCAT test can be quite useful. The ALCAT test is a novel method for assessing cellular response to antigenic challenge, ex vivo, in whole blood that is exposed to a battery of test substances. It has demonstrated not only a beneficial response to individually structured elimination of foods, but is also unique in that it exhibits a high correlation with double blind oral challenges with foods and food additives.

Allergy

The concept of allergy was fairly well understood when first introduce by von Pirquet, an Austrian physician, in 1906. It was intended to denote an altered reaction to a normally innocuous substance. As a matter of convention, Allergists later narrowed the definition of allergy to denote only such altered reactions that exhibit immediate and pronounced symptom onset.

It has been estimated that approximately 20% of the US population suffers from this form of allergy, also known as atopy, but this number seems to be growing rapidly. Reports suggest that as much as 54% of the population will show a positive skin test to at least one allergen. This is mainly in reaction to inhalant allergens, such as pollens, mites, and epidermals; occasionally some foods; peanuts and crustaceans being the most common, as well as some contactants. However, "true" food allergy, also know as classical food allergy; or a Gell and Coombs Type I reaction, rarely occurs, affecting less than 5% of the general population in the US.

Other reactions to foods and chemicals, reactions termed intolerances or sensitivities, where symptom onset is delayed and typically less acute in nature, occur considerably more often. Physicians distinguish between immediate allergic reactions, and adverse or toxic type altered reactions; referring to the latter as, "intolerance", "sensitivity" or, "hidden" food allergies. Although both involve abnormal immune reactivity, the mechanisms underlying each differ from one another. Broadly speaking, classical allergy is a function of the specific immune system while, intolerance or sensitivity, primarily involves the innate branch of the immune system.

Classical Allergy is a Function of Specific Immunity

The hallmark of specific immunity is memory; hence the rationale underlying vaccine immunizations. It is specific in that it makes use of pathogen or allergen-specific binding sites on immunoglobulins (Ig) and lymphocyte receptors in the process of recognition. Prior exposure to the activating substance is necessary in order to elicit a response. Re-exposure induces a response more rapidly and with greater efficiency, as affinity maturation, better antigen binding, occurs.

As early as 1920, American allergists Praustnitz and Kustner demonstrated that passive transfer of allergy may occur by injecting allergic serum into the skin of a non-allergic subject. In attempting to discover the factor causing such allergic reactions they injected allergic serum into the subcutaneous tissue of the arm of a non-allergic. Subsequent scratch testing at the injection site with specific allergen induced a characteristic allergic wheal and flare. Although unknown at the time, the causative serum factor was referred to as reagin.

Immunoglobulin E (IgE)

In 1967 two independent teams of investigators identified reagin as the rarest of the five basic antibody isotypes, IgE. One team comprising a husband and wife in Colorado named Ishizaka. The other, at the Karolinska Institute in Sweden, later developed an immunoassay for quantification of allergen specific IgE- the RAST, an acronym for Radio Allergo Sorbent Test, a sandwich immunoassay using a radiolabeled anti-IgE antibody tag, read with a gamma counter.

The role of IgE in the pathogenesis of allergy was later elucidated. An antigen capturing and presenting cell (usually a macrophage or dendritic cell) takes up the allergen and degrades it. It binds to a major histocompatibility complex molecule (MHC molecule) and the MHC/allergen complex then migrates to the cell surface membrane. (All somatic, nucleated, human cells express MHC molecules for recognition of, "self" tissue.) MHC class II molecules present allergens or pathogen components to CD4+ (Cell Determinate) lymphocytes. A T-Helper 2 (i.e., lymphocytes that mature in the thymus gland) lymphocyte, with a conforming receptor will recognize the antigen peptide/MHC complex. Activation of the T cell requires not only this interaction, but also a co-stimulatory signal, usually involving a B7 molecule on the APC, and a CD 28 receptor on the T-cell. The T-cells, once activated proceed to chemically "instruct" those few B-lymphocytes that also possess surface receptors conforming to the initiating allergen peptide sequence.

In this allergic pathway the chemical message from the T cell to the B cell is Interleukin 4 (IL4). Activated B-cells mature into plasmacytes, efficient antibody producing factories, and continue churning out thousands of antibody molecules specific to the initiating allergen peptides. These cells then clone themselves as rapidly as their genetic machinery and availability of nutrients will allow. Each new cell is now also secreting soluble forms of the specific receptor molecule; allergen specific IgE antibodies, conforming to the peptide structures of the initiating allergen. The T and B lymphocytes that persist in the circulation following the resolution of an infection (or, as in this case, allergenic exposure) are termed memory cells.

T and B cells are notably allergen or pathogen-specific in so far as their recognition mechanisms are concerned. Hence, there will be relatively few *memory* T and B cells that initially recognize the specific antigen; however, those that do are capable of cloning themselves as rapidly as the cell's genetic machinery and nutritional stores will allow upon repeated encounter with the pathogen. The key here is that the cells will require the appropriate signals (information) as well as the necessary store of nutrients to supply the needed building materials, as well as the enzymatic activity required by the synthesizing processes.

It is this capability of the memory cells to replicate and carry out their individual functions that underlies the human organism's ability to counter a subsequent invasion by a particular pathogen much more rapidly than the 7 to 14 days required to gear up following the initial infection. Of course, this is a good thing when it occurs at the appropriate time; but, considering that common allergens, such as pollen grains, do not have the ability to multiply inside the body and, therefore, do not inherently possess significant potential for harm, allergy, per se, would have to be regarded as an inappropriate and itself harmful altered reaction. It can even be fatal at times, i.e., anaphylactic shock. The prevalence of allergy as well as that of intolerance is increasing and should be taken seriously.

Once in circulation, IgE antibodies bind to surface *fc* receptors on mast cells in the connective tissue of the skin and mucosal linings of the respiratory, GI and genital-urinary tract; as well as with basophils in the circulation. These cells possess internal pre-formed mediator-containing granules, including histamine. When two or more cell-bound IgE antibodies subsequently encounter the specific allergen, their binding and "cross-linking" induces aggregation of cell membrane receptors, activating various enzymes and kinases, which in turn activate gene activation factors, such as NFκB, resulting in the release of these mediators, a process is known as degranulation (Figure 1). Inflammatory processes, including: increased blood vessel permeability, mucus secretion, irritation of nerve endings, and smooth muscle constriction – all common traits of "true" allergy, soon follow. The so-called late phase reaction, mediated by newly formed lipid mediators, products of arachidonic acid metabolism; leukotrienes, through the lipoxygenase pathway, and prostaglandins through the cyclo-oxygenase pathway, perpetuates the reaction and underlie what is referred to as the late phase.

The elucidation of this pathway is defined, and almost always involves IgE; thus, the RAST test can be quite useful in identifying these allergen triggers. However, as intolerance to foods or chemicals does not follow this pathway, RAST is of little benefit in identifying offending intolerogenic foods or ingested chemicals. Further, because IgE mediated symptom onset is rapid and dramatic, "true" allergic reactions to foods are usually obvious from the history thus obviating the need for testing. Intolerances to foods often produce delayed and less dramatic symptoms and are therefore less obvious.

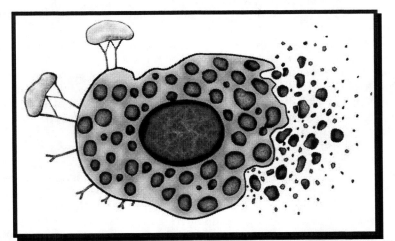

Figure 1. When two or more cell-bound IgE antibodies encounter the specific allergen, their binding and "cross-linking" induces a process known as degranulation.

Many "allergic conditions" that involve the immune system do not involve IgE antibodies. Recently, investigators from the University of Rome found that chronic fatigue patients had significantly higher levels of eosinophil cationic protein than did controls (18.0 +/- 11.3 micrograms/l vs. 7.3 +/- 2.1 micrograms/l (p≤0.01) yet, this was not related in a significant way to allergen specific IgE levels.[6]

Dermatologists from Humboldt University in Berlin previously reported that urticaria patients respond favorably to elimination diets, particularly to elimination of pureed tomato products, and exhibited recurrence of symptoms upon double blinded oral challenge, independently of the presence of IgE recptors.[7]

Dr. Lene Høj from Denmark also reported on a study of patients with chronic urticaria (CU), as well as angioedema (AE), that were tested for reactivity to both foods and airborne allergens using RAST to determine levels of allergen specific IgE, total IgE, and 100 common foods, using the ALCAT test. A test outcome driven elimination diet modification produced a positive outcome in 45 out of 51 of AE. "High clinical significance also at long-term follow-up was obtained in severe AE and CU by applying results of ALCAT test, whereas IgE-mediated allergy played a minor role.[8]

For this reason a lab test that can accurately identify offending foods and other environmental triggers, regardless of what the underlying mechanism may be, would be an invaluable tool for managing inflammatory conditions and would also trim health care costs. The ALCAT test is such a test.

In addition to the release of pre-formed mediators, particularly histamine, the cells will also synthesize prostaglandins, through the cyclo-oxygenase pathway, and leukotrienes, through the lipoxygenase pathway, which augment and prolong the reaction. Some leukotrienes can exert a constrictive effect on smooth muscles surrounding the bronchial tube many times more powerfully than histamine. The substrates of these pro-inflammatory lipid mediators derive from n6 fats which are incorporated into the phospholipids membrane, stored in peroxisomes in the cell, or, are present in the circulation.

At some point along the pathway of both n6 and n3 PUFA metabolism, competition exists for the same desaturation enzyme (Δ 5 desaturase). The n3 metabolites, in contrast to n6 metabolites, exert an anti-inflammatory effect. It is believed that during pre-industrial times the ratio of n3:n6 fats in the diet were in balance; something like a one to one balance ratio. Today, the standard American diet emphasizes consumption of the pro-inflammatory n6 substrates, products like corn oil, safflower oil, and rapeseed oil, also known as Canola oil, with a ratio of perhaps 20:1 Hence, dietary emphasis on fish oil consumption, to redress that imbalance, even more so than other foods containing n3's, has been shown, in several studies, to have some effect on moderating the inflammatory processes. Consumption of high amounts of fish oils can significantly alter the cell membrane composition by perhaps as much as 15%, thus diminishing the available substrate for pro-inflammatory mediator production.

Both pre-formed and newly synthesized lipid mediators, as well as other cytokines, including, IL3, IL5, and granulocyte macrophage-colony stimulating factor, attract inflammatory cells, primarily basophils and eosinophils, but not neutrophils, to the local site of the reaction. A chronic state of inflammation and allergic lesions may ensue. Although neutrophils are not directly involved in Type I allergy, they do, as we'll see, play a central role in intolerance reactions.

It is noteworthy that this pathway not only depends on the binding of the cell bound IgE antibodies with specific allergen, but also on a secondary or co-stimulatory signal by the antigen presenting cell. In fact, in the absence of this secondary signal the T-cell may undergo apoptosis or become anergic (unresponsive) to the specific antigen. Anergy is an important mechanism by which T-cells develop tolerance to self proteins whilst they are maturing in the thymus. That is, T cells, while maturing, if exposed to self proteins, will either become anergic; or, if reactive, apoptotic. A breakdown of this mechanism is likely to result in auto-immunity.

Therefore, claims that an in vitro lab test will detect either allergy, or intolerance, when a specific condition of the assay calls for the isolation of the lymphocytes in autologous serum (because; by definition, the antigen presenting cells and the necessary co-stimulatory signal they provide are absent), should be taken with skepticism. This is the case with the "ELISA-ACT Test" which neither has a sound scientific basis nor has ever been validated by comparing it to the "Gold Standard", a double blind oral challenge, because the promoters believe that no such standard exists.[9]

A useful lymphocyte proliferation assay should either be carried out on whole blood, where the normal cell to cell interactions are preserved, and growth factors are present; or, the sample should be enriched with macrophages or monocytes, to perform the role of antigen processing and presentation.

Modulation of the Specific Immune Response to Prevent Allergy

Thus there is clear evidence that IgE triggers allergy. A therapeutic strategy of injecting antibodies targeted against the cell binding *(fab)* portion of the IgE molecules appear to block the interaction at a critical point and thus prevents mast cell and basophil activation. In some test subjects, allergic subjects appear to have achieved tolerance to peanut under experimental conditions. However, there can be an untoward side effect of down regulating IgE, notably, compromising parasite defenses.

As the T-Helper 2 pathway is activated by parasitic infections the resulting explosive release of histamine is effective when confronting a pathogen of such relatively large size. Thus, non-specific blocking of the IgE mechanism may render the organism more susceptible to this form of infection.

A more specific therapy has been researched which, theoretically, will block a specific allergen reaction while leaving the general protective function of the immune system intact. This approach to classical allergy therapy lies with redirecting or modulation of this pathway to the non-allergy provoking T Helper 1 pathway.

When challenged with a viral or bacterial antigen instead of a parasite, T Helper 1, as opposed to TH 2 cell differentiation, is induced and the signals transmitted to B cells, notably, γ interferon (as opposed to IL 4), induces isotype switching to IgG, rather than the pathogenic IgE isotype. Instead of binding to mast cells and basophils and inducing them to release their deadly chemical arsenals, IgG antibodies, which are about 10,000 times more prevalent than IgE, opsonize the pathogen, enabling phagocytic binding and blocking of the pathogenic IgE antibodies.

This therapeutic effect is achieved by the use of injections of "immunostimulatory sequences" (ISS) of bacterial or viral nucleotides, covalently bound to the specific antigenic epitope. The bacterial or viral nucleotides induce a TH1 rather than the TH2 type response. Promising clinical results have been obtained using the specific allergenic epitope of ragweed pollen, Amb a 1, which will activate a TH 1 cell with a receptor molecule specific to that antigenic epitope. In this way, the non-allergy provoking TH1 response to the specific allergen is up-regulated, in direct proportion to the subsidence of the allergenic TH2 pathway.[10]

Hence, the reaction leads to the production of allergen specific IgG antibodies. In this fashion non allergy provoking, ragweed allergen specific IgG blocking antibodies are produced rather than the reaginic allergy provoking IgE antibodies.

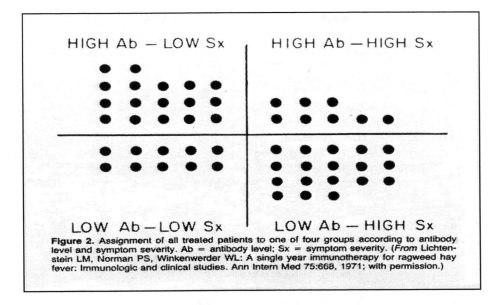

Figure 2. Assignment of all treated patients to one of four groups according to antibody level and symptom severity. Ab = antibody level; Sx = symptom severity. (*From* Lichtenstein LM, Norman PS, Winkenwerder WL: A single year immunotherapy for ragweed hay fever: Immunologic and clinical studies. Ann Intern Med 75:668, 1971; with permission.)

Figure 2. As immunotherapy for atopic allergy progresses allergen specific IgE antibody titers decline while allergen specific IgG antibodies increase.

The Protective Role of IgG

Frequent and high exposure to an antigen favors an IgG response, whereas low level and infrequent allergen exposure induces an IgE response. Herein lays the rationale underlying classical immunotherapy vaccines, referred to as "allergy shots", in use since 1911. The theory is born out by studies showing that as immunotherapy treatment for classical allergy progresses, allergen specific IgE titers decline, while titers of specific IgG increase (Figure 2). As the IgG increases, symptoms also abate (Figure 3). IgG is not an allergy provoking antibody; as in the case of viral or bacterial infection, it is protective.

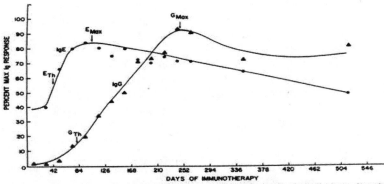

Figure 6. Kinetics of RW-IgE and RW-IgG antibody responses in 51 patients undergoing RW immunotherapy. Each point is the median antibody response expressed as the percentage of maximum response for all patients who were treated during progressive 21-day intervals of treatment. Median threshold and maximal antibody responses are indicated for IgE and IgG. The kinetic drawing demonstrates that RW-IgE threshold and maximum levels occurred earlier than the corresponding RW-IgG threshold and maximum levels. After maximum, the RW-IgG curve plateaued and the RW-IgE fell (45%) to baseline. (*From* Creticos PS, van Metre TE, Mardiney MR, et al: Dose response of IgE and IgG antibodies during ragweed immunotherapy. J Allergy Clin Immunol 73:102, 1984; with permission.)

Figure 3. As allergen specific IgG antibody titers increase, symptoms decline.

Just as IgG is not allergy provoking, a number of studies have also shown that IgG does not cause food intolerance related symptoms:

1. In their 1999 paper Keller *et al* write: *"the occurrence of IgG-cow's milk antibodies is a physiologic phenomenon without diagnostic significance"*. [11]

2. Hadjivassiliou *et al* conclude: *"IgG anti-gliadin antibodies have a high sensitivity not only for patients with celiac disease, but also for those with minimal or no damage…When the histological criteria of celiac disease are used as the gold standard IgG, anti-gliadin antibody has low specificity."* [12]

3. In their paper entitled *"Allergenicity of major cow's milk and peanut proteins determined by IgE and IgG immunoblotting"* Szabó and Eigenmann write: *"The presence of IgG antibodies in non-allergics was related to regular ingestion of food".* [13]

4. Jenkins and Vickers reported: *"We found no evidence that IgE/IgG4 antibody test…is a reliable diagnostic tool."* [14]

5. Zar, Kumar, and Benson sum up the situation in their paper, *Food hypersensitivity and Irritable bowel Syndrome (IBS)*: *"In fact, several studies have suggested that IgG and IgG4 production may be a normal immunological response to dietary antigens. It is probable that food hypersensitivity is a heterogeneous condition, and that more than one immunological abnormality may exist."* [15]

IgG maintains its protective role with respect to excess food antigens in the circulation by complexing with them and assisting the monocyte-macrophage system in their elimination; without inducing pathology. High IgG titers correlate with exposure, not sensitivity. Hence, allergen specific IgG testing is not of accurate in assessing food intolerance.

Thus, this specific branch of the immune system provides protection against specific foreign pathogens. It requires prior exposure to the pathogen in order to mount a targeted and specific response. Misidentification of normally non-pathogenic substances, such as pollens, mite feces, drugs, epidermals, and (occasionally) foods and other factors may induce an altered reaction, or allergy. Allergic reaction is very much a function of the specific immune system; it produces distinct symptomology and it follows a well defined and clearly understood pathway. Food intolerance, on the other hand, is induced by multiple pathogenic pathways – some immune and some non-immune, induces chronic and less acute symptomology, is not IgG related, is both genetically determined yet exposure related; and therefore is far less well understood and consequently, under-treated.

Innate Immunity

Despite the lack of supporting scientific evidence many labs promote allergen specific IgG testing for food intolerance. Confusing as it, the role of IgG in the pathology of food intolerance causes many clinicians, unsurprisingly, to misconceive that prior exposure to a food is necessary in order to develop sensitivity to that food, as indeed it would if food intolerance were a function of specific immunity. For instance, the late Robert Atkins of low-carbohydrate diet fame once questioned the author as to why all of his kosher pediatric patients were testing positive to pork on the ALCAT test, when, by definition, none of these patients had a prior exposure. A reasonable viewpoint if in fact food intolerance were a function of specific immunity. However, it is not. Rather, food intolerance is primarily a function of innate immunity.

Innate immunity may be activated by various factors, and priming, or previous exposure, is not a prerequisite. As Dr. Charles A Janeway, Jr., Professor of Immunobiology at Yale states, *"The innate immune system is born with the ability to recognize certain microbes...(and) can destroy many pathogens on first encounter."* (*How the immune system recognizes invaders, Scientific American, Sept. 1993*) The innate immune system also has an inborn ability to recognize offending foods.

The complement system, a major component of innate immunity, is a cascade of serum proteins first described by the Belgian bacteriologist, Jules Bordet in 1900. These proteins "complement" the activity of antibodies to opsonize the membranes of micro-organisms, thereby facilitating phagocytosis. Complement proteins are non-specific; they will bind indiscriminately. However, host cells secrete enzymes that normally inactivate complement; an example of self /non-self discrimination.

The complement system also protects from detrimental micro-organisms by attaching to their lipid membranes and assembling various components of the cascade called the membrane attack complex. This involves components C5 through C9, unimaginatively named in order of their discovery. They are capable of puncturing the membrane, thereby causing the inward rush of surrounding fluid and resultant destruction of the invader.

Some microbes, such as those causing pneumonia or streptococcus infections, wear a polysaccharide coat in an attempt to block the attachment of the complement proteins. This is dealt with in one of two ways: either the tissue macrophages, which have receptors for these sugars, can bind directly to the bacteria; or, the activated macrophage will release interleukin 6 inducing hepatic production of mannose binding protein, which will itself bind the bacterium, and then activate the complement cascade.

As mentioned, excess antigen is cleared from the circulation by complexing with IgG antibodies. Sometimes, a Gell and Coombs Type III immune reaction, also known as immune complex disease, may occur wherein immune complexes are deposited in tissue or joints and attract inflammatory cells to the site, as in rheumatoid arthritis and glomerulonephritis. But, these are usually IgM antibodies rather than IgG. In examining 1012 renal biopsies from patients with glomerulonephritis through electron microscopy, Dr. M Haas from the Department of Pathology at Johns Hopkins School of Medicine observed that such immune complexes were comprised of antibodies of the IgM isotype, and rarely of IgG. However the predominant component was C3, a key component of the complement cascade.

These findings are consistent with what researchers found while investigating the various mechanisms involved in food-induced asthmatic reactions (Figure 4). When the blood of nine asthmatic patients was analyzed to food reactions as measured by the ALCAT test, and compared to double-blinded oral challenge, there was a high level of correlation observed. Other immune parameters were measured. High correlation was also seen with activation of the complement cascade. Significant changes pre and post in vitro food challenges were also seen in levels of IgM antibodies, but not IgG antibodies. IgG antibodies do not appear to play a significant role in food sensitivity and are likely to be protective in that they block reaginic antibody action and facilitate natural clearance of excess antigen from the circulation without provoking symptoms. The cellular reactions (changes in cell size and/or count following in vitro challenge) seen by the ALCAT test, do appear to be clinically relevant and reflect a multitude of pathogenic mechanisms, often associated with complement activation.

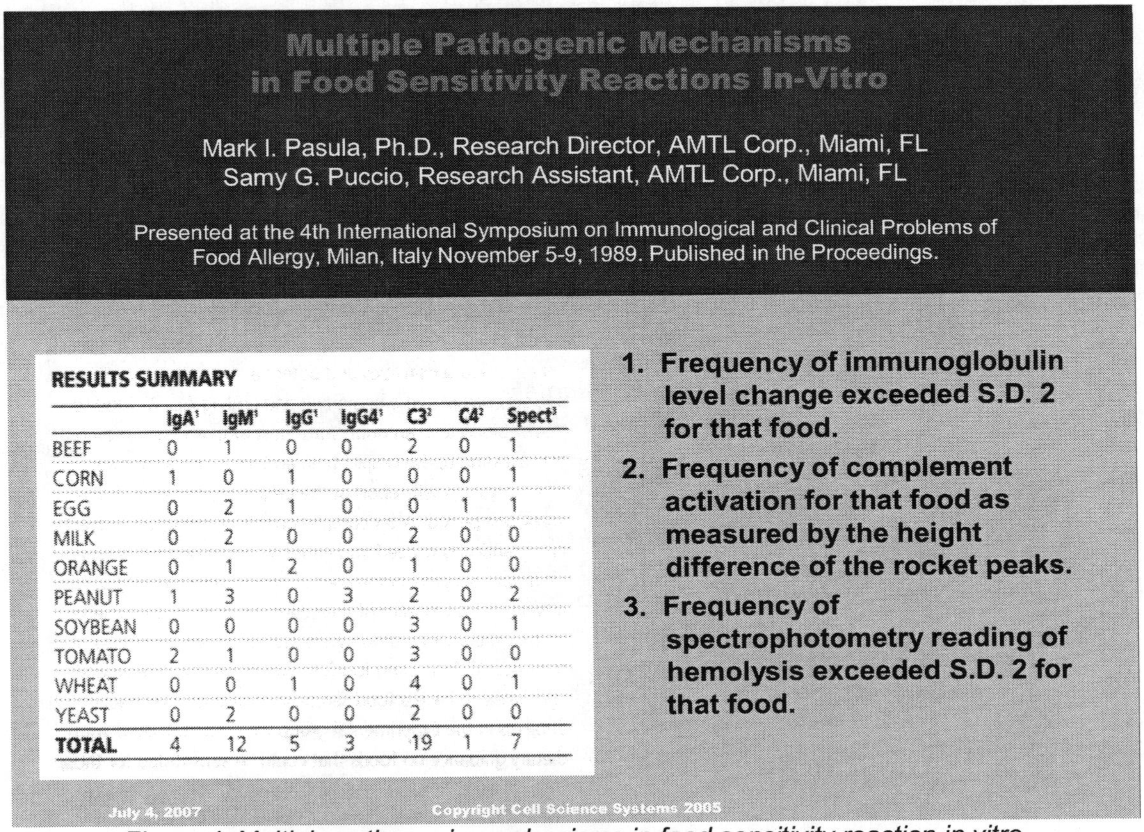

Multiple Pathogenic Mechanisms in Food Sensitivity Reactions In-Vitro

Mark I. Pasula, Ph.D., Research Director, AMTL Corp., Miami, FL
Samy G. Puccio, Research Assistant, AMTL Corp., Miami, FL

Presented at the 4th International Symposium on Immunological and Clinical Problems of Food Allergy, Milan, Italy November 5-9, 1989. Published in the Proceedings.

RESULTS SUMMARY

	IgA[1]	IgM[1]	IgG[1]	IgG4[1]	C3[2]	C4[2]	Spect[3]
BEEF	0	1	0	0	2	0	1
CORN	1	0	1	0	0	0	1
EGG	0	2	1	0	0	1	1
MILK	0	2	0	0	2	0	0
ORANGE	0	1	2	0	1	0	0
PEANUT	1	3	0	3	2	0	2
SOYBEAN	0	0	0	0	3	0	1
TOMATO	2	1	0	0	3	0	0
WHEAT	0	0	1	0	4	0	1
YEAST	0	2	0	0	2	0	0
TOTAL	4	12	5	3	19	1	7

1. Frequency of immunoglobulin level change exceeded S.D. 2 for that food.
2. Frequency of complement activation for that food as measured by the height difference of the rocket peaks.
3. Frequency of spectrophotometry reading of hemolysis exceeded S.D. 2 for that food.

July 4, 2007   Copyright Cell Science Systems 2005

Figure 4. Multiple pathogenic mechanisms in food sensitivity reaction in vitro.

The most common phagocytic cells of the innate immune system are the neutrophils. These are the one class of granulocytes that are not involved in the late phase reaction of type I allergy; however, they usually comprise more than 90-95% of the granulocytes in circulation. The overall system is an effective first line of defense in acute infection but chronic activation leads to disease. Unlike T or B cells, they have a short half life and are very aggressive.

As mentioned earlier, neutrophils destroy pathogens in various ways, but predominantly by generating highly toxic reactive oxygen and nitrogen species, and/or releasing powerful proteolytic enzymes. These include, superoxide anion, which will react with the neutrophil mediator, myeloperoxidase to form hypochlorous acid; peroxynitrate; hydrogen peroxide – which is not a free radical but is still highly toxic, and others.

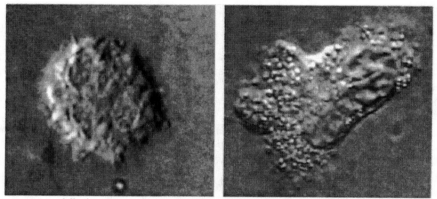

Figure 5. When neutrophils become activated they release toxic mediators of inflammation as well as reactive oxygen and nitrogen species, these are damaging to pathogens but also damaging to host molecules and tissues.

Inflammation and Oxidative Stress

This is where we see the link between chronic activation of the innate immune system and the degeneration described in Denham Harmon's free radical theory of aging.

William R Clark, Professor Emeritus of Immunology (UCLA) describes some of the effects of neutrophil activation in his book, *A Means to an End: The Biological Basis of Aging*, Oxford University Press, 1999: *"One of the more common sources of reactive oxygen species in the body as a whole is from cells that use the destructive power of these molecules as a natural defense against microbial infection. Phagocytes (literally, "eaters of cells") such as macrophages and neutrophils, purposely generate high levels of oxygen radicals, which they store in tightly sealed intracellular compartments.... Oxygen radicals released in this fashion can be taken up be adjacent cells, and once inside they cause the same sort of damage as radicals produced internally....in the case of prolonged infections a chronic inflammatory state may develop, and the repeated engorging and death of phagocytes can cause serious oxidative damage to nearby healthy cells. This is also a major source of damage in chronic inflammatory autoimmune reactions such as rheumatoid arthritis, and can lead to serious tissue loss.*

The damage done by reactive oxygen molecules needed to operate living cells can be enormous. No molecular species is immune. Oxygen radicals can attack and deform proteins molecules, disrupting structural complexes and inhibiting important enzymatic functions....Oxygen radicals also attack the individual nucleotide bases that make up both nuclear and mitochondrial DNA."

THE FREE RADICAL THEORY OF AGING

In 1956 Denham Harmon proposed the "The free radical theory of aging" in which he postulates that random deleterious tissue damage results from the generation of reactive oxygen species (ROS) and nitrogen species (RNS). Subsequent observational studies have lent support to this theory. As tissue deteriorates with age there may be a general increase in the level of ROS and RNS production. Of note is that aged rat mitochondria produce more superoxide anion than that of young rats suggesting 'leakier' electron transport and the ensuing mitochondrial damage. It is suspected that other ROS and RNS also exhibit increased production in other tissue as a function of age.

Further evidence of increased free radical activity and aging comes from the observation that larger animals consume less oxygen per unit of body mass than do smaller animals and exhibit a correspondingly longer lifespan. Similarly, cold blooded animals are more resistant to oxidative stress when maintaining a lower body temperature. Presumably, lower metabolic activity produces fewer free radicals and other ROS. Decreasing the flying activity of *drosophilae* by wing clipping or space restriction markedly increases survival time. Similarly, Queen Bees, which do not fly, live approximately 50 times longer than the worker bees that do.

Wolford has presented compelling evidence that caloric intake, which lowers metabolism and free radical production, is associated with increased lifespan across a range of species, including primates.

Mitochondrial DNA Disease	
This table lists only some of the disorders that can be caused by mutations in mitochondrial DNA. Certain of these conditions can also be caused by nuclear mutations or other proceses that hinder mitochondrial function.	
DISORDER	**FEATURES**
Alzheimer's Disease	Progressive loss of cognitive capacity
CPEO (chronic progressive external ophthalmoplegia)	Paralysis of eye muscles and mitochondrial myopathy [see below]
Diabetes mellitus	High blood glucose levels, leading to various complications
Dystonia	Abnormal movements involving muscular rigidity; frequently accompanied by degeneration of the basal ganglia of the brain
KSS (Kearns-Sayre syndrome)	CPEO combined with such disorders as retinal deterioration, heart disease, hearing loss, diabetes and kidney failure
Leigh's syndrome	Progressive loss of motor and verbal skills and degeration of the basal ganglia; a potentially lethal childhood disease
LHON (Leber's hereditary optic neuropathy)	Permanent or temporary blindness stemming from damage to the optic nerve
MELAS (mitochondrial encephalomyopathy, lactic acidosis	Dysfunction of brain tissue (often causing seizures, transient regional paralysis and dementia) combined with mitochondrial myopathy (see
MERRF (myoclonic epilepsy and ragged red fibers)	Deterioration of muscle, manifested by weakness and intolerance for exercise; muscle often displays ragged red fibers, which are filled with
NARP (neurogenic muscle weakness, ataxia and retinitis	Loss of muscle strength and coordination, accompanied by regional brain degeneration and deterioration of the retina
Pearson's syndrome	Childhood bone marrow dysfunction (leading to loss of blood cells) and pancreatic failure; those who survive often progress to KSS

Table 1. Diseases associated with mitochondrial DNA mutations.

The bulk of aerobic metabolism, and, therefore, oxygen consumption, occurs in the mitochondria. Hence, higher levels of damage occur to DNA in mitochondria, especially deletions, as compared to nuclear DNA. This is indicated by levels of 8-hydroxy-deoxyguanasine, observed in human brain, liver, and other tissues. It increases with age and produces a decline in the function of mitochondrion and the cells they provide energy to. A number of disorders are associated with mitochondrial damage (see Table 1).

CHRONIC INFLAMMATION AND DEGENERATIVE DISEASE

Many investigators have documented the role of neutrophil mediated inflammatory processes in a range of degenerative diseases. Crocker *et al* reported that peripheral blood neutrophils of pre-eclamptic woman are significantly more responsive to the agonists zymosan and fMLP, in terms of free radical production and the upregulation of other markers of cell activation, than are the cells of women with normal pregnancies or age-matched controls.[16] The authors conclude: "*Circulating neutrophils are neither activated nor primed in vivo, however the release of reactive oxygen species is diminished in normal pregnancy. In comparison, an elevation of reactive oxygen generation in preeclampsia may highlight a role for neutrophils in the oxidative stress and pathology of this disease.*" There are also anecdotal reports of previously infertile women becoming pregnant after following an ALCAT test directed diet for a few months.

Rheumatoid arthritis is clearly an inflammatory condition. Investigators from New Zealand reported a two to eight fold increase in phagocytic (neutrophils and monocytes) free radical production versus that of non-rheumatics and healthy controls. Notably, the increased levels of superoxide production seen in the rheumatic subjects correlated well with TNF-alpha, but there was no correlation with plasma levels of C-reactive protein and only slight correlation with erythrocyte sedimentation rate (ESR).[17]

Recently, investigators from Harvard observed that neutrophils of poorly managed diabetics released significantly higher levels of free radicals following stimulation than did those of patients whose blood sugar levels were well managed or normal controls. They also observed a significant correlation with blood sugar levels and severity of periodontal disease and postulated that high blood sugar levels induce priming of neutrophils.[18] Inflammation is increasingly being seen to be at the source of a diverse range of degenerative diseases. The authors conclude that, "*Inflammation and oxidative stress are important factors in the pathogenesis of diabetes and contribute to the pathogenesis of diabetic conditions.*"

Research has shown that when neutrophils adhere to cardiac myocytes the latter incur significant damage via the NADPH oxidase enzyme system mediated oxidative burst. Researchers from the Immunology Research Group at the University of Calgary investigated the role of the adhesion molecule alpha (4) integrin. They observed that neutrophils that left the circulation and adhered to cardiac myocytes quickly induce myocyte shortening by 30-50% and rates of contraction and relaxation by 30%, within the first ten minutes. Furthermore: "*An increased level of oxidative stress was detected in myocytes within 5 min of PMN (polymorphonuculear cells) adhesions.*" This effect was blocked by anti-alpha (4) integrin antibodies and also by extracellular superoxide dismutase (SOD) suggesting superoxide anion as the effector mechanism. The authors conclude: "*The results also provide pathological relevance as the emigrated PMN's have the capacity to injure cardiac myocytes through the alpha (4) integrin-coupled NADPH oxidase pathway that can be inhibited by extracellular, but not intracellular SOD.*"[19]

One of the most frightening of age-related diseases (for those who are aware of it) is cognitive decline. Proving once again what the legendary Indiana Jones stated to his much younger girlfriend: "*It's not the years, it's the mileage!*" French researches at the laboratory of Immunology (INSERM) investigating the role of neutrophil induced oxidative stress in Alzheimer's and Parkinson's patients, have indeed shown that levels of oxidative stress, and not chronological age, are most relevant to these conditions: "*As circulating neutrophils are the most powerful sources of reactive oxygen species, we measured oxidative stress levels in resting neutrophils from 44 Alzheimer's and Parkinson's disease patients and compared them to 40 healthy counterparts. Significantly increased oxidative stress levels were observed in patient's groups while control groups had very similar levels irrespective of age.*" They conclude, "*Our results indicate that oxidative stress levels in circulating neutrophils are of interest for further mechanistic studies of neurodegenerative diseases and might open the perspective of a diagnostic tool.*"[20] Indeed, the ALCAT test is such a diagnostic tool, as it measures the activation of circulating neutrophils when exposed to common foods and other environmental factors.

Atherosclerosis is the end point of an inflammatory process occurring within the intima of the artery mediated by chronic immune system activation. It occurs when oxidized cholesterol becomes a factor in the formation of plaque. As the oxidized cholesterol is consumed by macrophages they convert to foam cells. The result is stenosis of the artery, laying the basis for a stroke following a thrombotic event.

Investigators from Humboldt University in Berlin have measured plasma levels of fragments of the cell membrane lipid, phosphatidylcholine (PC) in blood plasma by HPLC and found significantly higher concentrations of PC in elderly coronary heart patients than in young healthy controls. Elevated fragmented PC was also seen following the smoking of even one cigarette and also during the reperfusion period following bypass surgery, which coincided with a surge in circulating neutrophils. These investigators also observed elevated PC levels in vitamin E deficient rats and concluded that plasma PC fragment levels increase following various forms of oxidative stress. Of course, fragmented cell membrane lipids may be metabolized to inflammatory eicosanoids.[21]

Dr. R Zhang and co-investigators reported in the *Journal of the American Medical Association* in November 2001, *Association between myeloperoxidase levels and risk of coronary artery disease,* a significant association between both blood and leukocyte levels of the neutrophil produced inflammatory mediator, myeloperoxidase (MPO) and the presence of coronary artery disease (CAD). They concluded: "*These findings support a potential role for MPO as an inflammatory marker in CAD and may have implications for atherosclerosis diagnosis and risk assessment.*"[22]

Another group from Shandong University very recently reported on the significance of MPO in cardiovascular disease by demonstrating a possible role for this neutrophil produced inflammatory mediator in the oxidation of low density lipoproteins. Referring to measurements of MPO and high sensitivity C-reactive protein in both cardiovascular patients and controls they find, "*MPO is a better marker for inflammation of local plaques. It may be one of the mechanisms that MPO induces the transforming from LDL to ox-LDL in plagues vulnerability.*"[23]

Also, In 2001, Duncan and Schmidt performed a meta analysis of the association of inflammatory markers of the innate immune system and diabetes, cardiovascular disease, and obesity. Their analysis revealed "*...evidence to suggest that chronic activation of the innate immune system may underlie the metabolic syndrome, characterizing the common soil for the causality of type 2 diabetes mellitus and cardiovascular disease.*" They conclude: "*Better understanding of the role of the innate immune system in these diseases may lead to important advances in the prediction and management of diabetes and cardiovascular disease.*"[24]

Similarly, obesity is a complicated and frustrating problem involving neurological and endocrine as well as immunologic components. In a study performed at Baylor Medical College, Sports Medicine and Performance Institute in Houston, reported in *The Bariatrician, Spring 1996,* entitled, *The Short term efficacy of the ALCAT Test of food sensitivities to facilitate changes in body composition and self-reported disease symptoms: a randomized controlled study,* it was found that overweight subjects following an eating plan eliminating foods suspected of activating innate immunity, based on laboratory analysis of whole blood samples, experienced a significant improvement in body composition and scale weight.

The effect of immune activating foods was distinct from that of caloric restriction, as a well matched control group that followed a calorie restricted diet was included in the study. The report, by Gilbert Kaats, PhD and co-workers states that "*80 percent of the subjects in the experimental group lowered their body fat during the study compared to 34 percent in the control group. 78 percent of the experimental group achieved an improvement in their body composition compared to 29 percent in the control group... and 98 percent of the subjects following the ALCAT plan either lost scale weight or improved their body composition.*"

Professor Cabo-Soler, Chief of Biochemistry at the University of Valencia reported in 1995 that iso-caloric food elimination diets, based on ALCAT test results, promoted enhanced weight loss, comprised more of adipose tissue, rather than muscle mass, as determined by DEXA studies.

One plausible interpretation of these data is that altered immune system reactions to the preponderance of artificial, genetically novel foods, and other environmental challenges, may overwhelm Phase I and Phase II detoxification capacity, thus triggering chronic innate immune activation. This, to a great extent, may account for the dramatic increase in metabolic syndrome and other chronic degenerative disorders seen in industrial societies. The lower nutritional value of commercially produced agricultural products is likely also a contributory factor.

POSSIBLE CAUSES OF FOOD INTOLERANCE

It appears that multiple mechanisms are involved in adverse reactions to foods. An enzyme deficiency, such as a lactase deficiency may manifest lactose intolerance. Whilst additives used in prepared foods have been found to be particularly problematic. Professor Brostoff, from the Middlesex Hospital Medical School of the University of London explains that azo dyes, used extensively in prepared foods, will inhibit the activity of phenyl-sulpanotransferase-P, which breaks down cresol-P in the gut. If cresol-P is not broken down it may become neurotoxic. Benjam Feingold warned about food colorings in the 60's with respect to hyperactivity in children. Results of a multi-disciplinary study of autistic children showed that all of the subjects had at least some reactivity to food colorings, as determined by our in vitro cellular assay.[26] Similarly, many foods contain chemicals, or have chemicals added to them, which are intolerogenic. Salicylates, for example, occur in many fruits and vegetables, and can induce a pharmacologically mediated adverse reaction in susceptible individuals.

Dietary lectins, which may be resistant to degradation through cooking and digestion, occur in numerous vegetables, fruits, grains, and some meats. All mammalian blood and tissue cells have membrane carbohydrate molecules that bind lectins and may cause reactivity. Some lectins can even bind to multiple fc receptors on mast cells, which triggers histamine release similar to that which is seen in classical allergic reactions. However, some lectin activity is actually beneficial, in that it may augment the normal immune response. This, as well as some other lectin activity, is not blood type specific. There is no convincing scientific evidence that blood type is associated with specific food induced pathologies.

Recently, Dr. Lu Shan and co-investigators from multiple departments at Stanford University and the Institute of Immunology from the Rikshopitalet in Oslo, reported in a paper entitled, *Structural basis for gluten intolerance in celiac sprue,* identifying a 33-mer peptide, rich in proline and glutamine, which was highly resistant to gastric, pancreatic, and small intestinal brush border membrane proteases. They also found that it occurs in all grains that are toxic to celiac sprue patients (wheat, rye, oats, and barley) but is absent in other grains. Additionally, the peptide was shown to be a potent stimulator of T cells (CD+, or helper type) in 14 out of 14 celiac sprue patients. However, in both in vitro and in vivo assays the peptide could be broken down by bacteria derived prolyl endopeptidase (PREP), thus suggesting a possible treatment strategy.[25]

Similarly, many naturopathic physicians and others have maintained for years that a gut dysbiosis or a "leaky gut" whose failure to degrade food components, may be an inciting factor when undigested proteins traverse the gut prematurely and enter the circulation.

Synergism

This model illustrates an adverse reaction to foods, in this case gliadin fractions occurring in grains, that involves activation of specific immunity; the T cells of celiac patients with a specific leukocyte antigen which then release potent cytokines, attracting inflammatory cells of the innate immune system which cause damage to local tissue through the release of their toxic mediators.

An additional feedback loop from innate immune reactivity to specific immune function is observed when activation of the innate immune system upregulates the expression of B7 molecules on antigen presenting cells, which, as seen in classical allergy, for example, provide the secondary signal necessary to turn on T helper cells. Thus, the co-ordination of the two branches of the immune system is suggestive of a complex synergistic function and it is often seen that treatment of allergy decreases food intolerance; and, conversely, the effective management of food intolerance, improves allergic states.

Nonetheless, classical allergy is mediated by the specific branch of the immune system and the broad category of adverse reactions to foods are mediated, primarily, by the innate branch of the immune system, secondary to gastrointestinal dysfunction and/or detoxification insufficiency. Although several factors can induce histamine release, usually it is IgE. Symptom onset is immediate and it requires a small dose of allergen to trigger symptoms.

Food Intolerance is Multi-Factorial

Multiple pathogenic mechanisms are involved in adverse reactions to foods, some of which are immunologic; others, toxic or pharmacologic. Symptoms are typically dose dependent, and symptom onset is delayed. Adverse reactions to foods are hard wired in our genes, but susceptibility is dependant upon many factors; such as the integrity of the natural barrier of the gut wall, the viability of phase I and phase II detoxification pathways, and the presence or absence of other co-factors. A combination of these conditions could push one over their level of tolerance at any given time. It should be borne in mind that the human lymphocyte possesses all of the enzymes and substrates that are involved in hepatic detoxification and therefore serves as a back up system, albeit, one that may provoke unwanted symptoms.

It is sometimes seen that reactions to apple do not occur unless airborne birch pollen, which cross reacts with apple, is high. A food which contains an intolerogenic chemical is tolerated in moderation; but over consumption of it, or it in combination with other food(s) dependent on the same detoxification pathway may overwhelm that pathway and produce symptoms when consumed on a more frequent basis. Therefore, nutritional status which supports detoxification can exert a significant impact on food intolerance states, thus meaning that rotational eating plans may be beneficial for food intolerant patients.

In exercised induced asthma, increased body temperature serves as a co-factor with antigen to induce the degranulation of basophils, and histamine release; not occurring at normal body temperature.

Stress produced cortisol will destroy secretory IgA antibodies in the gut (and at the site of other mucus membranes as well) allowing for the perfusion of undigested food macromolecules that may activate the immune system. Intestinal dysbioses, Type I allergy in the gut, prescribed cortisone, and other variables may also contribute to a leaky gut.

Given the complexity of food intolerance it is easy to appreciate the need for a rapid, cost effective and accurate laboratory test to substitute for the laborious process of elimination and challenge, which, if properly performed, would take months, and try the patience of even the most patient of patients, not to mention their health care provider.

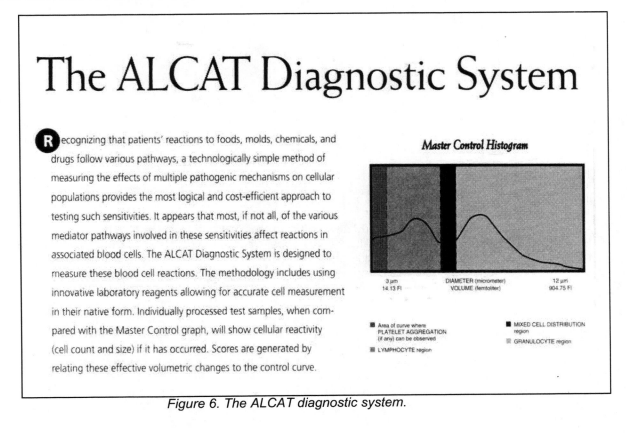

Figure 6. The ALCAT diagnostic system.

Laboratory Testing for Food Intolerance

We began our development of a reliable test for food intolerance in 1984. Previously, during the 1930's, allergists Cooke and Vaughn focused on changes in white blood cell counts following an in vivo challenge with a battery of foods. Initial successes encouraged others to continue this line of research utilizing microscopic observations of white cells following antigenic challenge in vitro. These methods offered some tantalizing results but were crude and results were not reproducible.

Our efforts focused on the utilization of electronic methods of cell measurement and computer analysis of the results following an ex vivo challenge of whole blood with food extracts and other substances suspected of association with non-IgE mediated hypersensitivity (Figure 7).

Analysis of whole blood offers a significant advantage in that it contains all of the immune factors, cellular elements and serum proteins that might be involved in an adverse reaction of this type, regardless of the underlying biological mechanism. Regardless of the various pathways that may underlie an adverse reaction to a food, the final common pathway will involve some mediator release. The cellular processes that occur; either swelling (vacuolization) decrease in number (destruction following de-granulation) or shrinking (probably partial de-granulation) are measurable through the ALCAT test.

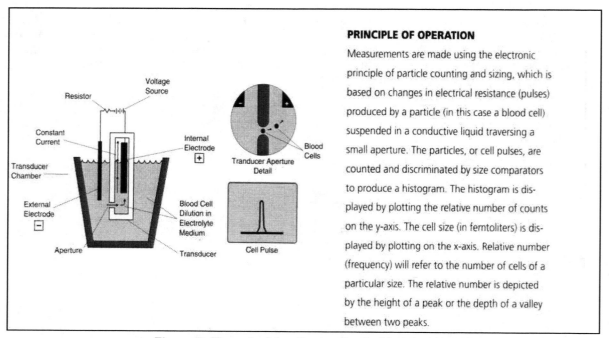

PRINCIPLE OF OPERATION

Measurements are made using the electronic principle of particle counting and sizing, which is based on changes in electrical resistance (pulses) produced by a particle (in this case a blood cell) suspended in a conductive liquid traversing a small aperture. The particles, or cell pulses, are counted and discriminated by size comparators to produce a histogram. The histogram is displayed by plotting the relative number of counts on the y-axis. The cell size (in femtoliters) is displayed by plotting on the x-axis. Relative number (frequency) will refer to the number of cells of a particular size. The relative number is depicted by the height of a peak or the depth of a valley between two peaks.

Figure 7. The principle of operation behind the ALCAT test.

It has been demonstrated by Mele *et al* from the Sacred Heart Catholic University of Rome that leukocytes which have reacted to ALCAT test positive food extracts in vitro, become incapable of releasing mediators when subsequently challenged by zymosan, an indication that the positive ALCAT test is associated with cell activation, and subsequent depletion of mediator stores.[28] Hence, a hypothesis that food intolerance reactions deplete immune resources and renders the subject more prone to infection, as has been observed, is not unreasonable. The method of measurement is the impedance or "Coulter" method that is used in routine hematology. It has demonstrated a high degree of correlation with clinical manifestations as confirmed through a rigorous double blind trial.

Drs. Peter Fell and Jonathon reported an 83.4% correlation with ALCAT test results and double blind oral challenges with foods. (45th Annual Congress of the American College of Allergy and Immunology). Whilst Hoj *et al* reported a 96% correlation with ALCAT test results and double blind placebo controlled oral challenges with food additives.[27] (*Journal of Allergy and Clinical Immunology*, Vol. 97 part 1, Jan., 1996). Hoj *et al* also reported a random sampling of clinical outcomes across a range of conditions suggesting the test results are accurate and useful in treating these conditions (Figure 8).

Outcome-study in 353 consecutive patients following the ALCAT diet plan

Main Complaints	Perennial Rhinitis / Sinusitis	Atopic Eczema	Urticaria	Irritable Colon	Migraine / Headache	Polyathrosis	Asthma	Angio-edema	Multo-organic syndrome
	(n=37)	(N=72)	(n=24)	(n=46)	(n=21)	(n=20)	(n=27)	(n=27)	(n=40)
Syptoms greatly improved	30	63	19	32	20	14	19	19	21
Improved	5	5	1	8		3	7	2	9
Little or no improvement	1	2	2	5	1	2	1		5
Worsening		2	2	1					3
No follow up	1					1			2
Total Improved %	95	94	83	87	95	85	96	100	75

L. Høj et al - 1998

Figure 8. Results of an outcome study by Hoj et al, of patients following the ALCAT diet plan.

ALCAT Nutritional Assessment (ANA)

Professor Roger Williams, in his 1956 classic book, *Biochemical Individuality*, wrote: "*Nutrition applied with due concern for genetic variations, which may be large, offers the solution to many baffling health problems.*"

The ALCAT test methodology can be adapted to perform a functional assessment of specific nutrient deficiencies. A functional test is superior to an assessment of levels of a specific nutrient in serum or other physical sample because an individual's level may fall within a "normal" range, but may be inadequate for that particular individual due to a number of factors. Some of these factors are genetically determined while others are phenomenological; such as, impaired absorption, increased requirements due to stress (i.e. pregnancy, drug use, impaired transport through the blood secondary to inadequate protein binding molecule function, inadequate cell uptake secondary to cell membrane abnormality, inadequate supply of co-factors) etc. Thus, serum tests may indicate normal levels, yet that particular individual, due to factors unique to them, is deficient.

Lymphocytes are metabolically active cells that are easily obtainable and reflect long term nutritional status, having an average life of approximately six to nine months. In this regard, measurement of nutrient impacted Lymphocyte growth and division will depict a more long term status, not one significantly impacted by vitamins or other supplements consumed just prior to testing. As such, this testing approach is analogous to how the measurement of Hemaglobin A1c represents long term (approx. 3 months) blood sugar balance.

Cell division and growth of lymphocytes represents metabolic pathways that are common to all reproducing cells and also indicates proficiency of immune system function. The lymphocytes that clone themselves to combat a specific pathogenic micro-organism, at the time of infection, leave behind a few examples of their type as memory cells to get a head start on combating the same pathogen on subsequent exposure. The success of the secondary immune response will depend on how quickly those memory cells can proliferate and produce specific antibodies upon re-exposure to the pathogen. That rate of proliferation will be limited by the intracellular stores of nutrients needed for new DNA synthesis and cell growth. The ALCAT Nutritional Assessment (ANA) is expected to indicate specific deficiencies that reflect the totality of cells but also those that are critical to the specific immune response.

The advantages of the ANA over other nutritional assays, even a cellular functional assay, is that testing whole blood preserves the normal cell to cell interactions and presence of the natural growth factors involved in cell division, and also eliminates a lot of cumbersome preparation procedures. It also allows for ease of measurement, avoids the requirement for radioactive material used in the old fashioned process of lymphocyte proliferation tests, and promises high accuracy, efficiency and reproducibility. The ALCAT method of measurement of lymphocyte proliferation may also be applicable to other uses, such as determination of vaccine efficacy (i.e. recall antigen induced proliferative response) and the monitoring of various immune proficiencies.

The assay will run on the current instrument platform with only minor software changes. Test kits can also be configured using the current ALCAT test kit cassettes.

CONCLUDING REMARKS

Measurement of immune function and response to dietary and other environmental factors using cellular laboratory assessment represents a viable and practical approach to optimization of immune function and normalization of the inflammatory response to the benefit of health and longevity.

REFERENCES

1. Harman D. Free radical involvement in aging. Pathophysiology and therapeutic implications. *Drugs Aging*. 1993;3:60-80. Review.
2. Morris BJ. A forkhead in the road to longevity: the molecular basis of lifespan becomes clearer. J Hypertens. 2005;23:1285-1309. Review.
3. O'Connell PJ, Wang X, Leon-Ponte M, Griffiths C, Pingle SC, Ahern GP. A novel form of immune signaling revealed by transmission of the inflammatory mediator serotonin between dendritic cells and T cells. *Blood*. 2006;107:1010-1017. Epub 2005 Oct 13.
4. Kelley DS, Taylor PC, Nelson GJ, Schmidt PC, Ferretti A, Erickson KL, Yu R, Chandra RK, Mackey BE. Docosahexaenoic acid ingestion inhibits natural killer cell activity and production of inflammatory mediators in young healthy men. *Lipids*. 1999;34:317-324.
5. Savill J, Dransfield I, Gregory C, Haslett C. A blast from the past: clearance of apoptotic cells regulates immune responses. *Nat Rev Immunol*. 2002;2:965-975. Review.
6. Conti F, Magrini L, Priori R, Valesini G, Bonini S.Eosinophil cationic protein serum levels and allergy in chronic fatigue syndrome. *Allergy*. 1996;51:124-127.
7. Henz BM, Zuberbier T. Most chronic urticaria is food-dependent, and not idiopathic. *Exp Dermatol*. 1998;7:139-142. Review.
8. Høj L. Food intolerance in patients with angioedema and chronic urticaria: An investigation by RAST and ALCAT Test. *Euro J of Allergy & Clin Immun*. 1995;50 (supplement No. 26).
9. Jaffe R. Delayed allergies in comprehensive care: Enhancing clinical outcomes through functional lymphocyte response assay in primary management of chronic ill health. *The Original Internist*. December 2003.
10. Marshall JD, Abtahi S, Eiden JJ, Tuck S, Milley R, Haycock F, Reid MJ, Kagey-Sobotka A, Creticos PS, Lichtenstein LM, Van Nest G. Immunostimulatory sequence DNA linked to the Amb a 1 allergen promotes T(H)1 cytokine expression while downregulating T(H)2 cytokine expression in PBMCs from human patients with ragweed allergy. *J Allergy Clin Immunol*. 2001;108:191-197.
11. Keller KM, Bürgin-Wolff A, Lippold R, Lentze MJ. [Quality assurance in diagnostics: are there normal values for IgG-antibodies to cow's milk proteins?] *Klin Padiatr*. 1999;211:384-388. [In German.]
12. Hadjivassiliou M, Grünewald RA, Davies-Jones GA. Gluten sensitivity: a many headed hydra. *BMJ*. 1999;318:1710-1711.
13. Szabó I, Eigenmann PA. Allergenicity of major cow's milk and peanut proteins determined by IgE and IgG immunoblotting. *Allergy*. 2000;55:42-49.
14. Jenkins M, Vickers A. Unreliability of IgE/IgG4 antibody testing as a diagnostic tool in food intolerance. *Clin Exp Allergy*. 1998;28:1526-1529.
15. Zar S, Kumar D, Benson MJ. Food hypersensitivity and irritable bowel syndrome. *Aliment Pharmacol Ther*. 2001;15:439-449. Review.
16. Crocker IP, Wellings RP, Fletcher J, Baker PN. Neutrophil function in women with pre-eclampsia. *Br J Obstet Gynaecol*. 1999;106:822-828.
17. Miesel R, Hartung R, Kroeger H. Priming of NADPH oxidase by tumor necrosis factor alpha in patients with inflammatory and autoimmune rheumatic diseases. *Inflammation*. 1996;20:427-438.

18. Karima M, Kantarci A, Ohira T, Hasturk H, Jones VL, Nam BH, Malabanan A, Trackman PC, Badwey JA, Van Dyke TE. Enhanced superoxide release and elevated protein kinase C activity in neutrophils from diabetic patients: association with periodontitis. *J Leukoc Biol.* 2005;78:862-870. Epub 2005 Aug 4.
19. Poon BY, Ward CA, Cooper CB, Giles WR, Burns AR, Kubes P. alpha(4)-integrin mediates neutrophil-induced free radical injury to cardiac myocytes. *J Cell Biol.* 2001;152:857-866.
20. Vitte J, Michel BF, Bongrand P, Gastaut JL. Oxidative stress level in circulating neutrophils is linked to neurodegenerative diseases. *J Clin Immunol.* 2004;24:683-692.
21. Frey B, Haupt R, Alms S, Holzmann G, König T, Kern H, Kox W, Rüstow B, Schlame M. Increase in fragmented phosphatidylcholine in blood plasma by oxidative stress. *J Lipid Res.* 2000;41:1145-1153.
22. Zhang R, Brennan ML, Fu X, Aviles RJ, Pearce GL, Penn MS, Topol EJ, Sprecher DL, Hazen SL. Association between myeloperoxidase levels and risk of coronary artery disease. *JAMA.* 2001;286:2136-2142.
23. Li L, Zhang Y, Chen YG, Li GS, Wang Y, Ma X, Li JF, Zhong M, Zhang W. [Changes of neutrophil myeloperoxidase in coronary circulation among patients with acute coronary syndrome.] Zhonghua Xin Xue Guan Bing Za Zhi. 2005;33:1106-1108. [In Chinese].
24. Duncan BB, Schmidt MI. Chronic activation of the innate immune system may underlie the metabolic syndrome. *Sao Paulo Med J.* 2001;119:122-127.
25. Shan L, Molberg Ø, Parrot I, Hausch F, Filiz F, Gray GM, Sollid LM, Khosla C. Structural basis for gluten intolerance in celiac sprue. *Science.* 2002;297:2275-2279.
26. Kotsanis, C. Paper presented to American Academy of Otolaryngic Allergy on a Multi-disciplinary treatment of autistic patients, combining allergy, nutrition, and auditory training. 1993; Data on file at CSS.
27. Høj L. Diagnostic value of ALCAT test in intolerance to food additives compared with double blind placebo controlled (DBPC) oral challenges. *J Alleg Clin Immun. 1996*: No 1, part 3.
28. Mele MC. Immune Cell Competence following In-Vitro challenge with ALCAT Positive Foods [English Translation]. Biotikos, Anno 1° – Numero 1, Giugno 2000.

ABOUT THE AUTHOR

Roger Deutsch has performed pioneering research in the field of food and chemical sensitivity testing for over 21 years. He was co-developer of the ALCAT test, a unique, patented method for identifying cellular reactions to foods, chemicals and other substances, though non- allergic pathways. He is co-author of the book series, *Your Hidden Food Allergies are Making You Fat*, as well as many scholarly and research papers on this topic. He is the CEO of Stem Cell Science Systems, Ltd. Corp. (and Alcat Europe, GmbH) which is a cutting edge company in the field of food intolerance diagnostics.

Chapter 10
The Role of Hormonorestorative Therapy in the Treatment of Major Illnesses

Sergey A Dzugan, M.D., Ph.D.*; George Rozakis, M.D.; R. Arnold Smith, M.D.
* Fountain Institute (Deerfield Beach, Florida); North Central Mississippi Regional Cancer Center (Greenwood, Mississippi)

ABSTRACT

Anti-aging medicine concepts and interventions are highly relevant to successful hormonorestorative therapy (HT). HT plays a critical role in the treatment of some major illnesses. HT was an effective approach in the control of hypercholesterolemia and was an effective adjuvant to conventional management for NSCLC. HT served as the core component of a successful multimodal migraine program.

KEYWORDS: hormonorestorative therapy, hypercholesterolemia, migraine, non-small cell lung cancer.

INTRODUCTION

Despite decades of research on prevention, detection, and management, coronary heart disease is still a number one cause of mortality and morbidity in the developed world for both men and women. Hypercholesterolemia is a major risk factor for coronary atherosclerosis and myocardial infarction.[1-3]

Migraine affects about 10-15% of the populations in different countries.[4-6] It has been known for many centuries, but remains a prevalent, disabling, underdiagnosed, and undertreated condition.[5] There are a number of theories and hypotheses concerning the pathogenesis of migraine, but they are frequently conflicting.[7] The pathophysiology of migraine is still incompletely understood.[8, 9]

Lung cancer remains the leading cause of cancer death in the United States. It is responsible for more than 150,000 deaths annually.[10] Lung cancer is the most common malignancy in males and kills more women than breast cancer. It costs the nation more than $4.9 billion/year. The most common type of lung cancer is NSCLC. The overall 5-year survival rate for non-small cell lung cancer (NSCLC) in the Surveillance, Epidemiology, and End Result Registry of the National Cancer Institute (SEER) is only 14%, and the probability of 5-year survival with unresected disease is less than 3%.[10,11]

In our article we describe hormonorestorative therapy (HT) and make a retrospective analysis evaluating the role and effect of HT in the treatment of these major illnesses.

CLINICAL EVIDENCE AND IMPLICATIONS
Study Summary

Purpose: to evaluate the role and effect of hormonorestorative therapy (HT) in the treatment of major illnesses such as hypercholesterolemia, migraine, and non-small cell lung cancer (NSCLC).

Materials and Methods: We analyzed three studies in patients with hypercholesterolemia (73 patients), migraine (30 patients), and advanced NSCLC (121 patients) where we used HT as the basic element of treatment. HT was a single element of hypercholesterolemia treatment and a basic element of a multimodal treatment program in migraine management, and immunorestorative therapy for NSCLC.

All patients were treated by HT with bioidentical hormones, which include a combination of several agents: pregnenolone, dehydroepiandrosterone (DHEA), triestrogen, progesterone, testosterone, hydrocortisone, Armour Thyroid and melatonin.

Serum levels of total cholesterol (TC), pregnenolone, dehydroepiandrosterone sulfate (DHEA-S), progesterone, total estrogen (for women), estradiol (for men), total testosterone levels, cortisol, and TSH, T3, T4 were done.

Results: In the group of patients with hypercholesterolemia all patients responded to HT. Mean serum TC dropped by 23.5% (from 252.0 mg/dL before to192.8 mg/dL after treatment), and completely normalized in 61.6% of patients. 38.4% of patients still had a minimal elevation of serum TC.

In the migraine group, all patients responded to the multimodal treatment program. No patients still had migraines after the program was initiated. Steroid hormone deficiencies were found in all patients. Pregnenolone and progesterone production was the most severely impaired.

In the lung cancer group, 9.9% of NSCLC patients who took radiation therapy with hormonorestoration were alive after 3.5 years and the survival curve was flat up to 70 months.

No adverse effects or complications related to HT were registered in all three studies. Most patients described a significant improvement in quality of life.

Conclusions: Anti-aging medicine concepts and interventions are highly relevant to successful hormonorestorative therapy. HT plays a critical role in the treatment of some major illnesses. HT was an effective approach in the control of hypercholesterolemia and was an effective adjuvant to conventional management for NSCLC. HT served as the core component of a successful multimodal migraine program.

Study Construct

This article is based on results of using of HT in three studies in patients with hypercholesterolemia, migraine, and NSCLC. A retrospective study of 73 patients with hypercholesterolemia, 30 patients with migraine, and 121 patients with advanced NSCLC where we used HT as basic element of treatment was performed. HT was a single element of hypercholesterolemia treatment, and a basic element of multimodal treatment program in migraine management and immunorestorative therapy for NSCLC.

All our patients were given HT. HT includes hormones that are chemically identical (bioidentical) to human hormones and administered in physiologic ratios with dose schedules intended to simulate natural human production cyclicity. Patients received HT with bioidentical hormones, which include a combination of several agents: pregnenolone, DHEA, triestrogen, progesterone, testosterone, Armour Thyroid, cortisol, and melatonin. We used oral and topical delivery systems for hormones. Oral form includes capsules (pregnenolone, DHEA, melatonin), tablets (Armour Thyroid, hydrocortisone), troche (progesterone –200 mg/troche), and drops [triestrogen – (E3:E2:E1- 80:10:10) - 5 mg/ml]. Topical form was used as a gel for triestrogen [(E3:E2:E1 – 90:7:3) - 1.25 mg/ml], progesterone (5% gel - 50 mg/ml), and testosterone (5% gel - 50 mg/ml).

The recommended doses for different patients during HT varied significantly and were determined by serum hormonal levels during serial testing. That is why we did not use a standard dose, rigid protocol, or traditional design for this study. Doses were individually selected during HT to produce youthful physiologic (not just "normal") serum levels. We administered hormones in doses sufficient to achieve circulating plasma levels observed in younger healthy individuals between the age of 20 and 30 for both genders. This level is at the high end of the normal range from the testing laboratory.

The preferable anatomic site of gel application was scrotum or vulva (excellent absorption), neck (areas of blushing), and the forearms.[12-14]

From our point of view there are a few important rules for using HT:
- Bioidentical structure of hormones
- Individually modified doses
- Cyclical manner
- Larger dose in the morning
- Treatment control by serum hormonal levels
- Mono- or bi-hormonal therapy is usually inadequate; poly-hormonal therapy is optimal

We believe that the problems found with conventional HRT were happening because:
- The majority of studies were performed with only one or two agents
- No physiological cyclicity
- Standard dose was used in most patients
- No bioidentical restoration attempted
- Serum hormonal levels not used clinically
- Mostly oral route of administration

When we talk about the cyclical manner for using hormones we must remember what normally happens with estrogen and progesterone production during the normal menstrual cycle.

Following initial consultation, a baseline lipid profile, pregnenolone, dehydroepiandrosterone sulfate (DHES), progesterone, total estrogen (for women), estradiol (for men), total testosterone, cortisol and TSH, T3, T4 levels were determined through routine blood testing, and serial determinations were made thereafter during treatment in all 3 groups of patients.

Hypercholesterolemia Study

In 2002 we suggested a new hypothesis of hypercholesterolemia.[15] This hypothesis implies that hypercholesterolemia is the reactive consequence of enzyme-dependent downregulation of steroid hormone biosynthesis and their interconversions. In short, hypercholesterolemia is the compensatory mechanism for declined production of steroidal hormones. We believe that a high cholesterol level is a consequence of a low production of steroid hormones and a low cholesterol level is a cause of low hormonal production. Considering this, if we restore a youthful level of hormones there is no reason for the extra production of cholesterol.

We decided to investigate our hypothesis and analyzed the role of HT in normalization of cholesterol levels. We studied 73 patients with hypercholesterolemia. Mean age – 56.7 (from 25 to 81yr). Male to female ratio – 1:1.7 (27-46). 56 patients (76.7%) had been taking one to three different steroid hormones prior to HT without any significant effect and still had hypercholesterolemia before starting our therapy. All agents such as equine conjugated estrogens, medroxyprogesterone acetate, methyl testosterone, etc., were changed during treatment. Nonphysiologic replacements such as estradiol alone were modified to physiologic estrogen ratios. Estrogen was always used with progesterone. The follow up period was from 5 to 79 months.

All patients responded to HT. Serum TC normalized in 45 patients (61.6%). 28 patients still have serum TC levels slightly higher then normal. The mean serum TC decreased from 252 mg/dL before treatment to 192.8 mg/dL after intervention. The average reduction was 23.5 %. The drop was from 262.7 mg/dL to 191.3 mg/dL (27.2%) in men and from 245.8 mg/dL to 193.7 mg/dL (21.2%) in women (Fig.1).

Serum HDL level decreased from 60.7 mg/dL to 48.8 mg/dL, (19.6% drop), but remained higher than undesirable levels in all cases. The serum HDL level decreased by 6.6% (from 45.7 mg/dL to 42.7 mg/dL) in men and 23.8% (from 66.2 mg/dL to 51.1 mg/dL) in women (Fig. 2). It is well known that HDL is the carrier that transports back cholesterol to the liver. Most studies of cholesterol-lowering drugs have shown the elevation of HDL after intervention. Our study shows that in the case of successful correction of cholesterol, HDL usually decreased with HT. We believe that a decreasing level of HDL is a good sign during treatment. If we normalize the level of TC, what reason exists for the extra production of HDL? If there is nothing to transport back to the liver, why produce an extra carrier? HDL, by this logic, should decrease.

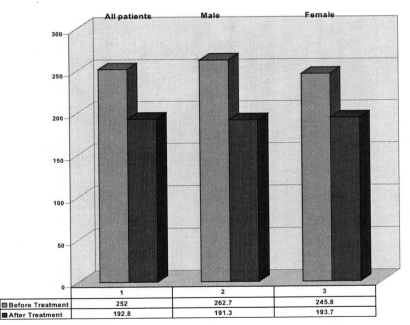

	1	2	3
▨ Before Treatment	252	262.7	245.8
■ After Treatment	192.8	191.3	193.7

Figure 1. Total cholesterol before and after hormonorestorative therapy.

Serial determinations for serum LDL exhibited a drop from 158.2 mg/dL to 123.8 mg/dL (21.7%). Serum LDL decreased by 34.8% in men (from 183.3 mg/dL to 119.5 mg/dL) and 15.7% in women (from 148.7 mg/dL to 125.4 mg/dL) (Fig. 3).

Serum triglycerides dropped from 203.6 mg/dL to 115.7 mg/dL (64.5%). A much larger drop in triglycerides was noted in men (58.5%) than in women (29.6%). In men triglycerides decreased from 334.3 mg/dL to 138.7 mg/dL and in women from 151.3 mg/dL to 106.5 mg/dL (Fig. 4).

During the follow up period no complications or serious side effects related to HT were registered. All patients described a significant improvement in quality of life.

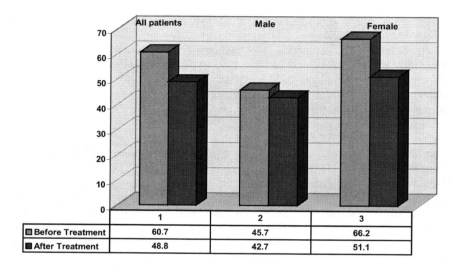

	All patients	Male	Female
	1	2	3
Before Treatment	60.7	45.7	66.2
After Treatment	48.8	42.7	51.1

Figure 2. HDL before and after hormonorestorative therapy.

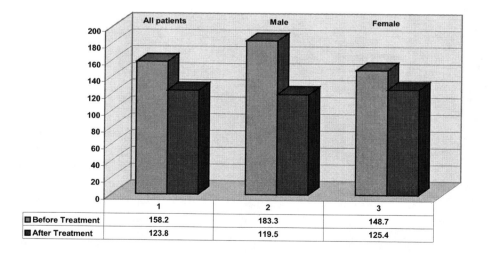

	All patients	Male	Female
	1	2	3
Before Treatment	158.2	183.3	148.7
After Treatment	123.8	119.5	125.4

Figure 3. LDL before and after hormonorestorative therapy.

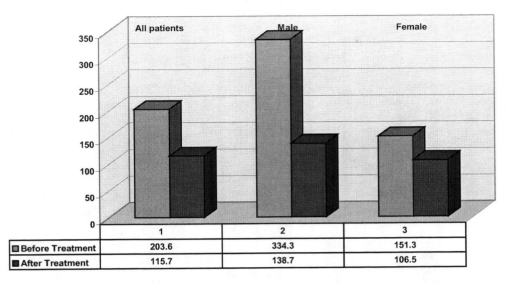

	1	2	3
■ Before Treatment	203.6	334.3	151.3
■ After Treatment	115.7	138.7	106.5

Figure 4. Triglycerides before and after hormonorestorative therapy.

The results of our study shows that the effect of HT versus cholesterol-lowering drugs on TC were comparable (Table 1),[16,17] but because of the adverse events, including poor quality of life, severe rhabdomyolysis, renal failure, and death from cholesterol-lowering drugs, HT could be a better treatment regimen for TC elevation. Side effects of cholesterol-lowering drugs were seen in 4-38% of patients resulting in discontinuation and dose reduction.[18]

Table 1. Effect of HT vs. cholesterol-lowering drugs on TC (mg/dL)

	before	after
NCMRCC[13]	252	192.8
Osaka University[14]	265	216

You have heard that if you keep your cholesterol under 200 mg/dl you will be safe against coronary heart disease (CHD). Right? This is the "conventional wisdom". But it is not necessarily so. We have to remember that a significant proportion of individuals with ischemic heart disease have desirable cholesterol concentrations. We know that plasma cholesterol level increases with age, as does the incidence of CHD. Also, we know that hypercholesterolemia was observed in 40-70% of patients with coronary artery disease.[19, 20] But, how can we explain that up to 60% of patients with myocardial infarction have documented "normal" level of cholesterol?

We are using in our practice the "relative hypercholesterolemia" term. What is relative hypercholesterolemia? We will take, for example, 2 patients and will observe the change of cholesterol during age.

Table 2. The change in total cholesterol level with age.

Age	25	40
Patient 1		
TC (nl <200 mg/dl)	130	190
Patient 2		
TC (nl <200 mg/dl)	180	240

As you can see in Table 2, life cycle related elevation of TC is 60 mg/dl in both cases. We hypothesize that TC elevation over time is a critical determinant of risk for CHD or myocardial infarction, not just an absolute number. In our opinion, the risk of heart attack in both cases was equal despite of a normal level of cholesterol in the first case. The term "relative hypercholesterolemia" was used for situations such as in the first case when cholesterol numbers are still in the normal laboratory range.

If we were right and our hypothesis is correct, the "normal" level of cholesterol during HT must decrease. We made an analysis of a small group of patients' so-called "relative hypercholesterolemia". As you can see, cholesterol level in all patients was decreased. The results are given in Fig. 5. It looks like our hypothesis is substantial.

The typical hypercholesterolemia case study (symptoms and blood results) was presented in Table 3.

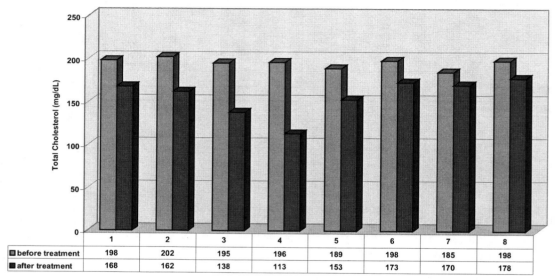

	1	2	3	4	5	6	7	8
before treatment	198	202	195	196	189	198	185	198
after treatment	168	162	138	113	153	173	170	178

Figure 5. "Relative" hypercholesterolemia before and after hormonorestorative therapy.

Table 2. Typical hypercholesterolemia case study (symptoms and blood results):

Patient E. 54 yr, male, first visit 08/31/00

Complaints: hypercholesterolemia, fatigue, severe erectile dysfunction, depression, short-term memory problems, and insomnia.

	DHEAS (280-640)	Pregn (10-200)	Estradiol (0-53)	Progest (0.3-1.2)	Test (280-830)	Cortisol (4.3-22.4)
08/31/00	93	24	56	0.3	186	0.9
09/09/03	540	159	30	1.3	496	15.6

	TC	TRG	HDL	LDL	VLDL	TC/HDL
08/31/00	330	216	54	233	43	6.1
09/09/03	187	138	40	119	28	4.7

	DHT (30-85)	Free Test (9.3-26.5)	PSA (0-4)
08/31/00	44	1.01	1.1
09/09/03	38	19.6	0.8

Follow-up 09/09/03 – no complaints

Migraine Study

From the traditional point of view migraine appears to be a primary disorder of the cerebral vessels. We believe that migraine is not a primary disorder, but that it is a consequence of neurohormonal and metabolic disorders. In 2002 we suggested a new hypothesis of migraine.[21] This hypothesis implies that migraine is a consequence of a loss of neurohormonal and metabolic integrity. From our point of view migraine is a complex disorder in several systems:

- Neurohormonal system – includes hypothalamus, pituitary gland, and glands that produce steroid hormones;
- Sympathetic-parasympathetic nervous systems – imbalance leads to decreased pain threshold of brain nociceptive system;
- Calcium-magnesium ion system – imbalance can change electricity of cells membrane, and condition of calcium channels;
- Pineal gland – decreased function of pineal gland with lower production of melatonin or decreased sensitivity of cells membrane to melatonin;
- Digestive system – abnormal absorption related to changed intestinal flora.

All these systems and changes within them are closely interrelated, and each can be a trigger mechanism for migraine.

We investigated our new hypothesis and analyzed the role of HT as part of a multimodal method of migraine treatment in 30 patients with severe migraine. Mean age is 46.4 (from 16 to 66 yr) years. Male to female ratio is 1:9 (3-27). Prior to our program all patients have used for prophylaxis and treatment of migraine several drugs and/or tried different supplements without any significant effect. Illness duration was from 2 to 46 years. 21 women (77.8%) had used HRT or oral contraceptive (OC). Most frequent concurrent illnesses such as fatigue, depression, lipid disorders, insomnia, gastrointestinal (GI) disorders, and fibromyalgia, were seen in 93.3%, 93.3%, 90.0%, 86.7%, 70%, and 16.7% respectively (Fig. 6). Lipid abnormalities were found in 27 (90%) patients. Most patients have a hypercholesterolemia - 24 (80%) patients (highest level - 360 mg/dL). 3 patients (10%) with lowest level – 86 mg/dL suffered from hypocholesterolemia. The follow up period ranged from 5 to 77 months.

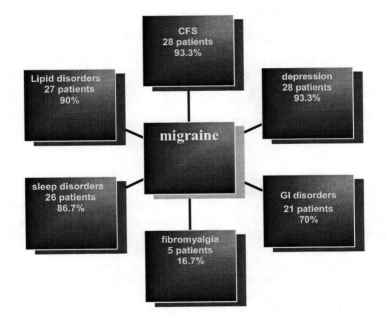

Figure 6. Most Frequent Migraine Concurrent Illnesses

A multimodal treatment program was administered to all patients in this group. The program incorporated the following basic four components:

- Hormonorestorative therapy (HT) – includes a combination of several agents: pregnenolone, dehydroepiandrosterone (DHEA), triestrogen, progesterone, testosterone, Armour thyroid, and hydrocortisone;
- Simultaneous correction of the imbalance between sympathetic and parasympathetic nervous systems and the ratio of calcium to magnesium;
- "Resetting" the pineal gland (melatonin);
- Improvement of intestinal absorption through restoration of normal intestinal flora.

It is necessary to stress the fact that the parts mentioned above cannot be separated.

Laboratory finding prior to HT shows the significant deficiency in production of all steroid hormones. Pregnenolone levels were extremely low in many patients. 29 (96.7%) patients had a low level of pregnenolone, and 18 (60%) of them had less than the minimal detectable level (less then 10 ng/dL). 27 (90%) patients had levels of DHEA sulfate less than optimal level, 13 (43.3%) of them had less than minimal normal level (less than 65 ug/dL for female, and less than 280 ug/dL for male). Not optimal was defined as a level of hormones below one third of the highest normal range for all steroid hormones. Testosterone level in 22 (73.3%) patients was below optimal; 9 (30%) patients had a very low level. Progesterone production was significantly declined in 24 (80%) patients. Only 3 (10%) persons had a good level of progesterone. 9 (30%) patients had a normal level of total estrogen (or estradiol); 8 (26.7%) – a very high, and 13 (43.3%) – a very low level.

All patients who participated in this study responded to migraine management. None of the patients who participated still suffered from migraine after they initiated this program. All patients were free of concurrent illnesses. Total cholesterol completely normalized in 22 (91.7%) patients. Acute morbidity of a multimodal program was zero. The typical migraine case study (symptoms and blood results) is presented in Table 4.

Table 4. Typical Migraine Case Study (symptoms and blood results):

Patient L. 30 y.o., female first visit 12/10/03
Complaints: hypercholesterolemia, migraine (2-3 times weekly) since age 15, fatigue, insomnia, constipation, PMS, no libido, poor sex drive, overweight.

	TC (<200)	DHEAS (65-380)	Pregnenol. (10-230)	Estr (total) (61-437)	Progest (0.2-28)	Testoster. (14-76)	
12/10/03	207	81	87	128	0.8	42	
10/18/04	178	205	172	274	17.7	47	

(blood was drawn on 21 day of menstrual cycle in both cases)

Follow-up 10/18/04 – no complaints
Follow-up 07/17/07 – no complaints

Non-Small Cell Lung Cancer Study

It is well known that five-year survival rate for conventional NSCLC treatment has remained almost the same since 1950. Why? From our point of view it happens because the popular treatment paradigm has remained similar: surgical resection, debulking with irradiation, and cellular poisons (chemotherapy). Chemotherapy, radiation, and surgery do nothing to change the age-related underlying condition, which allowed NSCLC to activate. All of them depress immunity and ignore anti-aging science.

It is widely recognized that dramatic acceleration in epithelial cancer incidence including NSCLC occurs around age 40. We suggested our own hypothesis of NSCLC development and possible cancer correction. This hypothesis includes the following assumptions:

- The documented life cycle NSCLC inflection with increased age is caused by a loss of immune surveillance;
- Loss of surveillance is driven by hormone decline;
- Loss of surveillance can be hormonally corrected;
- HT is a key to successful systemic therapy of NSCLC treated with radiation therapy.

In our clinical work we are using so-called Comprehensive Integrative Cancer Treatment. This combines Integrative Anti-Cancer Strategy and Integrative Anti-Aging Strategy. The following Anti-Cancer Strategy has been used for management of NSCLC:

- Tumor removal – surgery;
- Enhanced direct killing – radiation therapy with sensitization;
- Restoration of youthful immunity– hormones, antioxidants, cimetidine;
- Judicious use of chemotherapy to avoid damaging host immunity;
- Immune hyperstimulation – IL-2, Transfer Factor, interferon, mushroom extracts;
- Tumor biological manipulation – tumor angiogenesis inhibitors, epidermal growth factor (EGF) blockers, etc.

The Anti-Aging Strategy (also we used the term "immunorestorative therapy or IRT") includes:

- Hormonorestorative therapy (HT);
- Antioxidant therapy;
- Correction of protein malnutrition;
- Miscellaneous.

The goal of IRT was to stimulate the recognition of cancer by macrophages, to stimulate natural killer (NK) cell production, and to restore the youthful physiology with anti-aging medicine. We believe that IRT becomes efficacious after bulk reduction. It can be potentially more efficient than radiotherapy, surgery, or chemotherapy for small disease volume.

In our NSCLC study we analyzed 121 NSCLC patients with extensive disease, who were treated with radiotherapy and IRT (87 male and 34 female), and 283 patients who received radiotherapy without IRT (197 male and 86 female). Only 0.8% of patients were under age 40. Our results show that 12 of 121 patients (9.9%) irradiated with IRT were alive after 3.5 years and survival curve was flat up to 70 months. Only 5 of 283 (1.8%) irradiated patients without IRT are still alive 2.5 years or more. The comparison of statistical survival of NSCLC patients in our study (North Central Mississippi Regional Cancer Center - NCMRCC) and SEER is shown in Figure 7.

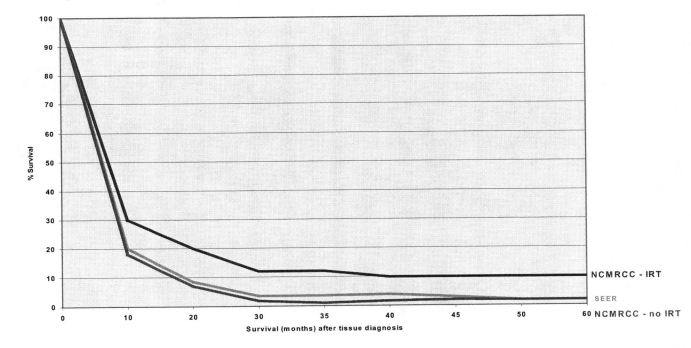

Figure 7. Comparison of statistical survival: NSCLC.

We believe that HT is the core element of IRT. Is it any wonder why women placed on high doses of uninterrupted and unopposed estrogen get more cancers rather than less? Nothing is simple, or as Albert Einstein once said, "*Things should be made as simple as possible but not one bit simpler.*" We think that no cyclicity during estrogen replacement may be dangerously simple. That is why we must remember that when the express intention of a pharmacological intervention is the re-creation of youthful immune system function, one should be cautious with non-physiologic chronicity in the strategy.

Also we have never had an extraordinary responder with NSCLC who did not take either testosterone or progesterone. There is direct experimental evidence that progesterone and testosterone are co-stimulants of NK activity.[22-24]

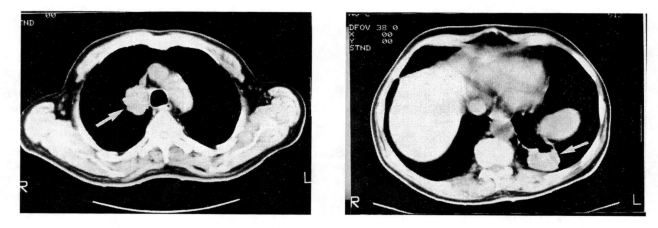

Figure 8. CT scan of bilateral NSCLC before treatment

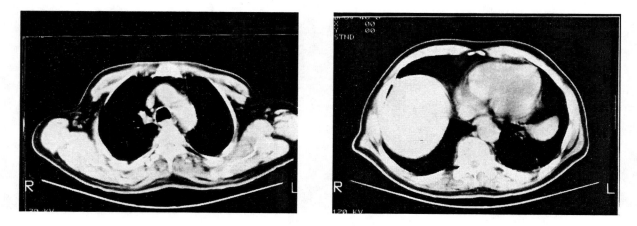

Figure 9. CT Scan of bilateral NSCLC 3 years after radiation therapy and immunorestorative therapy (IRT)

Figures 8 and 9 show a CT scan of a 80-year-old male (5-years survivor) with bilateral NSCLC before treatment and 3 years after radiation therapy with IRT.

CORTISOL AND AGING

There is a lot of talk in medical literature about the elevation of cortisol during aging. Our results did not show the similar pattern in our patients. That is why we decided to launch the cortisol study. We analyzed 246 patients - 158 men and 88 women (Fig. 10). Their age ranged from 16 to 93 years. We found that the average morning cortisol levels did not increase with age. Percentage of people with high cortisol (over 22.4) was only 7.7%. The majority of patients (46.3%) possessed a less than optimal level (10.4- 16.4).[25]

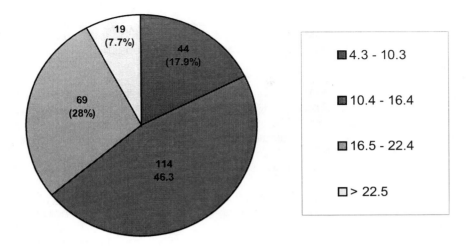

Fig.10. Average Distribution of Cortisol Ranges

CONCLUDING REMARKS
The results of our studies allows us to make the following conclusions:

- Hormonorestorative therapy is an effective approach in the control of hypercholesterolemia.
- Hormonorestorative therapy as part of a multimodal method of migraine treatment was a very effective treatment approach and was typically associated with a complete management of migraine.
- Hormonorestorative therapy as a key element of immunorestorative therapy was an effective adjuvant to conventional management for NSCLC. IRT should be considered in all NSCLC patients.

Finally, it is important to remember when you are doing hormonorestoration that the program cannot be rigid and needs to be individualized according to each patients' clinical symptoms and blood results.

REFERENCES
1. Starfield B. Is US health really the best in the world? *JAMA.* 2000;284:483-485.
2. American Heart Association. Heart and stroke statistical update. Dallas, Texas: American Heart Association, 2001.
3. Lewis V, Hoeger K. Prevention of coronary heart disease: a nonhormonal approach. *Semin Reprod Med.* 2005;23:157-166.
4. Mathew NT. Pathophysiology, epidemiology, and impact of migraine. *Clin Cornerstone.* 2001;4:1-17.
5. Gazerani P, Pourpak Z, Ahmadiani A, Hemmati A, Kazemnejad A. A correlation between migraine, histamine and immunoglobulin e. *Scand J Immunol.* 2003;57:286-290.
6. Lampl C, Buzath A, Baumhackl U, Klingler D. One-year prevalence of migraine in Austria: a nation-wide survey. *Cephalalgia.* 2003;23:280-286.
7. Rajda C, Tajti J, Komoroczy R, Seres E, Klivenyi P, Vecsei L. Amino acids in the saliva of patients with migraine. *Headache.* 1999;39:644-649.
8. Welch KM. Concepts of migraine headache pathogenesis: insights into mechanisms of chronicity and new drug targets. *Neurol Sci.* 2003;24 Suppl 2:S149-153.
9. Prusinski A, Sokolowski P. Current views on pathophysiology of migraine. Part II: Further development and current status of the vascular theory. Migraine and allergy. *Neurol Neurochir Pol.* 1995;29:857-866.
10. National Cancer Institute's Cancer Progress Report 2001 at: http://progressreport.cancer.gov
11. SEER Registry.

12. Wester RC, Noonan PK, Maibach HI. Variations in percutaneous absorption of testosterone in the rhesus monkey due to anatomic site of application and frequency of application. *Arch Dermatol Res*. 1980;267:229-235.

13. Wester RC, Noonan PK, Maibach HI. Percutaneous absorption of hydrocortisone increases with long-term administration. In vivo studies in the rhesus monkey. *Arch Dermatol*. 1980;116:186-188.

14. Oriba HA, Bucks DA, Maibach HI. Percutaneous absorption of hydrocortisone and testosterone on the vulva and forearm: effect of the menopause and site. *Br J Dermatol*. 1996;134:229-233.

15. Dzugan SA, Smith RA. Hypercholesterolemia treatment: a new hypothesis or just an accident? *Med Hypotheses*. 2002;59:751-756.

16. Dzugan SA, Smith RA., Kuznetsov AS. A new statin free method of hypercholesterolemia. *Health Don*. 2004;4:19-25.

17. Morimoto S, Koh E, Fukuo K, Mikami H, Ikegami H, Miki T, *et al*. Effects of pravastatin administration for 12 months on serum lipid levels in aged patients with hypercholesterolemia. *Nippon Ronen Igakkai Zasshi*. 1994;31:310-317.

18. Law MR, Thompson SG, Wakd NJ. Assessing possible hazards of reducing serum cholesterol. *BMJ*. 1994;308:373-379.

19. Ladeia AM, Guimaraes AC, Lima JC. The lipid profile and coronary artery disease. *Arq Bras Cardiol*. 1994;63:101-106.

20. Bratus' VV, Talaieva TV, Lomakovs'kyi OM, Tretiak IV, Radalovs'ka NV. Modified lipoproteins – their types and role in atherogenesis. *Fiziol Zh*. 2000;46:73-81.

21. Dzugan SA, Smith RA. The simultaneous restoration of neurohormonal and metabolic integrity as a very promising method of migraine management. *Bull Urg Rec Med*. 2003;4:622-628.

22. Genazzani AR, Petraglia F, Silferi M, Latessa AM, Coukos G, Genazzani AD, *et al*. Progestins modulate the action of estrogen on gonadotropin-releasing hormone, luteinizing hormone and prolactin in the rat. *Gynecol Obstet Invest*. 1990;29:197-202.

23. Schuiling GA, Moes H, Koiter TR. Interdependence of oestradiol and 5 alpha-dihydrotestosterone in modulating LH and FSH secretion in rats. *J Endocrinol*. 1989;123:257-262.

24. Stimson WH, Crilly PJ. Effects of steroids on the secretion of immunoregulatory factors by thymic epithelial cell cultures. *Immunology*. 1981;44:401-407.

25. Dzugan, S.A., Scipione A. Cortisol misconceptions. *SAJNM*. 2006;27:45-47.

ABOUT THE AUTHOR

Dr. Sergey A Dzugan is President of the Fountain Institute. He was formerly a heart surgeon and Chief of Cardiovascular Surgery at the Donetsk Regional Medical Center in Donetsk, Ukraine. His PhD in cardiovascular surgery was received in 1990 and pertained to heart rhythm disorders. Dr. Dzugan's current primary interests are anti-aging and natural therapy for cholesterol, fatigue, migraine, fibromyalgia, behavioral and hormonal disorders.

Dr. Dzugan has suggested a new hypothesis on hypercholesterolemia and has worked out an original statin-free method regarding hypercholesterolemia treatment. He has also introduced a new approach to the treatment of migraine. Dr. Dzugan was accepted (June, 30 2006) to the International Academy of Creative Endeavors (Moscow, Russia) as a Corresponding Member of the Academy for the outstanding contribution to the development of new methods of hypercholesterolemia and migraine treatment.

Dr. Dzugan is the author of 132 publications in medical journals and these publications include surgical, oncological, academic, and anti-aging topics. He has also had several articles published in *Life Extension Magazine* and the *South African Journal of Natural Medicine*. He is the author of *Migraine Cure* and the holder of 3 patents (all related to heart surgery). Dr. Dzugan is a member of the Medical Advisory Board at Life Extension Magazine.

Chapter 11
The Risks Associated with Electromagnetic Fields (EMFs):
A Literature Review
Howard W. Fisher, B.Sc., B.Ed., D.C.

ABSTRACT

Electromagnetic fields (EMFs) of assorted strengths and frequencies abound in our environment as they are produced by the creation, transmission, and subsequent use of electricity by any device. The startling reality is that most of us will be affected by magnetic fields virtually twenty-four hours per day for our entire lives. There are electromagnetic fields created in houses, cars and of course from the cell phone you are using while walking down the street. Eastern Bloc scientists have been studying the health risks associated with EMFs for over fifty years, and there is now a wealth of medical literature documenting the risks associated with these magnetic fields. The aim of this paper is to review the medical literature surrounding the risks associated with EMFs.

INTRODUCTION

Humans are electrical creatures. Our neurological systems function by using electrical currents (cerebral cortex, cortical tracts) and we are able to create our own endogenous electricity with no outside mechanisms involved (sino-atrial node of the heart).

Electromagnetic fields of assorted strengths and frequencies abound in our environment. When electricity leaves the energy production plant, it is clean 50 or 60 Hertz sine wave energy; however along the way it is affected by power surges (transients), radio frequencies (RF), and harmonics as it passes through electronic resistances and devices. The electricity gets chopped up into smaller segments, gathers high frequencies (RF), and spreads out to flow across wires, pipes, and even the ground. The energy leaves the generating facility and travels across high-voltage power lines and is then routed through transformers (which lower the voltage) and into individual homes. Electric and magnetic fields surround every aspect of this energy transmission.

EMFs (electromagnetic fields) are produced by the creation, transmission, and subsequent use of electricity by any device. In other words, power lines, electrical wiring, transformers, wireless, and electrical equipment create this hazard, although the actual fields in your home are dependent upon many factors. EMFs include Electro-Static Fields (fields that surround direct current), Radio Frequency (RF), and Electrical Noise. EMFs are also created by a transient phenomenon, which occurs whenever there is a dramatic burst of energy, such as a spark plug firing, lightning, or the motor brushes in an induction load (refrigerator, furnace fan, air conditioning compressor). These fields are the area of concern and more appropriately referred to as high-frequency, microsurge transients or 'dirty' electricity. The intensity of these currents fluctuates with the conductivity of the organ or tissue, but this energy can produce ionization of serum or cellular electrolytes and change body chemistry. EMFs' effects are on a cumulative basis, so awareness of one's environment can help you make wise decisions.

THE EFFECTS OF EMFS ON THE BODY

Information started to come out of the Eastern Bloc, where scientists have been studying about increased incidences of cancer and other health disturbances among the population affected by EMFs for over fifty years. According to Yuri Grigoriev, Chairman of the Russian National Committee on Non-Ionizing Radiation Protection, research on the biological effects of EMFs in the former Soviet Union has been ongoing for fifty years. Mr. Grigoriev advocates the belief that exposure to magnetic fields (EMFs) greater than two milliGauss (mG.) causes cancer.

In North America, one of the first investigations to publicly report an association between cancer and power lines was published in 1979 by Wertheimer and Leeper. They reached the conclusion that children who died from cancer were two to three times more likely to live within forty meters of a power transmission line. EMFs (magnetic fields) were linked as a possible reason.[1]

After attending a major symposium on the health effects of electromagnetic fields held in Kazakhstan, American engineer Dr, Karl Maret commented, *"There appears to be some confirmation that EMFs can have a significant impact on metabolic systems including elevated blood glucose levels, elevations in lipid levels, increased neuro-regulatory disturbances, decreased testosterone levels in males, and impacts on the CNS, cardiovascular, and immune systems. In general, it appears that EMF stress leads to conditions of more rapid aging and the current proliferation of EMFs, especially the increased use of low-level microwave devices such as cell phones by our children, may have important socio-economic consequences.*[2]

The startling reality is that most of us will be affected by magnetic fields virtually twenty-four hours per day for our entire lives. There are electromagnetic fields created in houses, cars and of course from the cell phone you are using while walking down the street. EMFs are everywhere and to ignore the apparent relationship is paramount to negligence. No one has really told us exactly what potential threat EMFs possess. Many of us believe that headaches, heart disease, ADD, fatigue, aches, pains, allergies, digestive difficulties, mucus build-up, and chemical sensitivities that affect a large percentage of the population are due to other causes. From an epidemiological perspective, the evidence is irrefutable. There are too many studies with positive findings for this health issue to be overlooked.

EMFs may manifest in a two hundred to four hundred percent (200% to 400%) greater risk of diseases such as cancer, leukemia, lymphoma, brain tumors, spontaneous abortions, Alzheimer's disease, or suicide (of electrical workers).[3-5]

A prominent Russian researcher, Nikitina Valentina, author of, *"Occupational and Population Health Risks of Radio Frequency Electromagnetic Fields,"* states that EMFs can cause central nervous system, blood chemistry, and cardiovascular system damage, with symptoms including angina, atherosclerosis, chest pain, digestive disorders, fatigue, headache, hypertension, insomnia, irritability, low blood pressure, sleep disturbances, and many other cardiac and neurological pathologies.[6] She went on to indicate that the clinical findings from prolonged EMF exposure look like premature aging.

EMFs and Cancer

A group of international researchers combined their efforts to provide conclusive evidence that cells inside electromagnetic fields can activate certain signaling pathways that have been associated with cancer.[7-8] Their results demonstrate that EMFs may change the biochemistry of the immune system that affects our degree of resistance to pathogens. The body of research consistently finds strong associations of EMF effects beyond random chance.[9-13]

A Swedish study in the early 1990's by Feychting and Ahlbom (1993) demonstrated a 1.7 times higher risk for leukemia in adults and a 2.7 times higher risk for childhood leukemia.[14] Several studies indicate an increased incidence of cancer due to EMFs.[15-17] Savitz and Loomis observed a strong exposure-response relationship for brain tumors.[18] Several other researchers have found an increased risk of brain tumors linked to EMFs as a suspected agent.[19-25] There has been an increasing amount of associated evidence linking residential exposure to magnetic fields and both leukemia and childhood leukemia.[26-30]

Pregnancy and EMFs

Many of the investigators have found a definite association between miscarriage (spontaneous abortion) and magnetic fields.[31, 32] Whether this is deemed to be spontaneous abortion, miscarriage, or early pregnancy loss, too many researchers have found results to dismiss this finding.[33] Correlations as to the cause of miscarriage have been drawn from computers,[34-37] electric blankets,[38, 39] and EMFs from various sources.[40-43]

Dr. De-Kun Li, an epidemiologist at the Kaiser Institute in Oakland, conducted a study in which approximately one thousand women in the first trimester of pregnancy wore a magnetic field meter around their waists for a day. He concluded that women exposed to an intermittent 16 mG magnetic field had an one hundred and eighty percent (180%) increased risk for spontaneous abortion.[44] Furthermore, even higher risks were found for women at less than ten weeks (220%) and women who had previously miscarried (310%).

Dr. Neil Cherry (2000) summarizes the general consensual findings, *"Animal studies show that chromosome aberrations and single and double strand DNA breakage occurs with EMR (electromagnetic radiation) exposure; mice and rats have pregnancy, birth, and fertility problems associated with EMR exposure, which are also found in exposed human populations. There is consistency within human studies and between human studies and animal studies."*[45] He went on to conclude after much research, *"Electromagnetic fields and radiation, damage DNA and enhance cell death rates and therefore they are a Ubiquitous Universal Genotoxic Carcinogen that enhances the rates of cancer, cardiac, reproductive, and neurological disease and mortality in human populations. Therefore there is no safe threshold level. The only safe exposure level is zero, a position confirmed by dose-response trends in epidemiological studies.*"

The Impact of EMFs on Neurological Tissues

In 1983 the work of Dr. AS Davydov, of the Ukrainian Academy of Sciences, was released, indicating that cellular chemistry in the brain could be affected by extremely low frequency radiation which he found could cross the blood brain barrier. According to the Defense & Foreign Affairs Daily, June 7, 1983, the Soviets have been conducting research on RF radiation since 1960.

The impact of EMFs being able to affect neurological tissues such as the brain, makes the findings of the researchers, who have found neurodegenerative disorders such as decreased cognitive functions and Alzheimer's Disease, fall into the realm of not only being plausible, but totally credible as well. The question of the relationship between EMFs and neurological degeneration and cognitive function has been examined by many researchers. Many of them have found such a relationship.[46, 47]

Alzheimer's Disease (AD) is a progressive, irreversible, brain disorder with no known cause or cure, affecting more than four and a half million Americans. Unfortunately this disease leads to a rapid functional decline. The clinical cause of Alzheimer's disease is related to amyloid peptide microtubule deposits (tau), neurofibril entanglement and inflammation (neuronal toxicity).[48]

In 1994, Dr. Eugene Sobel, USC School of Medicine, and colleagues found an association between occupational exposure to EMFs and Alzheimer's disease. Sobel's team found that subjects occupationally exposed to "high" and "medium" levels of EMFs risk of developing Alzheimer's was three times (300%) greater than those exposed to "low" levels of EMFs.[49] Some researchers look for factors that create increased risk while other look for those that create decreased risk. This was the case for a Turkish research group. Harmanci et al (2003) studied the risk factors for Alzheimer's disease and came up with some particularly interesting findings. The research subjects with college or university degrees had a ninety percent (90%) decreased risk of AD. People who had electric heating in their homes had a two-hundred and seventy-seven percent (277%) increased risk for Alzheimer's disease and people who were exposed to EMFs occupationally had a four hundred and two percent (402%) increased risk for being affected by this neurodegenerative disorder.[50]

Strickland (1996) and other investigators have found relationships between occupations and an increased incidence of amyotrophic lateral sclerosis (ALS),[51-52] some of which were found to involve consistently elevated EMFs (welding, soldering, electrical utility).[53-54] Schulte et al (1996) studied the incidence of neurodegenerative disorders and found that three of these diseases, Alzheimer's, Parkinson's and motor neuron disease (ALS) had increased incidence in occupations involving pesticides, solvents, and electromagnetic fields.[55] Ahlbom (2001), after a review of the relationship between neurodegenerative diseases and electromagnetic fields, concluded that there is *"relatively strong data indicating that electric utility work may be associated with an increased risk for amyotrophic lateral sclerosis."*[56]   Hakansson et al (2003) examined the relationship between extremely low frequency magnetic fields from occupational exposure and the mortality from neurodegenerative diseases. The conclusions support previous researcher's findings, demonstrating an increased risk of AD and ALS among employees occupationally exposed to EMFs.[57]

In case studies by Havas and Stetzer, an EMF-sensitive student's classroom behavior was positively affected by the removal of EMF radiation.[58] Several studies have linked decreased cognitive function,[59] dementia, depression,[60-63] and Alzheimer's disease to increased exposure to EMFs.[64]

Childhood Cancer and EMF – The Power Line Controversy

Childhood cancer concerns and the relationship to electromagnetic radiation have been an issue for more than twenty-five years. One of the first published studies into EMF affects was the research out of the University of Colorado which noted a 200% to 300% increase in the cancer deaths of children living near power transmission lines in Denver, Colorado.[65] A point of interest in a Danish study found that children living near power lines emitting a 4 mG EMF had a five hundred percent (500%) increase in lymphomas, brain tumors and childhood leukemia.[66]

Another proposed mechanism for EMF exposures increasing the risk of cancer was given credibility by a recent study by Juutilainen (2006). This paper demonstrates that *in vitro* and animal experiments show that EMFs increase the effects of known carcinogens.[67]

Reported Effects of EMFs on the Cardiovascular System

Dr. Antonio Sastre of the Midwest Research Institute observed that EMFs caused changes in heart rhythms (endogenous electrical impulses) that have been linked to increased risks of heart disease.[68] His conclusions led him to forecast that utility workers would have a higher rate of two types of cardiovascular disease. An epidemiological study corroborated Sastre's prediction that workers with high EMF exposure could show increased cardiovascular risk from arrhythmia and myocardial infarctions (heart attacks).[69]

Hypertension affects a broad segment of the population. The effects of EMFs on raising blood pressure, pulse rate, and affecting other dynamics of cardiovascular function have been well documented.[70-74]

EMFs Linked to Increased Cortisol Levels

Cortisol decreases the effectiveness of the immune system by affecting leukocytes, eosinophils, neutrophils, phagocytes, and T-lymphocytes.[75] These components are integral to defending the body against invading microorganisms and internal threats. As an example, investigators studying the ability of T-lymphocytes to destroy lymphoma cells found that a 450MHz magnetic field was able to inhibit the lymphocyte activity.[76] Higher and more sustained serum cortisol levels, (such as those found in chronic stress or similar conditions) have been shown to have negative effects, such as decreased cognitive function, thyroid function, immune function, bone density and muscle tissue. Furthermore, increased serum cortisol also leads to hyperglycemia, hypertension, and increased abdominal fat. EMFs cause increased serum cortisol levels[77, 78] and that increases serum glucose levels.[79] As a result of cortisol's influence on liver glycogen more glucose is released into the bloodstream. In other words, cortisol acts to inhibit the effects of insulin, predisposing an individual to diabetic serum glucose values. Insulin secretion by the pancreatic islets was decreased by exposure to EMFs, thus increasing serum glucose levels.[80] Furthermore, EMFs also impair insulin's ability to bind to its receptor.[81] Increased serum cortisol can also cause mood swings, depression, insomnia, decrease memory and memory functions.[82]

The Melatonin Theory

Research has indicated that chronic exposure to EMFs can affect adrenal, pituitary, and pineal gland function.[83, 84] Serotonin production and serotonin receptors can be affected by EMFs.[85]

Suppression of the secretion of melatonin by the pineal gland has been suggested as a pathway for EMF effects on health. Henshaw and Reiter (2005) propose "*that the melatonin hypothesis, in which power frequency magnetic fields suppress the nocturnal production of melatonin in the pineal gland, accounts for the observed increased risk of childhood leukemia.*"[86] The pineal gland is an endocrine organ located in the brain that secretes the hormone melatonin, which appears to play a major role in sexual development, metabolism,[87] antioxidant functions,[88] and many other physiological activities.

Serum melatonin is reputed to be responsible for antioxidant, immunological, and anti-tumor functions.[89-93] The evidence that EMFs affect serum melatonin and pineal gland function is absolutely overwhelming.[94-98] Researchers have demonstrated that electric fields and ELFs (extremely low-frequency magnetic fields) as well as static magnetic fields depress melatonin secretion.[99-108] Dr. Russell Reiter suggests that the suppression of melatonin by magnetic fields could result in a higher incidence of cancer in any tissue,[109] and certainly predispose one to neurodegenerative disorders and dementia.[110]

The work of Dr. Eva Schernhammer not only corroborates the melatonin theory but suggests that other cancers, aside from breast cancer, such as colorectal cancer may be related to decreased serum melatonin.[111, 112] The fact that EMFs can affect a broad range of hormonal secretions[113] may, in fact, be the solution to one of the mysteries of the magnetic field/cancer diversity issue.[114]

Electrical Hypersensitivity

There is a certain segment of the population that suffers from a condition known as electrical hypersensitivity. Although Hillert *et al* (2002) has found only one to two percent (1%-2%) of the Swedish population to be electromagnetically hypersensitive,[115] current estimates reveal that approximately three percent (3%) of the population has this sensitivity and another thirty-five percent have some symptoms of EHS.[116]

What about Cell Phones?

Electromagnetic fields are produced by so many of our modern conveniences that most of us cannot revert back to a simpler, perhaps somewhat less convenient lifestyle. There are currently more than two billion, seven hundred million cell phones in use on the planet and of course the millions of cell phone towers (masts) that allow these phones to function. The real question we should be asking is how safe are they, because these devices totally fill our environment, and then to top it off, we hold them beside our largest collection of neurological tissue... our brain. One of the problems that we are all currently facing is the fact that there is virtually no place left on the planet where we can be free of the radio frequency wavelengths that now transmit information.

In 1998 Hocking published his findings related to the symptoms associated with analog and digital cellular phones. These symptoms included discomfort, dizziness, difficulty concentrating, memory loss, fatigue, headache, burning skin sensations (a sensation of warmth on or near the ear), and tingling and tightness of the skin near the phone.[117] In that same year, Dr. Kjell Mild examined 11,000 cell phone users and corroborated all of the symptoms found by Hocking, and stated that fatigue, headaches, and burning sensations are more frequent symptoms of those people who make longer phone calls.[118]

Since those initial findings the association and dose-relationships between cell phones and disease place cell phone users into a high-risk health group.[119] Cell phones can cause DNA damage, headaches, blurred vision, dizziness, fatigue, short term memory loss, neuralgias, tumors, and sleep disturbances to name a few.[120-125]

In the early 1990's, Lai and Singh developed a technique to determine genetic damage in peripheral blood lymphocytes called single cell gel electrophoresis. This technique was able to recognize DNA fragments that represented the appearance of a 'comet' under the scrutiny of a microscope. The increased length of the 'comet's' tail represented an increased degree of DNA damage.[125]

Aside from his numerous investigations into melatonin, Vijayalaxmi (1997) irradiated transgenic (predisposed to developing tumors) mice to a continuous cell phone signal and found a forty-one percent (41%) increase in tumor growth and twelve and a half per cent (12.5%) increase in chromosome damage in bone and blood.[126] Meanwhile, Dr. Leif Salford and his group of Swedish researchers found that cell phone radiation at all levels causes significant blood brain barrier leakage.[127, 128] Cell phones have also been shown to decrease cognitive function by increasing reaction time[129] and decreasing performance in memory testing.[130, 131]

When we bear in mind the fact that so little is known about the bioaccumulation effects of EMFs or, in fact, what portion of these fields is capable of causing health issues, there might be an element to further investigate. To indicate that cell phone use and rapidly expanding wireless technology do not have health consequences is simply a blatant denial of the fact that researchers have found mutagenic and genotoxic effects.[132]

The theoretical possibility of the existence of an accumulated EMF threshold that predisposes any individual to a diseased state when surpassed seems to validate the risk factor and incidence of disease that so many researchers have found as an associative or causal relationship.

CONCLUDING REMARKS

The majority of us will be affected by magnetic fields virtually twenty-four hours per day for our entire lives. EMFs are everywhere and to ignore the medical literature that links them to miscarriage, cancer, and a whole host of other health risks is paramount to negligence. No one has really told us exactly what potential threat EMFs possess. From an epidemiological perspective, the evidence is irrefutable. There are too many studies with positive findings for this health issue to be overlooked.

REFERENCES

1.   Wertheimer N, Leeper E. Electrical wiring configurations and childhood cancer. *Am J Epidemiol.* 1979;109:273-284.
2.   Maret K. *Electromagnetic Fields and Human Health.* National Foundation for Alternative Medicine. Washington, D.C: 2003;17.

3. Villeneuve PJ, Agnew DA, *et al*. Non-Hodgkin's lymphoma among electric utility workers in Ontario: the evaluation of alternative indices of exposure to 60Hx electric and magnetic fields. *Occup Environ Med*. 2000;57:349-357.

4. Hillman D. Exposure to electric and magnetic fields (EMF) linked to neuro-endocrine stress syndrome: increased cardiovascular disease, diabetes and cancer. *Shocking News*. 2005;8:2.

5. Wertheimer N, Leeper E. Adult cancer related to electrical wires near the home. *Int J Epidemiol*. 1982;11:345-355.

6. Maret K. Electromagnetic Fields and Human Health. National Foundation for Alternative Medicine. Washington, D.C: 2003;13.

7. Dibirdik I, Kristupaitis D, Kurosaki T, Tuel-Ahlgren L, Chu A, Pond D, Tuong D, Luben R, Uckun FM. Stimulation of Src family protein tyrosine kinases as a proximal and mandatory step for SYK kinase-dependent phospholipase C Gamma 2 activation in lymphoma B-cells exposed to low energy electromagnetic fields. *J Biol Chem*. 1998;273:4035-4039.

8. Kristupaitis D, Dibirdik I, Vassilev A, Mahajan S, Kurosaki T, Chu A, Tuel-Ahlgren L, Tuong D, Pond D, Luben R, Uckun FM. Electromagnetic field-induced stimulation of Bruton's tyrosine kinase. *J Biol Chem*. 1998;273:12397-12401.

9. Wertheimer N, Leeper E. Adult cancer related to electrical wires near the home. *Int J Epidemiol*. 1982;11:345-355.

10. Poole C, Trichopoulis D. Extremely low-frequency magnetic fields and cancer. *Cancer Causes Control*. 1991;2:267-276.

11. Adey WR. Evidence for tissue interactions with microwave and other nonionizing electromagnetic fields in cancer promotion. In: Fiala J, Pokorny J, eds. *Biophysical Aspects of Cancer*. Prague, Czech Republic: Charles University; 1987.

12. Draper G, Vincent T, Kroll ME, Swanson J. Childhood cancer in relation to distance from high voltage power lines in England and Wales: a case controlled study. BMJ. 2005; 330:p1290-1295.

13. Baris D, Armstrong BG, Deadman J, Theriault G. A mortality study of electrical utility workers in Quebec. *Occupational and Environmental Medicine*. 1996;53:25-31.

14. Feychting M, Ahlbom A. Magnetic fields and cancer in children residing near Swedish high voltage power lines. *Am J Epidemiol*. 1993;138:467-481.

15. Washburn EP, Orza MJ, Berlin JA, Nicholson WJ, Todd AC, Frumkin H, Chalmers TC. Residential proximity to electric transmission and distribution equipment and risk of childhood leukemia, childhood lymphoma, and child hood nervous system tumors: Systematic review, evaluation, and meta-analysis. *Cancer Causes Control*. 1994;5:299-309.

16. Trichopoulos D. Epidemiologic studies of cancer and extremely low-frequency electric and magnetic field exposures. In: Health Effects of Low-Frequency Electric and Magnetic Fields. Report to the Committee on Interagency Radiation Research and Policy Coordination; Oak Ridge Associated Universities Panel. NTIS Publication #029- 000-00443-9: V-1-58. 1992.

17. Savitz DA, Pearle NE, Poole C. Methodological issues in the epidemiology of electromagnetic fields and cancer. *Epidemiol Rev*. 1989;11:59-78.

18. Savitz DA, Loomis DP. Magnetic field exposure in relation to leukemia and brain cancer mortality among electric utility workers. *Am J Epidemiol*. 1995;141:123-124.

19. Kheifets LI, Afifi AA, Buffler PA, Zhang ZW. Occupational electric and magnetic field exposure and brain cancer: a meta analysis. *J Occup Environ Med*. 1996;38:655-658.

20. Sorahan T, Nichols L, van Tongeren M, Harrington JM. Occupational exposure to magnetic fields relative to mortality from brain tumours: updated and revised findings from a study of United Kingdom electricity generation and transmission workers. *Occupational Environmental Medicine*. 2001;58:626-630.

21. Guenel P, Nicolau J, Imberon E, Chevalier A, Goldberg M. Exposure to electric filed and incidence of leukemia, brain tumors, and other cancers among French electric utility workers. *Am J Epidemiol*. 1996;144:1107-1121.

22. Kheifets LI. Electric and magnetic field exposure and brain cancer: A review. *Bioelectromagnetics*. 2001;Suppl 5:S120-131.

23. Schlehofer B, Kunze S W, Blettner M, Niehoff D, Wahrendorf J. Occupational risk factors for brain tumors: results from a population-based case-control study in Germany. *Cancer Causes Control*. 1990;1(3):209-215.

24. Villeneuve PJ, Agnew DA, Johnson KC, Mao Y, Canadian Cancer Registries Epidemiology Group. Brain cancer and occupational exposure to magnetic fields among men: results from a Canadian population-based case control study. *Int J Epidemiol*. 2002;31:210-217.

25. Wei M, Guizzetti M, Yost M, Costa LG. Exposure to 60-Hz magnetic fields and proliferation of human astrocytoma cells in vitro. *Toxicology and Applied Pharmacology*. 2000;162:166-176.

26. Feychting M, Ahlbom A. Childhood leukemia and residential exposure to weak extremely low frequency magnetic fields. *Environ Health Perspect*. 1995;103 Suppl 2:59-62.

27.	Miller MA, Murphy JR, Miller TI, *et al*. Variation in cancer risk estimates for exposure to powerline frequency electromagnetic fields: A meta-analysis comparing EMF measurement methods. *Risk Analysis*. 1995;15:281-287.

28.	Coleman MP, Bell CMJ, Taylor H, *et al*. Leukemia and residence near electricity transmission equipment: A case control study. *Br J Cancer*. 1989;60:793-798.

29.	Linet MS, Hatch EE, Kleinerman RA, Robison LL, Kaune WT, Friedman DR, Severson R K, Haines CM, Hartsock CT, Niwa S, Wacholder S, Tarone RE. Residential exposure to magnetic fields and acute lymphoblastic leukemia in children. *N Engl J Med*. 1997;337:1-7.

30.	Feychting M, Ahlbom A. Magnetic fields, leukemia, and central nervous system tumors in Swedish adults residing near high-voltage lines. *Epidemiology*. 1994;5:501-509.

31.	Shaw GM, Croen LA. Human adverse reproductive outcomes and electromagnetic field exposures: review of epidemiological studies. *Environ Health Perspect*. 1993;101 (Suppl 4):107-119.

32.	Wertheimer N, Leeper E. Fetal loss associated with two seasonal sources of electromagnetic field exposure. *Am J Epidemiol*. 1989;129:220-224.

33.	Juutilainen J, Matilainen P, Saarikoski S, Laara E, Suonio S. Early pregnancy loss and exposure to 50Hz magnetic fields. *Bioelectromagnetics*. 1992;14:229-236.

34.	McDonald AD, Cherry NM, Delorme C, McDonald JC. Visual display units and pregnancy: evidence from the Montreal survey. *J Occup Med*. 1986;28:1226-1231.

35.	Goldhaber MK, Polen M, Hiat R. Miscarriages of women using computers in the workplace. *Amer J Industrial Med*. 1988;13:695.

36.	Schnorr TM, Grajewski Hornung RW, Thun MJ, Egeland GM, Murray WE, Conover DL, Halperin WE. Video display terminals and the risk of spontaneous abortion. *N Engl J Med*. 1991;324:727-733.

37.	Lindbohm ML, Hietanen M, Kyyronen P, Sallmen M, Von Nandelstadh P, Taskinen H, Pekkarinen M, Ylikoski M, Hemminki K. Magnetic fields of video display terminals and spontaneous abortion. *Am J Epidemiol*. 1992;136:1041-1051.#

38.	Belanger K, Leaderer B, Kellenbrand K, Holford T, *et al*. Spontaneous abortion and exposure to electric blankets and heated water beds. *Epidemiology*. 1998;9:36-42.

39.	Wertheimer N, Leeper E. Possible effects of electric blankets and heated waterbeds on fetal development. *Bioelectromagnetics*. 1986;7;13-22.

40.	Hocking B, Joyner K. Re: *Miscarriages among female physical therapists who report using radio- and microwave frequency electromagnetic radiation*. A letter to the Editor. *Am J Epidemiol*. 1995;141:273-274.

41.	Ouellet-Hellstrom R, Stewart WF. Miscarriages among female physical therapists who report using radio- and microwave-frequency electromagnetic radiation. *Am J Epidemiol*. 1993;138:775-786.

42.	Larsen AI, Olsen J, Svane O. Gender specific reproductive outcome and exposure to high frequency electromagnetic radiation among physiotherapists. *Scand J Work Environ Health*. 1991;17:324-329.

43.	Taskinen H, Kyyronen P, Hemminki K. Effects of ultrasound, shortwaves, and physical exertion on pregnancy outcome in physiotherapists. *J of Epidemiology and Community Health*. 1990;44:196-210.

44.	Li DK, Odouli R, Wi S, *et al*. A population-based prospective cohort study of personal exposure to magnetic fields during pregnancy and the risk of miscarriage. *Epidemiology* 2002;13:9-20.

45.	Cherry N. Critcism of the health assessment in the ICNIRP guidelines for radiofrequency and microwave radiation (100 kHz-300GHz). Lincoln University. 2000;87.

46.	Savitz D, Checkoway H, Loomis D. Magnetic field exposure and neurodegenerative disease mortality among electric utility workers. *Epidemiology*. 1998;9:398-404.

47.	Savitz D, Loomis D, Tse CK. Electrical occupations and neurodegenerative disease: Analyisis of U.S. mortality data. *Archives of Environmental Health*. 1998;53:1-5.

48.	Zlokovic BV, Deane R, Sallstromm J, Chow N, Miano JM. Neurovascular pathways and Alzheimer amyloid beta peptide. *Brain Pathol*. 2005;15:78-83.

49.	Sobel E, Davanipour Z, Sulkava R, Erkinjuntti T, Wikstrom J, Henderson VW, Buckwalter G, Bowman JD, Lee PJ. Occupations with exposure to electromagnetic fields: A possible risk factor for Alzheimer's disease. *Am J Epidemiol*. 1995;142:515-524.

50.	Harmanci H, Emre M, Gurvit H, Bilgic B, Hanagasi H, Gurol E, Sahin H, Tinaz S. Risk factors for Alzheimer disease: a population-based case-control study in Istanbul, Turkey. *Alzheimer Dis Assoc Disord*. 2003;17:139-145.

51.	Strickland D, Smith SA, Dolliff G, Goldman L, Roelofs RI. Amyotrophic lateral sclerosis and occupational history. A pilot case-control study. *Archives of Neurology*. 1996;53:730-733.

52.	Gunnarsson LG, Lindberg G, Soderfeldt B, Axelson O. Amyotrophic lateral sclerosis in Sweden in relation to occupation. *Acta Neurologica Scandinavica*. 1991;83:394-339.

53.	Davanipour Z, Sobel E, Bowman JD, Qian Z, Will AD. Amyotrophic lateral sclerosis and occupational exposure to electromagnetic fields. *Bioelectromagnetics*. 1997;18:18-28.

54.	Johansen C, Olsen JH. Mortality from amyotrophic lateral sclerosis, other chronic disorders and electric shocks among utility workers. *Am J Epidemiol*. 1998;148:362-368.

55. Schulte PA, Burnett CA, Boeniger MF, Johnson J. Neurodegenrative diseases: occupational occurrence and potential risk factors. *Am J Public Health*. 1996;86:1281-1288.

56. Ahlbom A. Neurodegenarative diseases, suicide and depressive symptoms in relation to EMF. *Bioelectromagnetics*. 2001;Suppl 5:S132-143.

57. Hakansson N, Gustavsson P, Johansen C, Floderus B. Neurodegenerative diseases in welders and other workers exposed to high levels of magnetic fields. *Epidemiology*. 2003;14:420-426.

58. Havas M, Stetzer D. Dirty Electricity and Electrical Hypersensitivity: Five Case Studies. World Health Organization Workshop on Electrical Hypersensitivity, 25-26 October, Prague, Czech Republich, 2004.

59. Lyskov E, Juutilainen V, Jousmaki V, Hanninen O, et al. Influence of short-term exposure of magnetic field on the bioelectric processes of the brain and performance. *Int J Psychophysiol*. 1993;14:227-231.

60. Verkasalo PK, Kaprio J, Varjonen J, Romanov K, Heikkila K, Koskenvuo M. Magnetic fields of transmission lines and depression. *Am J Epidemiol*. 1997;146;1037-1045.

61. Poole C, Kavet R, Funch DP, et al. Depressive symptoms and headaches in relation to proximity of residence to an alternating-current transmission line right-of-way. *Am J Epidemiol*. 1003;137:318-330.

62. Perry S, Pearl L, Binns R. Power frequency magnetic field: depressive illness and myocardial infarction. Public Health. 1989; 103:p177-180.

63. Beale IL, Pearce NE, Conroy DM, Henning MA, Murrell KA. Psychological effects of chronic exposure to 50 Hz magnetic fields in humans living near extra high voltage transmission lines. *Bioelectromagnetics*. 1997;18:584-594.

64. Sobel E, Davanipour Z. Electromagnetic field exposure may cause increased production of amyloid beta and may eventually lead to Alzheimer's disease. *Neurology*. 1996;47:1591-1600.

65. Wertheimer N, Leeper E. Electrical wiring configurations and childhood cancer. *Am J Epidemiol*. 1979;109:273-284.

66. Olsen JH, Nielsen A, Schulgen G. Residence near high voltage facilities and risk of cancer in children. *British Medical Journal*. 1993;307:891-895.

67. Juutilainen J, Kumlin T, Naarala J. Do extremely low frequency magnetic fields enhance the effects of environmental carcinogens? *Int J Radiat Biol*. 2006;82:1-12.

68. Sastre A, Cook MR, Graham C. Nocturnal exposure to intermittent 60 Hz magnetic fields alter human cardiac rhythm. *Bioelectromagnetics*. 1998;19:98-106.

69. Savitz DA, Liao D, Sastre A, Kleckner RC. Magnetic field exposure and cardiovascular disease mortality among electric utility workers. *Am J Epidemiol*. 1999;149:135-142.

70. Braune S, Wrocklage C, Raczek J, Gailus T, Lucking CH. Resting blood pressure increased during exposure to a radio-frequency electromagnetic field. *Lancet*. 1998;351:1857-1858.

71. Braune S, Reidel A, Schulte-Monting J, Raczek, J. Influence of a radio-frequency magnetic field on cardiovascular and hormonal parameters of the autonomic nervous system in healthy individuals. *Radiat Res*. 2002;158:352-356.

72. Sait ML, Wood AW, Sadafi HA. A study of heart rate and heart rate variability in human subjects exposed to occupational levels of 50 Hz circular polarized magnetic fields. *Med Eng Phys*. 1999;21:361-369.

73. Huber R, Schudererm J, Grat T, Jutz K, Borbely AA, Kuster N, Achermann P. Radio frequency electromagnetic field in humans: Estimation of SAR distribution in the brain, effects on sleep and heart rate. *Bioelectromagnetics*. 2003;24:262-276.

74. Sastre AM, Cook R, Graham C. Nocturnal exposure to intermittent 60 Hz magnetic fields alters human cardiac rhythm. *Bioelectromagnetics*. 1998;19:98-106.

75. Lyle DB, Ayotte RD, Sheppard AR, Adey WR. Suppression of t-lymphocyte cytotoxicity following exposure to 60-Hz sinusoidal electric fields. Bioelectromagnetics. 1988;9:303-313.

76. Lyle DB, Schecter P, Adey WR, Lundak RL. Suppression of t-lymphocyte cytotoxicity following exposure to sinusoidally amplitude-modulated fields. *Bioelectromagnetics*. 1983;4:281-292.

77. Hillman D. Exposure to electric and magnetic fields (EMF) linked to neuro-endocrine stress syndrome: increased cardiovascular disease, diabetes and cancer. *Shocking News*. 2005;(8):2.

78. Becker RO. *Cross Currents: The Perils of Electropollution- the Promise of Electromedicine*. New York: Putnam Publishers; 1990.

79. Berne RM, Levy MN, Koeppen BM, Stanton BA. *Physiology*. Fifth Edition. Philadelphia: Mosby; 1998.

80. Sakurai T, Sataka A, Sumi S, Inoue K, Miyakoshi J. An extremely low magnetic field attenuates insulin secretion from the insulinoma cell line, RIN-m. *Bioelectromagnetics*. 2004;25:160-166.

81. Li L, Dai Y, Xia R, Chen S, Qiao D. Pulsed electric field exposure of insulin induces anti-prolifeative effects on human hepatocytes. *Bioelectromagnetics*. 2005;26:1-9.

82. Hillman D. Exposure to electric and magnetic fields (EMF) linked to neuro-endocrine stress syndrome: increased cardiovascular disease, diabetes and cancer. *Shocking News*. 2005;(8):p4.

83. Kavet R, Zaffanella LE, Daigle JP, Ebi KL. The possible role of contact of contact current in cancer risk associated with residential magnetic fields. *Bioeletromagnetics*. 2000;21:538-553.

84. Kavet R. Review: Contact current hypothesis: Summary of results to date. *Bioelectromagnetics*. 2005;7 (supplement):S75-S85.

85. Sieron A, Labus L, Nowak P, Cieslar G, Brus H, Durczok A, Zagzit T, Kostrzewa T, Brus R. Alternating extremely low frequency magnetic field increases turnover of dopamine and serotonin in rat frontal cortex. *Bioelectromagnetics.* 2004;25:426-430.

86. Henshaw DL, Reiter RJ. Do magnetic fields cause increased risk of childhood leukemia via melatonin disruption? *Bioelectromagnetics.* 2005;Suppl 7:S86-97.

87. Axelrod J. The pineal gland. *Endeavour.* 1970;29:144-148.

88. Pappola MA, Chyan YJ, Poeggeler B, Frangione B, Wilson G, Ghiso J, Reiter RJ. An assessment of the antioxidant and the antimyloidogenic properties of melatonin: implications for Alzheimer's disease. *J Neural Transm.* 2000;107:203-231.

89. Hillman D. Exposure to electric and magnetic fields (EMF) linked to neuro-endocrine stress syndrome: increased cardiovascular disease, diabetes and cancer. *Shocking News.* 2005;(8):5.

90. Badr FM, El Habit OHM, Harraz MM. Radioprotective effect of melatonin assessed by measuring chromosomal damage in mitotic and meiotic cells. *Mutation Research.* 1999;444:367-372.

91. Vijayalaxmi, Reiter RJ, Sewerynek E, Poeggeler B, Leal BZ, Meltz ML. Marked reduction of radiation-induced micronuclei in human blood lymphocytes pretreated with melatonin. *Radiation Research.* 1995;143:102-106.

92. Vijayalaxmi, Reiter RJ, Herman TS, Meltz ML. Melatonin and radioprotection from genetic damage: In vivo/in vitro studies with human volunteers. *Mutation Research.* 1996;371:221-228.

93. Vijayalaxmi, Thomas CR Jr, Reiter RJ, Herman TS. Melatonin: From basic research to cancer treatment clinics. *J Clin Oncology.* 2002;20:2575-2601.

94. Wilson BW, Anderson LE, Hilton DI, Phillips RD. Chronic exposure to 60-Hz electric fields: Effects on pineal function in the rat. *Bioelectromagnetics.* 1981;2:371-380.

95. Grota LJ, Reiter RJ, Keng P, Michaelson S. Electric field exposure alters serum melatonin but not pineal melatonin synthesis in male rats. *Bioelectromagnetics.* 1994;15:427-437.

96. Reiter RJ, Anderson LE, Buschbom RL, Wilson BW. Reduction of the nocturnal rise in pineal melatonin levels in rats exposed to 60-Hz electric fields in utero and for 23 days after birth. *Life Science.* 1988;42:2203-2206.

97. Wilson BW, Chess EK, Anderson LE. 60-Hz electric-field effects on pineal melatonin rhythms: Time course for onset and recovery. *Bioelectromagnetics.* 1986;7:239-242.

98. Yellon SM. Acute 60 Hz magnetic field exposure effects on the melatonin rhythm in the pineal gland and circulation of the adult Djungarian hamster. *Journal of Pineal Research.* 1994;16:136-144.

99. Wilson BW, Stevens RG, Anderson LE, eds. Extremely *Low Frequency Electromagnetic Fields: The Question of Cancer.* Columbus, OH: Battelle Press; 1990.

100. Brady JV, Reiter RJ. Neurobehavioral effects. In: *Health Effects of Low-Frequency Electric and Magnetic Fields. Report to the Committee on Interagency Radiation Research and Policy Coordination;* Oak Ridge Associated Universities Panel. NTIS Publication #029-000-00443-9: VII-1-VII-56. 1992.

101. Stevens RG. Re: Risk of postmenopausal breast cancer and use of electric blankets. *Am J Epi.* 1995;142:146.

102. Burch JB, Reif JS, Noonan CW, Yost MG. Melatonin metabolite levels in workers exposed to 60 Hz magnetic fields: work in substations and with 3-phase conductors. *J Occup Envir Med.* 2000;42:136-142.

103. Arnetz BB, Berg M. Melatonin and adrenocorticotropic hormone levels in video display unit workers during work and leisure. *J Occup Med.* 1996;38:1108-1110.

104. Selmaoui B, Touitou Y. Sinusoidal 50-Hz magnetic fields depress rat pineal NAT activity and serum melatonin. Role of duration and intensity of exposure. *Life Science.* 1995;57:1351-1358.

105. Kato M, Honma K, Shigemitsu T, Shiga Y. Effects of exposure to a circularly polarized 50-Hz magnetic field on plasma and pineal melatonin levels in rats. *Bioelectromagnetics.* 1993;14:97-110.

106. Truong H, Yellon SM. Effect of various acute 60 Hz magnetic field exposures on the nocturnal melatonin rise in the adult Djungarian hamster. *Journal of Pineal Research.* 1997;22:177-183.

107. Kato M, Honma K, Shigemitsu T, Shiga Y. Circularly polarized 50-Hz magnetic field exposure reduces pineal gland melatonin and blood concentrations of long-evans rats. *Neuroscience Letters.* 1994;166:59-62.

108. Wilson BW, Wright CW, Morris JF, Buschbom RL, Brown DP, Miller DL, Sommers-Flannigan R, Anderson LE. Evidence for an effect of elf electromagnetic fields on human pineal gland function. *Journal of Pineal Research.* 1990;9:259-269.

109. Rogers WR, Reiter RJ, Smith HD, Barlow-Walden L. Rapid-onset/offset, variably scheduled 60 Hz electric and magnetic field exposure reduces nocturnal serum melatonin concentration in nonhuman primates. *Bioelectromagnetics.* 1995;S3:119-122.

110. Reiter RJ, Tan DX, Pappolla MA. Melatonin relieves the neural oxidative burden that contributes to dementias. Ann N Y Acad Sci. 2004;1035:179-196.

111. Schernhammer ES, Hankinson SE. Urinary melatonin levels and breast cancer risk. *J Natl Cancer Inst.* 2005;97:1084-1087.

112. Schernhammer ES, Laden F, Speizer FE, Willett WC, Hunter DJ, Kawachi I, Fuchs CS, Colditz GA: Night-shift work and risk of colorectal cancer in the Nurses' Health Study. *J Natl Cancer Inst.* 2003;95:825-828.

113. Davis S, Mirick DK, Chen C, Stanczyk FZ. Effects of 60-Hz magnetic field exposure on nocturnal 6-Sulfatoxymelatonin, estrogens, luteinizing hormone, and follicle-stimulating hormone in healthy reproductive age women: Results of a crossover trials. *Ann Epidemiol.* 2006;16(8):622-631.

114. Stevens RG, Wilson BW, Anderson LE. *The Melatonin Hypothesis: Breast cancer and the use of electric power*. Columbus, Ohio: Battelle Press; 1997.

115. Hillert L, Berglind N, Arnetz BB, Bellander T. Prevalence of self-reported hypersensitivity to electric magnetic fields in a population-based questionnaire survey. *Scand j Work Environ Health*. 2002;28:33-41.

116. Philips A, Philips J. *The Power Watch Handbook*. London: Piatkus Books; 2006: 294.

117. Hocking B. Preliminary report: Symptoms associated with mobile phone use. *Occ Med*. 1998;48:357-360.

118. Mild KH, Oftedal G, Sandstrom M, Wilen J, Tynes T, Haugsdal B, Hauger E. Comparison of symptoms by users of analogue and digital mobile phones - A Swedish-Norwegian epidemiological study. National Institute for Working Life, Umea, Sweden. 1998;23:84.

119. Gandhi GA, Singh P. Mobile phone users: Another high health risk group. *J Hum Ecol*. 2005;18:85-92.

120. Lai H, Singh NP. Acute low-intensity microwave exposure increases DNA single-strand breaks in rat brain cells. *Bioelectromagnetics*. 1995;16:207-210.

121. Hamblin DL, Wood AW. Effects of mobile phone emissions on human brain activity and sleep variables. *Int J Radiat Biol*. 2002;78:659-669.

122. Gandhi GA, Singh P. Mobile phone users: Another high health risk group. *J Hum Ecol*. 2005;18:85-92.

123. Ahlbom A, Green A, Kheifets L, Savitz D, Swerdlow A. Epidemiology of health effects of radiofrequency exposure. *Environ Health Perspect*. 2004;112:1741-1754.

124. Mild KH, Oftedal G, Sandstrom M, Wilen J, Tynes T, Haugsdal B, Hauger E. Comparison of symptoms by users of analogue and digital mobile phones - A Swedish-Norwegian epidemiological study. National Institute for Working Life, Umea, Sweden. 1998;23:84.

125. Lai H, Singh HP. Single and double strand DNA breaks in rat brain cells after acute exposure to radiofrequency electromagnetic radiation. *Int J Radiat Biol*. 1996;69:513-521.

126. Vijayalaxmi BZ, Frei MR, Dusch SJ, Guel V, Meltz ML, Jauchem JR. Frequency of micronuclei in the peripheral blood and bone marrow of cancer-prone mice chronically exposed to 2450 MHz radiofrequency radiation. *Radiation Research*. 1997a;147:495-500.

127. Salford LG, Brun A, Sturesson K, Eberhardt JL, Persson BR. Permeability of the blood-brain barrier induced by 915 MHz electromagnetic radiation, continuous wave and modulated at 8, 16, 50, and 200 Hz. *Microsc Res Tech*. 1994;27:535-542.

128. Carlo G, Schram M. *Cell Phones: Invisible Hazards in the Wireless Age*. New York, NY: Carroll & Graf Publishers; New York: 2001; 111.

129. Hamblin DL, Wood AW, Croft RJ, Stough C. Examining the effects of electromagnetic fields emitted by GSM mobile phones on human event-related potentials and performance during an auditory task. *Clin Neurophysiol*. 2004;115171-178.

130. Krause CM, Harrala C, Sillanmäki L, Koivisto M, Alnko K, Reyonsuo A, Laine M, Hämäläinen H. Effects of electromagnetic field emitted by cellular phones on the EEG during an auditory memory task: a double blind replication study. *Bioelectromagnetics*. 2004;25:33-40.

131. Koivisto M, Revonsuo A, Krause C, Haarala C, Sillanmäki L, Laine M, Hämäläinen H. Effects of 902 MHz electromagnetic field emitted by cellular telephones on response times in humans. *Neuroreport*. 2000;11:413-415.

132. Heynick LN, Johnston SA, Mason PA. Radio frequency electromagnetic fields: Cancer, mutagenesis and genotoxicity. *Bioelectromagnetics*. 2003;Suppl 6:S74-100.

Chapter 12
Use of Iodine in Clinical Practice
Jorge D. Flechas, M.D., MPH
Medical Director, Flechas Family Practice (Hendersonville, North Carolina USA)

ABSTRACT
This paper will discuss the importance of iodine for health and its use in clinical practice. The incidence of iodine deficiency in the United States and its consequences will be discussed, as will the inadequacy of the current RDA.

INTRODUCTION

Iodine is a member of the halogen family, which also includes fluorine, chlorine, bromine, and astatine. Chlorine was the first member of the halogen family to be discovered back in 1809, followed by iodine in 1811, bromine in 1826, fluorine in 1886, and astatine in 1940. The use of iodine for the treatment of goiter was the first time that a single item (iodine) was used to treat a specific illness (goiter). Interestingly, many doctors today incorrectly believe that iodine is a cause of goiter, and many will try to discourage people from taking iodine.

WHERE IS IODINE FOUND IN THE BODY?

Every cell in the body contains and utilizes iodine. White blood cells cannot effectively guard against infection without adequate amounts of iodine. Iodine is concentrated in the glandular systems of the body. The thyroid gland contains the largest amount of iodine, although it is also concentrated in breast tissue, salivary glands, parotid glands, pancreas, cerebrospinal fluid, brain, stomach, skin, lacrimal glands, and etc. all have the ability to concentrate iodine. The absence of iodine is known to be a promoter of cancer.

How do organs and tissue concentrate iodine? In 1995 it was found that the body uses a type of channel called the sodium/iodide symporter pump to concentrate iodine. The calcium channel, sodium channel, and chloride channel, only allow one type of ion to pass through them. However, symporters are channels that allow two different types of ions to pass through the channel. Furthermore, the sodium/iodide symporter is a pump, which means that it has the ability to pump iodine against a gradient.

What is the difference between iodine and iodide? Iodide is the salt. Breast tissue, prostate tissue and stomach prefer iodine, whilst the thyroid, the salivary glands, and the skin prefer iodide. To sit and say that you need one or the other is ludicrous. The body needs both iodine and iodide in order for it to function correctly, which is why we prefer to use Lugol's solution when treating patients, as it contains both iodine and iodide.

Iodine is essential for the normal growth and development of children. It is crucial for the development of the central nervous system development. A baby's IQ is set by the age of two, and iodine is what sets that IQ. A deficiency in iodine can result in cretinism, mental deficiency and deafness, delayed physical and intellectual development. Research suggests that mild iodine deficiency in early fetal life may be a cause of attention deficit disorder. Attention deficit disorder is not associated with the thyroid T4 levels or thyroid stimulating hormone (TSH) levels at the time of birth, but it is related to the amount of iodine in a mother's diet and her body at the time that she gets pregnant.

In Japan, the average individual eats 13.8 milligrams of iodine per day, whilst the average American eats around 168 micrograms, of iodine per day. Interestingly, the US has the highest incidence of breast cancer in the world, whilst Japan has the lowest. It is a similar story with life expectancy; in the US the average life expectancy is 77.85 years, whereas in Japan it is 81.25 years, and infant mortality, in the US there are 7 deaths under age 1 per 1000 live births whereas in Japan it is 3.5, which is the lowest in the world.

IODINE DEFICIENCY

Iodine deficiency is thought to be present in approximately 128 countries. It is associated with a number of disorders, including goiter, mental retardation, and cretinism. We have known for many years that people who have a goiter are at increased risk of developing thyroid cancer, breast cancer, stomach cancer, esophageal cancer, ovarian cancer, and endometrial cancer.

During the time of the First World War a lot of young men that tried to join the military were rejected because they had goiters. We looked at the data that shows where these men with goiters came from and then went to check the soil. We found that the soils of the Great Lakes region were depleted of iodine, but also noticed that the soils along the Northern United States and along the West Coastline are very depleted. There is a lot more Iodine in the soil and the water in the south and a lot less of it as you go north.

In the 1900s, goiter was very prevalent among the people living in the Great Lakes region – approximately 40% of school-aged children had goiters. In 1924 in Akron, Ohio, 56% of the population had goiter, with a ratio of six women to one male. Health officials began to investigate the problem and a research study found that iodized salt seemed to prevent goiter, and as a result the US government decreed that iodine should be added to salt to help prevent this major public health problem.

The iodine loading test is a very useful test for determining whether or not a patient has an iodine deficiency. This test works on the principle that iodine binds to receptors throughout the body, and if there is sufficient iodine present in the body, the iodine will then be excreted. However, if an iodine deficiency is present, then iodine will not be excreted. The test is conducted by giving the patient 50 mg of iodine-iodide mixture (Lugol's solution), collecting their urine for 24-hours, and then measuring iodine excretion. A patient is deemed to have sufficient levels of iodine when they excrete 90% or more of the iodine administered.

Results of an iodine loading study of more than 2500 patients conducted at FFP Labs in 2004 revealed that 98% of participants had significantly low iodine levels. We are taking the iodine out of bread, we are taking the iodine out of milk, and we have taken the iodine out of salt. Half of cooking salt now contains no iodine. Furthermore, the first thing patients are told to do if they have high blood pressure is decrease the total salt in their diet. So, they take away the cooking salt that contains iodine. Where do we expect our patients to get the iodine they need?

IODINE INTAKE IN THE UNITED STATES

The first National Health and Nutrition Examination Survey (NHANES), which took place between 1971 and 1974, revealed that the average intake of iodine in the US was 320 mcg per liter (mcg/l). By the time the third NHANES survey was conducted (between 1988 and 1994) the average iodine intake had fallen to 145 mcg/l. Thus, within a period of approximately twenty years the average iodine intake in the US dropped by more than 50%. However, data from a NHANES conducted between 2001 and 2002 showed that iodine intake appeared to have risen, albeit slightly, to approximately 168 mcg/l. Results of a nationwide study of women by my own laboratory, FPP labs, during 2004 and 2006 found that the average intake of iodine nationwide is approximately 175 mcg/l.

Data reveals that in 1997 approximately 11.4% of the population had a severe iodine deficiency, and the later studies that we conducted between 2004 and 2006 show that 16.5% of men and 17.6% of women in the US now have a severe iodine deficiency. Thus, suggesting that the problem of iodine deficiency has increased over the last decade.

During 1971 and 2000, the period when the NHANES data showed that average iodine intake in the US fell by more than 50% there was an increase in thyroid illnesses and cancer of the breast, prostate, endometrium, and ovaries. All of these conditions are associated with goiter caused by iodine deficiency.

HOW MUCH IODINE DOES THE BODY NEED?

The total amount of iodine present in the body is 30 to 50 mg. However, studies have shown that the human body can hold up to as much as 1500 mg of iodine. The average thyroid holds around 9 mg of iodine, but with iodine supplementation the thyroid, at its maximum, can hold 50 mg of iodine. 20% of all the body's iodine is found in the sweat glands of the skin.

How much iodine does the body need? First and foremost, the thyroid needs about 6 mg of iodine per day in order to function properly. Breast tissue needs approximately 5 mg of iodine per day in order to maintain the health of the breast. Larger women and women with large breasts therefore have an increasing requirement for iodine, and men have lower iodine requirements. Other tissues, such as the adrenals, thymus, ovaries, hypothalamus, and pituitary, are very dependent upon the presence of iodine and require approximately 2 mg per day in total.

The RDA for iodine is set at 150 mcg/day for adult males and females, 220 mcg/day for pregnant women, and 290 mcg/day for women who are breastfeeding. However, the RDA was set to prevent goiter. It was not set to prevent other diseases that can be caused by a lack of iodine. At the time that the RDA was set, there was no real concern about the rest of the body's need for iodine. Thus the RDA is inadequate not only for the needs of the thyroid but also for those of the rest of the body as well. Furthermore, it does not address the problem of increased exposure to goitrogens in the environment. Goitrogens are chemicals that compete with iodine for absorption in the body and thus reduce the body's ability to absorb iodine. Common goitrogens include: bromine, chlorine, and fluoride.

IODINE AND BREAST TISSUE

Breast tissue needs both iodine and iodide in order to remain healthy. During lactation the breast is more effective in capturing iodide via the sodium/iodide symporter pump of iodine. When a woman is not lactating, the capture occurs via the pendrin (chloride) transporter.

Iodine deficiency results in fibrocystic breast disease and dysplastic changes of the breast. In breast cancer cells, the activity of an enzyme called lactoperoxidase (lpa) is inversely related to estrogen receptor concentration and tumor size. Iodine replacement significantly increases the action of lpa.

Iodine treatment of benign breast disease (fibrocystic breast disease) is accompanied by reduced breast size and remission of disease symptoms. In fact, 50 mg of iodine a day will resolve breast pain within a few weeks, and if you keep the patient on iodine for three to four years, her mammograms will show that the amount of scar tissue and pathology in the breast tissue will drop significantly with time.

Iodine helps to reduce the risk of breast cancer by inducing apoptosis by the formation of iodolactones of arachidonic acid in both thyroid and breast tissue. Therefore iodine takes away the immortality of cancer cells. Studies in rats with DMBA-induced breast cancer showed that Lugol's solution exerted a suppressive effect on the development and size of the neoplasias.

Subtle defects in thyroid function are a feature of breast cancer. Breast cancer rates are higher in areas of endemic goiter in the US. In countries where goiter is rarely seen, for example Japan, Iceland, and Chile, breast cancer rates are also low.

Low iodine intake leads to a hyperestrogenic state. Hypothyroidism is associated with up to 80 to 90% free estrogen levels, compared to a normal value of 40 to 60%. In contrast, hyperthyroidism is associated with only 20% free estrogen levels. Furthermore, thyroid hormone induces sex hormone binding globulin (SHBG). Thyroid hormone, or triiodothyronine (T3), has the ability to regulate cellular oxidation and calorigenesis, thermoregulation, and intermediary metabolism. It is needed for protein synthesis and promotes nitrogen retention, glycogenesis, intestinal absorption of glucose and galactose, lipolysis, and the uptake of glucose by adipocytes.

THE REAL TRUTH ABOUT IODINE

The real truth about iodine is that you need micrograms of iodine for the body to produce adequate amounts of thyroid hormone, you need milligrams of iodine to achieve optimum health, prevent cancer, and to prevent and treat fibrocystic breast disease, and you need grams of iodine to treat dermatological, pulmonary, and cardiovascular diseases.

So, the medical establishment is saying that you need may be 150 mcg of iodine per day, however I am saying that you need 50 mg. A lot of people would query that amount. They would say that there is a big difference between 150 mcg and 50 mg. However, the average pulmonologist will prescribe some of his pulmonary patients between 300 and 400 mg of SSKI (potassium iodide oral solution) three or four times a day. And few people will query that. This is a very good example of one of the inconsistencies that exist in medicine. We will quite happily prescribe iodine at extremely high levels for the treatment of certain diseases, but yet if we try to give our patients 50 mg for preventative purposes people will start to question your judgment.

GIVING PATIENTS IODINE
There are several different kinds of iodine:
- Inorganic non-radioactive (^{127}I) iodine: KI, SSKI, Lugol's solution, Iodoral, tincture of iodine, Povidone-Iodine
- Organic iodine:
  - Endogenous – thyroid hormones
  - Synthetic – Amiodarone, radiocontrast media (iopanoic acid, meglumine iotroxate, propyliodone, etc.)
- Inorganic radioactive isotopes.

You will find that the vast majority of people who say that they have an allergy to iodine, will actually have an allergy to organic iodine. Most of these people can take inorganic iodine or elemental iodine and do fine with that. You will also find that the vast majority of patients who say they have "iodine sensitivity" can eat iodized salt, and if they can eat iodized salt, they can take these other types of elemental iodines. There is a very, very, very small percentage of the population who cannot eat iodized salt, and they are obviously the patients that you cannot treat with iodine.

The body needs about 50 mg of Lugol's solution or iodine per day. Lugol's solution irritates the stomach of about 20% of patients. However, it is now possible to give Lugol's in a tablet format, which should significantly reduce this problem. Body saturation can be achieved by initially prescribing 100 mg of Lugol's for six weeks and then dropping the dose down to about above 50 mg a day.

Once you start treating a patient with iodine it is likely that their TSH levels will go up for a few weeks or a few months while the sodium/iodide symporter system is being stimulated. You will also usually see a slight increase in thyroid T4. T3 should remain stable. We have now found that different hormones in the body that have the ability to stimulate the sodium/iodide symporter. One of these hormones is TSH. So, as soon as you give a patient iodine their TSH is being used to stimulate the body to absorb iodine through the sodium/iodide symporter. Other hormones that are involved in this include: prolactin, progesterone, and oxytocin.

Before you start treating a patient with iodine it is important to check their thyroid levels (T4, T3, and TSH). If, once they have started treatment, their T4 and T3 levels go down, you should consider an organification defect with either a vitamin B2 or vitamin B3 defect being present. What that means is that you need to give the patient riboflavin or niacin so that they can absorb, organify, and bind iodine to the tissues of the body.

Some people complain of developing a metallic flavor in their mouth when being treated with iodine. This can easily be gotten rid of with chlorophyll. Patients who complain of this should be given one tablet of chlorophyll four times a day and within two or three days the metallic flavor will have gone. They should continue to take the chlorophyll for a few weeks, and then stop taking it, the metallic flavor will not return. Iodine and chloride both take bromide out of the body, so it is important to warn patients that they may see a brown discharge in their urine or sweat.

CONCLUDING REMARKS
Iodine is becoming depleted in the population and as it becomes depleted, we are seeing more and more problems. Within the last five or six years, the incidence of attention deficit disorder in United States has gone up by almost 500%, and the reason why is because so many pregnant women are iodine deficient. I implore you to think very carefully about using iodine in your medical practice not only for the treatment of fibrocystic breast disease but also for the treatment and prevention of other diseases.

Remember, iodine deficiency in the thyroid gland leads to the development of cysts, nodules, scar tissue, and enlargement, and we call that goiter. And we have known for many years that people who have goiter are at increased risk of developing thyroid cancer, breast cancer, stomach cancer, esophageal cancer, ovarian cancer, and endometrial cancer. Similarly, a lack of iodine in the breast tissue leads to the development of cysts, nodules, scar tissue, and enlargement, and we call that fibrocystic breast disease. Recent research has shown that women with fibrocystic breast disease have a higher incidence of breast cancer. So, we go from normal breast to fibrocystic breast disease to breast cancer. Why? Simply, a lack of iodine in the breast tissue. The ovaries have the second highest ability to concentrate iodine in the body. If you have a lack of iodine in the ovaries, you get what? You get cysts, nodules, scar tissue, and enlargement of the ovaries, and we call it polycystic ovary syndrome (PCOS).

By the time women with PCOS get into their 40s and 50s they have a higher rate of ovarian cancer. Can you see what is going on? There is a clear link between iodine deficiency and increased risk of cancer.

REFERENCES

1. Abraham GE, Flechas JD, Hakala JC. Optimum Levels of Iodine for Greatest Mental and Physical Health. *The Original Internist.* 2002; 9:5-20.

2. Abraham GE, Flechas JD, Hakala JC. Orthoiodosupplementation: Iodine sufficiency of the whole human body. *The Original Internist.* 2002;9:30-41.

3. Abraham GE. Serum Inorganic Iodide levels following ingestion of a tablet form of Lugol solution: Evidence for an Enterohepatic Circulation of Iodine. *The Original Internist.* 2004;11(3):29-34.

4. Abraham GE. The Effect of Ingestion of Inorganic, NonRadioacive Iodine/Iodide in Patients with Simple Goiter and in Graves' Disease: A Review of Published Studies Compared with Current Trends. *The Original Internist.* 2004;11(1):17-36.

5. Abraham GE. The Concept of Orthoiodosupplementation and Its Clinical Implications. *The Original Internist.* 2004;11(2):29-38.

6. Abraham GE, Brownstein D. Evidence That the Administration of Vitamin C Improves a Defective Cellular Transport Mechanism for Iodine: A Case Report. *The Original Internist.* 2005;12(3):125-130.

7. Abraham GE. The Wolff-Chaikoff Effect: Crying Wolf? *The Original Internist.* 2005;12(3):112-118.

8. Abraham GE, Brownstein D. Validation of the Orthoiodosupplementation Program: A Rebuttal of Dr. Gaby's Editorial on Iodine. *The Original Internist.* 2005;12(4):184-196.

9. Abraham GE, Brownstein D, Flechas JD. The Saliva/Serum Iodide Ratio as an Index of Sodium Iodide Symporter Efficiency. *The Original Internist.* 2005; 12(4):152-156.

10. Abraham G. Iodine Supplementation Markedly Increases Urinary Excretion of Fluoride and Bromine. Townsend Letter for Doctors and Patients 2000.

11. Abraham G. The Historical Background of the Iodine Project. *The Original Internist.* 2005;12(2):57-66.

12. Cann SA, van Netten JP, van Netten C. Hypothesis: Iodine, selenium and the development of breast cancer. *Cancer Causes and Control.* 2000;11:121-127.

13. Eskin BA. Iodine Metabolism and Breast Cancer. *Trans New York Acad of Sciences.* 1970;32:911-947.

14. Eskin BA. Iodine and Mammary Cancer. *Adv Exp Med Biol.* 1977;91:293-304.

15. Eskin BA. Dynamic Effects of Iodine Therapy on Breast Cancer and the Thyroid. *Proc Int Thyroid Symposium.* 1996;6:192-197.

16. Foster HD. The Iodine-Selenium connection: Its Possible Roles in Intelligence, Cretinism, Sudden Infant Death Syndrome, Breast Cancer and Multiple Sclerosis. *Medical Hypotheses.* 1993;40:61-65.

17. Kilbane MT, Ajjan RA, Weetman AP, Dwyer R, McDermott EWM, O'Higgins NJ et al. Tissue iodine content and serum-mediated I-uptake blocking activity in breast cancer. *Journal of Clinical Endocrinology & Metabolism.* 2000;85(3):1245-1250.

18. Stadel BV. Dietary Iodine and Risk of Breast, Endometrial, and Ovarian Cancer. *Lancet.* 1976;1:890-891.

19. Talamini R, Franceschi S, Favero A, *et al.* Selected medical conditions and risk of breast cancer. *British Journal of Cancer.* 1997; 75(11):1699-1703.

20. Venturi S, Donati FM, Venturi M, *et al.* Role of Iodine in Evolution and Carcinogenesis of Thyroid, Breast, and Stomach. *Adv Clin Path.* 2000;4:11-17.

21. Wiseman RA. Breast cancer hypothesis: a single cause for the majority of cases. *J Epiderniol Community Health.* 2000;54:851-858.

22. Aceves C, Anguiano B, Delgado G. Is Iodine a gatekeeper of the integrity of the mammary gland? *Journal of Mammary Gland Biology and Neoplasia.* 2005;10:189-196.

23. Garcia-Solis P, Alfaro Y, Anguiano B, Delgado G, Guzman RC, Nandi S, Diaz-Munoz M, Vazquez-Martinez O, Aceves C. Inhibition of N-methyl-N-nitrosourea-induced mammary carcinogenesis by molecular iodine (I2) but not by iodide (I-) treatment Evidence that I2 prevents cancer promotion. *Mol Cell Endocrinol.* 2005;236:49-57.

ABOUT THE AUTHOR

Dr. Jorge Flechas is the medical director of Flechas Family Practice in Hendersonville, NC, specializing in hormonal therapy for the treatment of fibromyalgia and chronic fatigue and immune dysfunction syndrome (CFIDS). He also specializes in iodine therapy for hypothyroidism and fibrocystic breast disease. He is on the family practice staff of Park Ridge Hospital in Fletcher, NC, and is a member of the American College of Nutrition. Four years ago, Dr. Flechas learned the technique to measure urine iodide levels and the iodine/iodide loading test at Dr. Abraham's Laboratory. He has since performed over 20,000 tests.

Chapter 13
Mesotherapy in Sports Medicine
Janine Gaston Nhan, MD, DIU Mesotherapy
President, 2FAME (French Functional Aromatherapy Anti-Aging Mesotherapy Medicine)

ABSTRACT

Mesotherapy is an efficient medical technique for pain control and energy production for athletes. Almost all French soccer clubs have a mesotherapist physician to treat their members, and all French athletes are treated with mesotherapy. This is because mesotherapy treats inflammation, controls pain, and aids recovery, thus providing fast and efficient pain relief with low doses of injected drugs and few side effects.

In order to protect tissue integrity and to guarantee cellular energy production and mitochondrial function we have developed a specific glutathione protocol for use in sports mesotherapy. Intake of nutritional supplements by athletes does not mean that their tissues get optimal levels of these nutrients. Mesotherapy enables optimal levels of these nutrients to be delivered to the tissues where they are needed. Our protocols in mesotherapy do not include drugs which are on the International Olympic Committee (IOC) doping list.

Keywords: mesotherapy, pain control, intradermal, glutathione, overtraining

INTRODUCTION

Dr Michel Pistor invented mesotherapy in 1952, and in 1987 mesotherapy was recognized by the French Academy of Medicine as a specialty of medicine. Domains in which mesotherapy has expanded most successfully are pain management, sports medicine, and aesthetic medicine. The technique of mesotherapy is held in high regard in France. All French athletes are treated with mesotherapy, and all French sports teams, from the French Olympic Team to local swimming, skiing, and handball teams have a mesotherapist physician to care for them. In France, all soccer and rugby clubs require their doctors in charge to be qualified in mesotherapy. The INSEP (National Institute for Sports France) has a mesotherapy department, and all rehabilitation centers and hospital pain units have a mesotherapy clinic. Many French medical universities offer postgraduate degrees in Sports Medicine and Mesotherapy.

A French national epidemiology investigation conducted in 2006 revealed that mesotherapy comprises 19-20% of the total treatments used to treat all kinds of sports injuries. Mesotherapy enables athletes to return to training earlier as it speeds healing and recovery from injury. It also removes the need for athletes to take oral drugs and have corticoid injections. Mesotherapy can be completed with physiotherapy and osteopathy.

Mesotherapy is used in sports medicine for pathologies of muscle (elongation, cramps), tendon (tendonitis of calcaneum, patella, and ankle, knee, shoulder, wrist, and finger sprains), bone (osteochondroses of Osgood-Schlatter, Sever's disease, and Sinding-Larsen-Johansson syndrome), the periosteum (periostitis), and joints. Mesotherapy is particularly useful in the treatment of young athletes and women athletes presenting with osteochondrosis, periostitis, and fatigue fracture. It is also used to treat back pain.

In addition to pain control, the intradermal use of glutathione and other nutrients can help to protect tissue integrity and to guarantee cellular energy production and mitochondrial function, promote healing, control oxidative stress, and aid recovery in overtrained athletes.

MESOTHERAPY

Mesotherapy is a medical intradermal injection technique. It delivers the required nutrients and medications, at reduced doses, direct to the site of injury. Mesotherapy is a therapeutic concept that aims to improve the efficacy of treatment by delivering treatment closer to the site of injury via the intradermal and subcutaneous pathways. Mesotherapy is very useful in sports medicine as injuries are typically peripheral and therefore accessible with short (4 mm) needles.

Oral intake of nutritional supplements by athletes does not mean that their tissues get optimal levels of these nutrients. Mesotherapy enables optimal levels of these nutrients to be delivered to the tissues where they are needed, and is an alternative to corticoid injections for treatment of injuries.

Before carrying out any mesotherapy treatments the mesotherapist will also conduct a through clinical exam. Determining the primary cause of injury is vital as treatment of obvious, but secondary causes, could alleviate but not cure the problem. It is important to remember that the primary cause of injury could be extrinsic (lack of physical fitness, lack of hydration, gait problems, drug intake) or intrinsic (disc and joint disorders).

In Good Practice Mesotherapy (GPM), there is no use of corticoids due to the risk of necrosis associated with their use. Mesotherapy is not associated with any adverse drug reactions or morbidity and mortality when it is administered by a properly trained mesotherapist. Mesotherapy should not be performed within the 24 hours prior to an event. All drugs used in academic mesotherapy are not on the International Olympic Committee (IOC) doping list. The mesotherapist should provide the athlete with a certificate detailing all the injected drugs and their dosages.

Mesotherapy Techniques
Depth of Injection
It is important never to use more than three products in the same syringe. If necessary, use two or more syringes.

- Intra-EpiDermis (IED): 1 mm depth: 30G ½ 13 mm needle: 2/3 liquid loss no pain, no haematoma.
- Intra-Dermal Superficial (IDS): 2 mm depth: 30G ½ 13 mm needle: 2/3 liquid loss no pain, no haematoma.
- Intra-Dermal Profound (IDP): 4 mm depth: 0.3 to 0.5 ml/point injection with a 30G ½ 4mm or 6 mm needle: occasional pain, haematoma, flush, allergy.
- Dermal-Hypo Dermal (DHD):10 mm depth: 0.5 to 1 ml/point injection with a 30G ½ 13 mm needle: minor pain, no haematoma, point by point
- Intra-Dermal Profound (IDP): 4 mm depth: 30G ½ 4 mm or 6 mm needle: 0.3-0.5 ml/point injection: frequent pain, risk of haematoma (rarely), flush, and allergy (rarely)
- Dermal-Hypo Dermal (DHD): 10 mm depth: 30G ½ 13 mm needle: 0.5 to 1 ml liquid volume injection per point: possible minor pain, no haematoma; point by point.

All preparations must be EXTEMPORANEOUS
All injectable solutions should be HYDROSOLUBLE

Specific Pharmacokinetics of the Intradermal Pathway
The deeper the injection is, the faster, the stronger, and the shorter the pharmacological effect is. The more superficial the injection is, the slower, the weaker, and the longer the pharmacological effect is. IED and IDS have slower, weaker, and longer pharmacological effects than IDP, which has a slower, weaker, and longer pharmacological effect than DHD. An injection in DHD has a fast, intense, and short pharmacological effect compared to IED, IDS, and IDP. It is important to be aware that you can mix techniques simultaneously: superficial and deep for fast, efficient, and long-acting relief. Mesotherapy suppresses the first hepatic and renal passages, therefore the drugs are more available and more efficient and their metabolism is better tolerated.

Frequency of Treatment
Sessions should be once weekly, for example day 1, day 8, and day15. After the third session it is important to re-evaluate the patient. If the patient has made a good improvement they should receive a fourth session on day 30, however if they have only made a moderate improvement the fourth session should take place on day 20.

For the treatment of acute pain, patients should be treated on day 1 and day 3. If the injury is very new the patient will probably require 1-2 sessions, however if the injury is 2-3 weeks old they will require at least 3 sessions at weekly intervals (day 1, day 8, and day 15) and evaluation at day 30.

Drugs and Combination of Drugs Used in Mesotherapy

Local anaesthetics

- Lidocaine without paraben (WP): 25 mg/5 ml or 5 mg/5 ml vial. Mesotherapy indication: vasodilatation & membrane permeability modulator; when suspicion of allergy to procaine exists. Compatible with nearly all mesotherapy products. Local injection of lidocaine is authorized by the Sports Ministry and the IOC.
- Procaine: 100 mg/5 ml vial. Mesotherapy indication: vasodilatation. Contraindications: epilepsy, allergy to procaine, pregnancy. Undesirable effects: allergy, cardiovascular collapses.

NSAID (Non steroidal anti-inflammatory drugs)

- Piroxicam injectable: 20 mg/2 ml vial. Mesotherapy indication: inflammatory rheumatism, tendonitis, ligamentitis, sprains, osteoarthritis. Contraindications: allergy, gastric ulcer, kidney liver insufficiencies, disorders of hemostasis, use of blood thinners, children under 15, pregnant women over 6 months. Mesotherapy technique: **IED, IDP, DHD** point by point. Never in papules, on injection 1-3 mm deep. Diluted with lidocaine 5ml.
- Calcitonin (Hemi-Synthetic Salmon Calcitonin): 50 UI (for small areas, e.g., fingers and toes) or 100 UI (for larger areas). Mesotherapy indication: powerful analgesic for the treatment of nociceptive and neuropathic pain, vasomotor properties, anti-oedema, vascular modulator. Contraindication: allergy to calcitonin. Mesotherapy technique: **IED IDS IDP DHD**. Undesirable effects: nausea, flush, pruritus. The undesirable effects associated with are particularly reduced in mesotherapy, especially by **IDS** or **IED**. If necessary add an antihistamine. Salmon calcitonin is more potent than human calcitonin.

Muscle Relaxant

- Thiocolchicoside: 4 mg/2 ml vial. Mesotherapy indication: all painful muscular contractions, smooth muscle relaxant. Mesotherapy technique: IED, IDS, IDP, DHD. To be diluted with 5ml lidocaine.

Calcium Chelator

- EDTA

Vasodilators

- Buflomedil: 50 mg/5 ml vial. Mesotherapy indication: powerful vasodilator. Mesotherapy technique: **IED, IDS, IDP, DHD,** coating, point by point. Buflomedil is a phosphodiesterase enzyme inhibitor which directly stimulates cyclic AMP and acts as a biological vasodilator by blocking calcium channels in the vascular smooth muscles. It does not block adrenergic fibers nor does it have any systemic hemodynamic action.
- Pentoxyfilline: 100 mg/5 ml vial. Mesotherapy indication: antioxidant, immunomodulator, and peripheral vasodilator.
- Etamsylate: 250 mg/2 ml vial. Mesotherapy indication: local oedemas, vein toner. Mesotherapy technique: **IED, IDS, IDP, DHD**. Cutaneous allergy (sulfite).

Neurology Products

- Benzodiazepine (Clonazepam) is a muscle relaxant, anticonvulsant, and minor tranquilizer. It is an agonist of some specific GABA receptors.
- Amitriptyline: 50 mg/2 ml vial. Mesotherapy indication: fibromyalgia, muscle pain. Mesotherapy technique: **IED, IDS** only, no more than 0.5 ml to be diluted in 5 ml lidocaine.

Nutrients, Vitamins, and Minerals

- Polyvitamins: 2 ml vial. Mesotherapy indication: antioxidants. Contraindication: allergy to some of the components (vitamin B1), hypercalcemia, calcium stone, pregnant women. Mesotherapy technique: **IED, IDS, IDP,DHD**.
- Retinol: antioxidant and membrane messenger prohormone.
- Cholecalciferol: a bone and immunity modulator prohormone.
- Tocopherol: antioxidant.
- Thiamine: involved in glucose and energy metabolism.

- Riboflavin: glutathione recycling and mitochondrial function.
- Nicotinamide or niacin: fat metabolizer.
- Pantothenic acid: coenzyme A converter and hormone production.
- Piridoxin: amino acid, fatty acid, and neurotransmitter metabolism.
- Biotin: cocarboxylase and glucose metabolism.
- Folic acid: DNA methylation and homocysteine metabolism.
- Cyanocobalamin: nucleic acid metabolism and nerve function.
- PABA: protein metabolism and a metabolite of procaine.
- Ascorbic acid: antioxidant and collagen synthesis.
- Magnesium pidolate: 1 g/10 ml vial. Mesotherapy indication: Anti-spasm, anti-stress Mesotherapy technique: **IED, IDS, IDP, DHD**.
- Zinc gluconate: nucleic acid synthesis and neurosensory activity.
- Selenium sodium: antioxidant.

Biological compounds
- Glutathione: the most important antioxidant.
- N-acetyl cysteine: promotes endogenous glutathione synthesis.
- Ambroxol: 15 mg/2 ml vial. Antioxidant for NOS, boosts endogenous glutathione synthesis.
- Non cross-linked hyaluronic acid
- Co-enzyme Q10
- Lipoic acid
- Amino acids (carnitine, taurine...)
- Placenta extracts
- Growth factors

Injectable homeopathic drugs
- Arnica, equisetum arvense.

Materials
Single Use
- Antiseptic: chlorhexidine spray
- Compresses (Gauze) 10 X 10 cm
- Gloves
- Syringes: Luer cone excentered 10 ml
    Insulin injection 1 ml
- Needles: Pink 18 G X 1½ X 1.2 mm X 40 mm
    Yellow 30G X ½: X 0.3 mm X 13 mm
    Yellow 30 G X 0, 30 mm X 4 mm
- Mesorollers 0.2/0.3 mm

Guns

Guns are useful for large areas for fast work, but they are not mandatory. The best are those with an integrated compressor, so as to maintain a regular pressure, however they are not mandatory. Mesotherapy guns are usually made in France; however some are made in Korea.

Mesotherapy – The Golden Rules
How to Do It: The Choice of Products

For the first session, choose the product related to the signal symptom (for example, pain); use only one syringe, and only one chemical. At the second session choose the products related to the pathology and the physiopathogenesis (for example, osteoarthritis). You have to choose biological compounds either for nutritional purposes (vitamins, minerals, and etc.), for biological process (glutathione, etc.), or for hormonal action (calcitonin, etc.). You may choose a synthetic drug (chemical) for example, piroxicam.

For chemicals (local anaesthetic included) it is best to use one syringe. Two is OK, but you must not use three. For biological compounds you may use two or three syringes – it is fine to combine up to three nutritional substances in the same syringe, however only one or two nutrients can be mixed with one chemical only.

It is important to be aware that glutathione should not be injected with any other nutrients or chemical to avoid oxidation, with the exception of lidocaine or procaine, in order to relieve the injection pain.

For subsequent session, products related to the patient's chronic "milieu" (stressed patients, old patients, chronic inflammatory diseases and etc.) should be used.

How to Do It: The Choice of Techniques
- For a fast, immediate and intense action, choose a 10 mm depth injection (DHD).
- For a slow release and a long lasting effect, choose a 4 mm depth injection (IDP). However, this depth of injection carries a greater risk of an arteriole breaking and its consequences (allergy, haematoma, flushes, and etc.).
- For a very slow release and a very long lasting effect, choose a 1 mm depth injection (IDS or coating). However, you will loose two-thirds of the product.
- Techniques can be mixed simultaneously, for example, superficial and deep for fast, efficient, and long acting relief.

How to Do It: Where to Inject
- On painful points
- The Power Zones – The basis for the Power Zones is to be found in Traditional Chinese Medicine. Acupuncture and Energy Channels, these key areas on the body map are primary zones to enter the body circuits in order to penetrate the web of interconnectedness. The goal is to improve energy flow and blood flow_through endothelial function, and to achieve optimal function and organ reserve.

MESOTHERAPY IN PAIN MANAGEMENT
The majority of acute sports injuries are treated by surgery, however pain, oedema, and inflammation will benefit from Mesotherapy. Mesotherapy is very useful in the management of acute, rebel, and chronic forms of pain, as it can deliver an optimal concentration of the products to the site of injury. This method avoids systemic side effects and removes the need for the athlete to take oral NSAIDs, pain killers, and injectable corticoids. Mesotherapy can be used to treat inflammation, to control pain, to aid recovery, to protect tissue integrity, and to guarantee cellular energy production and mitochondrial function.

The pathological structures to be treated include: bursa, synovium, cartilage, tendon, ligaments, muscles, bones, and the vascular system. Before treating the athlete a number of factors have to be taken into consideration, including: the age of the athlete, the age of the injury, the quality of the skin and the muscle contraction, the pain as expressed by the patient, specific tender and trigger points and areas of radiation identified by the physician, the mechanical disruption responsible for the ailment, the type of inflammation present – acute, subacute, or chronic, and the pathology behind the injury – mechanical, sports, degenerative, or wear and tear.

Choice of Drugs
The choice of drugs used is dependent upon the type of pain:
- Nociceptive moderate pain: arnica 4 DH.
- Nociceptive pain with tense muscles: thiocolchicoside and/or calcitonin 100 UI.
- Strong, nociceptive pain: calcitonin 100 UI, piroxicam

The stage of the injury:
- Acute inflammation: piroxicam.
- Subacute inflammation with tense muscle: thiocolchicoside +/- magnesium pidolate.
- Degenerative pathology: procaine 2% + pentoxifilline +/- calcitonin 100 UI.
- Anti-oedema: etamsylate.

Protocol I for Acute Pain:
- lidocaine WP   1% 2 ml
- piroxicam   1 ml
- calcitonin   100 UI 1 ml

Protocol II for Acute Pain and Muscle Soreness:
- lidocaine WP   1% 2 ml
- piroxicam   1 ml
- thiocolchicoside   1 ml

Protocol III for Chronic Pain:
- lidocaine WP   1% 2 ml
- or procaine   2 ml
- calcitonin   100 UI 1 ml
- pentoxyfilline   2 ml

Choice of Depth of Injections

Depends upon the site of the pain :
- Small joints (fingers, toes): **IED, IDS** (coating).
- Major joints (shoulders, knees):**IED, IDS, IDP, DHD.**
- Spine, neck, lumbar: **IED, IDS, IDP,DHD**

TISSUES AND PATHOLOGY-ORIENTED MESOTHERAPY

- Muscles: cramps
- Ligaments and tendons: tendonitis
- Carpal tunnel syndrome
- Joints: osteoarthritis
- Bones: trauma

Muscles

- Cramps, aching, no lesion: lidocaine without paraben 1% 2 ml, thiocolchicoside 3 ml: (**IED, IDS, IDP, DHD**) 0.1ml-0.5ml /Pt.
- Torn muscle lesion: D 1-10: thiocolchicoside 3 ml, etamsylate 2 ml, or lidocaine without paraben 1% 2 ml, thiocolchicoside 3 ml: (**IED, IDS, IDP, DHD**) 0.1ml-0.5ml /Pt.

Tendons

- On nodes: piroxicam 1 ml, etamsylate 1 ml, pentoxyfilline 1 ml.
- On tendons insertion; piroxicam 1 ml, etamsylate 1 ml, calcitonin 100 IU 1 ml.
- On muscle and junction muscle –tendon: thiocolchicoside 1 ml, pentoxyfilline 1 ml.
- Tenosynovitis:
  - exsudation phase: lidocaine without paraben 1% 2 ml, piroxicam 1 ml, etamsylate 1 ml.
  - crepitus phase; lidocaine without paraben 1% 2 ml, piroxicam 1 ml, calcitonin 100 IU 1 ml.
  - constriction phase: procaine 2% 1 ml, pentoxifylline 1 ml.
- D 10-21: piroxicam 1 ml, pentoxyfilline 2 ml.
- D 21-45: procaine 2% 1 ml, pentoxifylline 3 ml, Multiple Vit 1 ml

All **IED, IDS, IDP, DHD** 0.1ml-0.5ml /Pt.

SPORTS PATHOLOGIES

The most common site of injury in sport is the lower limb and knee (24%), followed by the ankle (15%), spine (14%), and thigh (9%). The following is a list of sports and injuries and pathologies associated with that sport.

- Rowing: spine disorders, tendonitis.
- Basketball: ankle, finger, and wrist sprains.
- Boxing: head trauma – eye, retina, and brain, and neurodegenerative disorders.
- Cycling: iliotibial band syndrome, saddle pathologies.
- Football: ankle sprain, knee meniscitis, athletic pubalgia.
- Golf: golf elbow.
- Gym: risk of fall.
- Handball: sprains.
- Judo and Sumo: risk of fall.
- Throwing: tendonitis of the shoulder.
- Rugby: fractures
- Jumping: tendonitis
- Ski: risk of fall, knee sprain.
- Ice sports: fatigue fractures.
- Tennis: tennis elbow, tennis leg, peroneal artery occlusion syndrome.

CLINICAL APPLICATIONS OF MESOTHERAPY

Neck Pain & Post Traumatic Cervical Syndrome

Sports associated with: shooting, American football, boxing, jumping, hurdling,
Occupations associated with: racing drivers, mechanics, and plumbers.
Mechanical disorders of superficial structures of the disks – cervical, dorsal, lumbar.
Degenerative

Protocol for Neck Pain
Protocol I for Acute Pain on Ligaments and Tendons:
- lidocaine WP   1% 2 ml
- piroxicam   1 ml
- calcitonin   100 UI 1 ml
- **(IDP DHD)** 0.1ml-0.5ml /Pt

Protocol II for Neck Pain with Spasmodic Torticollis:
- lidocaine WP   1% 2 ml
- thiocolchicoside   2 ml
- magnesium pidolate   2 ml
- **(IED, IDS, IDP, DHD)** 0.1ml-0.5ml /Pt

Protocol III for Chronic Pain and Osteoarthritis:
- lidocaine WP   1% 2 ml
- piroxicam   1 ml
- calcitonin   100 UI 1 ml
- **(IED, IDS, IDP, DHD)** 0.1ml-0.5ml /Pt

Protocol for Dorsolumbar Pathologies

Sheuerman epiphysitis, spondilolysis, and spondylolysthesis are associated with sports that involve rotation (tennis, throwing, rowing) and sports with risk of fall (gymnastics, judo, parachuting, weightlifting, jumping).

Back Pain
Protocol for Moderate Pain:
- lidocaine WP   1% 2 ml
- thiocolchicoside   2 ml
- piroxicam   1 ml
- **(IED, IDS, IDP, DHD)** 0.1ml-0.5ml /Pt.

Protocol for Intense Pain:
- lidocaine WP   1% 2 ml
- calcitonin   100 IU 1 ml
- **(IED, IDS, IDP, DHD)** 0.1ml-0.5ml /Pt

Protocol for Neurogenic Pain:
- Injectable water   2 ml
- lidocaine WP   1% 3 ml
- calcitonin   100IU 1 ml
- Only **IED**

Protocol for Mixed Pain:
- lidocaine WP   1% 2 ml
- piroxicam   1 ml
- calcitonin   100 IU 1 ml
- **(IED, IDS, IDP, DHD)** 0.1ml-0.5ml /Pt

Protocols for the Upper Limb – Shoulder

Pathologies of the shoulder, the elbow, the wrist, the hand, and the fingers, can occur as a result of all sports that involve arming, throwing, and lifting. The shoulder is particularly vulnerable. Subacromial conflict and rotator cuff rupture are associated with sports that involve arming, throwing, lifting. For example: tennis, badminton, table tennis, javelin, hand ball, volley ball, baseball. Certain swimming styles (crawl and butterfly stroke) can also cause shoulder pathologies. Secretaries, gardeners, and mechanics are also prone to shoulder pathologies.

Protocol for Tendonitis of Long Biceps:
- lidocaine WP   1% 2 ml
- piroxicam   1 ml
- etamsylate   1 ml

or:
- lidocaine WP   1% 2 ml
- thiocolchicoside   3 ml
- **(IED, IDS, IDP, DHD)** 0.1ml-0.5ml /Pt and on irradiations

Protocol for Subacromial Conflicts:
On tendon insertion:
- lidocaine WP   1% 2 ml
- piroxicam   1 ml
- etamsylate   1 ml
- **(IED, IDS, IDP, DHD)** 0.1ml-0.5ml /Pt and on irradiations.

On ligament:
- lidocaine WP   1% 2 ml
- piroxicam   1 ml
- etamsylate   2ml
- **(IED, IDS, IDP, DHD)** 0.1ml-0.5ml /Pt and on irradiations.

On muscle:
- lidocaine WP   1% 2 ml
- thiocolchicoside   3 ml
- **(IED, IDS, IDP, DHD)** 0.1ml-0.5ml /Pt and on irradiations

Protocol for Calcification-Related Shoulder Pain:
- Syringe 1:xylocaine   2% 1 ml
- Syringe 2:EDTA   0.5 ml
- **DHD** 0.5ml /Pt

Protocols for the Upper Limb – Elbow

Tennis elbow (epicondylitis) is the most common problem seen with the elbow. Epitrochleitis is associated with golf.

Protocol for Epicondylitis and Epitrochleitis:
On tendon insertion:
- lidocaine WP   1% 2 ml
- piroxicam   1 ml
- calcitonin   100IU 1 ml
- **(IED, IDS, IDP, DHD)** 0.1ml-0.5ml /Pt on painful points

On muscle:
- lidocaine WP   1% 2 ml
- thiocolchicoside   3 ml
- etamsylate   2 ml
- **(IED, IDS, IDP, DHD)** 0.1ml-0.5ml /Pt and on irradiations on D 1,7,15,30.

Protocols for the Upper Limb – Wrist

Skiing and volley ball are associated with pathologies of the wrist. Secretaries are particularly are risk of wrist pathologies. Common problems with the wrist include: tendonitis, tenosynovitis stenosus, sprain of the ligaments of the wrist, and carpal tunnel syndrome.

Protocol for Carpal Tunnel Syndrome:
- lidocaine WP   1% 4 ml
- piroxicam   1 ml
- calcitonin   100IU 1 ml
- Pinch the skin, 3 points
- **IDP DHD** 0.1ml /Pt on painful points
- **IED** on palmar site of wrist and fingers

Protocol for Tenosynovitis:
Acute stage:
- lidocaine WP   1% 2 ml
- piroxicam   1 ml
- calcitonin   100IU 1 ml
- 0.1 ml /Pt **IDP & IED**

Chronic stage:
- procaine   2% 1 ml
- pentoxyfilline   1 ml
- multiple Vit   1 ml
- 0.1 ml /Pt **IDP & IED**

Protocols for the Upper Limb – Hands and Fingers

Common pathologies of the hands and fingers include: ligamentitis: sprains, micro trauma, arthropathies.

Protocol for Osteoarthritis of the Fingers:
- procaine   2% 1 ml
- pentoxyfilline   1 ml
- multiple Vit   1 ml
- 0.1 ml /Pt **IDP**

Protocol for Dupuytren's disease:
Specific technique on fibrous nodes:
- lidocaine   WP 1% 4 ml
- thiocolchicoside   1 ml
- calcitonin   100 UI 1ml
- Injection in the node **IDP**

Pathologies of the Lower Limb – Hip

Joggers, dancers, soccer players, and cyclists are particularly at risk of hip pathologies. Common pathologies include: adductors medial side – pubalgia, injuries of muscles (quadriceps, sartorius, gluteus medius, tensor facia lata, rectus femoris), ligamentitis of the iliofemoral and ischiofemoral sacrotuberous ligaments, tendonitis of the biceps femoris, and arthritis of the hip.

Protocol for Soccer Players Pubalgia:
6 mm needle, perpendicular
On painful tendons opposite and facing the pubic symphysis
Acute phase:
On tendon insertion:
- lidocaine WP   1% 2 ml
- piroxicam   1 ml
- calcitonin   100 IU 1 ml
- **(IED, IDS, IDP, DHD)** 0.1ml-0.5ml /Pt

On muscles:
- lidocaine WP   1% 2 ml
- thiocolchicoside   1 ml
- calcitonin   100 UI 1 ml
- **(IED, IDS, IDP, DHD)** 0.1ml-0.5ml /Pt

Chronic phase:
On tendons insertions:
- calcitonin   100IU 1 ml
- pentoxifylline   2 ml
- multiple Vit   2 ml
- **(IED, IDS, IDP, DHD)** 0.1ml-0.5ml /Pt

On muscles:
- procaine   2% 1 ml
- pentoxyfilline   1 ml
- thiocolchicoside   2 ml
- **(IED, IDS, IDP, DHD)** 0.1ml-0.5ml /Pt
- Sessions 1/week until no pain and negative clinical tests

Pathologies of the Lower Limb – Knee

Football, skiing, high jump, long jump, somersault, hurdling, racing, and parachuting are sports that are associated with a high risk of knee injury. Common pathologies include: tendonitis and myalgia of the quadriceps, gracilis, semitendonosus, and sartorius tendons, and ligamentitis of the medial tibial collateral ligament and patella ligament.

Protocol for Acute Pain on Ligaments and Tendons:
- lidocaine WP   1% 2 ml
- piroxicam   1 ml
- calcitonin   100IU 2 ml
- **(IED, IDS, IDP, DHD)** 0.1ml-0.5ml /Pt

Protocol for Patella Chondropathy, Plica, and Popliteal Cyst:
- lidocaine WP   1% 2 ml
- piroxicam   1 ml
- calcitonin   100IU 2 ml
- **(IED, IDS, IDP, DHD)** 0.1ml-0.5ml /Pt

Protocol for Patella Tendonitis:
D1-D1-D14:
- lidocaine WP   1% 2 ml
- thiocolchicoside   3 ml
- etamsylate   2 ml
- **(IED, IDS, IDP, DHD)** 0.1ml-0.5ml /Pt and on irradiations
D 30:
- procaine   2% 1 ml
- buflomedil   1ml
- calcitonin   100IU 2 ml
- **(IED, IDS, IDP, DHD)** 0.1ml-0.5ml /Pt

Protocol for Tensor Fascia Lata Syndrome and Lateral Ligaments Sprains:
- lidocaine WP   1% 2 ml
- piroxicam   1 ml
- etamsylate   2 ml
- **(IED, IDS, IDP, DHD)** 0.1ml-0.5ml /Pt and on irradiations

Protocol for Anterior Tibial Compartment Syndrome:
Note: Mesotherapy should be tried before surgery.
- procaine   2% 1 ml
- etamsylate   2 ml
- multiple Vit   3 ml
- **(IED, IDS, IDP, DHD)** 0.1ml-0.5ml /Pt

Pathologies of the Lower Limb – Ankle and Foot

Skiing, tennis, jogging, dancing, basket ball, and soccer are all high risk sports for ankle and foot pathologies. The most common problem is ligamentitis (tibialis posterior anterior, posterior flexor digitorum longus, fibularis longus, front extensors of the foot, and back calcaneal tendon).

Protocol for the Treatment of Sprains:
On the injured tendon:
Phase I – within 3 days:
- lidocaine WP   1% 2 ml
- piroxicam   1 ml
- arnica   5 CH 1 ml
- **(IED, IDS, IDP, DHD)** 0.1ml-0.5ml /Pt and on irradiations
Phase II – 7 till 14 days:
- lidocaine WP   1% 2 ml
- piroxicam   1 ml
- etamsylate   2 ml
- **(IED, IDS, IDP, DHD)** 0.1ml-0.5ml /Pt and on irradiations

Phase III – 2 to 3 weeks:
- lidocaine WP   1% 2 ml
- etamsylate   2 ml
- (**IED, IDS, IDP, DHD**) 0.1ml-0.5ml /Pt and on irradiations

There are numerous other painful conditions where mesotherapy is more effective than conventional medicine, for example: calcaneum spur.

Protocol for Calcaneum Spur or Plantar Aponeurositis:
1° Double disinfection
2° Liquid Nitrogen or menthol spray
3° Combination of drugs in 10 ml syringe
- lidocaine WP   1% 2 ml
- piroxicam   20 mg/1 ml 1 ml
- salmon calcitonin   100 U.I./1 ml 1 ml
4° **DHD** on three to five main painful points
5° The use of the gun is especially recommended for a fast pain-free procedure
6° Up to three sessions at one week interval

Protocol for Periostitis:
(In young athletes periostitis commonly affects the tibia).
- lidocaine WP   1% 2 ml
- etamsylate   2 ml
- calcitonin   100 UI 1 ml
- (**IED, IDS, IDP, DHD**) 0.1ml-0.5ml /Pt and on irradiations. Mostly located about the tibial, fibula, and cubital crests.

Miscellaneous

Protocol for the Treatment of Fatigue Fractures:
Mesotherapy is to be performed after rest and discharge. The purpose of mesotherapy in the treatment of fatigue fractures is to ensure a good quality of the callus.
- pentoxyfilline   3 ml
- calcitonin   100 UI 1 ml
- equisetum arvens   4 DH 2 ml
- or organic silicium   2 ml
- (**IED, IDS, IDP, DHD**) 0.1ml-0.5ml /Pt and on irradiations

Mostly lower limbs (95%): **IDP DHD** facing the fracture area

Protocol for the Treatment of Osteochondrosis:
Mostly seen in young athletes.
Epiphysis (vascular defect).
Apophysis (mechanical stress about the growth cartilage and traction excess of insertions tendons): tibial tuberosity (Osgood-Schlater disease), calcaneum (Sever's disease), patella (Sinding-Larsen-Johansson syndrome).

Acute stage: D1 to D8:
- lidocaine WP   1% 2 ml
- piroxicam   1 ml
- etamsylate   2 ml

or:
- arnica 4 DH 1 ml
- B complex 1 ml
- (**IED, IDS, IDP, DHD**) 0.1ml-0.5ml /Pt and on irradiations

Facing the growth cartilage:
- lidocaine WP   1% 2 ml
- etamsylate   2 ml
- calcitonin   100 UI 1 ml
- **(IED, IDS, IDP, DHD)** 0.1ml-0.5ml /Pt and on irradiations

Around the growth cartilage:
- lidocaine WP   1% 2 ml
- pentoxyfilline   2 ml
- **IED**

Chronic stage: D 15-30:
- lidocaine WP   1% 2 ml
- calcitonin   100 UI 1 ml
- silicium   1 ml
- 0.1 ml/Pt **IDP**

Chronic stage: D 31:
- lidocaine WP   1% 2 ml
- multiple Vit   2 ml
- Mg   2 ml
- 0.1 ml/Pt **IDP IED**

Protocol for Scheuermann Disease:
On vertebrae:
- lidocaine WP   1% 2 ml
- calcitonin   100 UI 1 ml
- multiple Vit   1 ml
- **(IED, IDS, IDP, DHD)** 0.1ml-0.5ml /Pt and on irradiations

On muscles:
- lidocaine WP   1% 2 ml
- thiocolchicoside   3 ml
- etamsylate   2 ml
- **(IED, IDS, IDP, DHD)** 0.1ml-0.5ml /Pt and on irradiations

Protocol for Bursitis:
- lidocaine WP   1% 2 ml
- piroxicam   1 ml
- calcitonin   100IU 1 ml
- 0.1 ml /Pt **IDP**

Protocol for Cyst:
- procaine   2% 1 ml
- pentoxyfilline   1 ml
- 0.1 ml /Pt **IDP & IED**

MESOTHERAPY FOR OVERTRAINED ATHLETES

Overtraining induces significant oxidative stress leading to mitochondrial membrane depolarization and elevated cytosolic cytochrome C (mitochondrial leakage). This pathological biochemical process is associated with a depletion of intracellular glutathione. Type II fibers are associated with mitochondria depletion related to oxidation (ROS, NOS, H2O2 production). Overtraining in athletes is associated with local and systemic inflammation reactions, related to cytokine overproduction, which are responsible for the impairment of IGF-1-induced protein synthesis in skeletal muscle myoblasts. Therefore resulting in immune imbalances, because of lymphocyte and thymocyte apoptosis and ATP-depleted muscles.

Clinical findings of overtraining syndrome in athletes include: alteration of physiological functions, altered performance (fatigue and underperformance), impairment of psychological processing, immunological imbalance, and biochemical abnormalities. Common symptoms of oxidative stress in sports medicine include: anxiety, depression, irritability, poor mental function, digestive symptoms, dizziness, fatigue, headaches, hypoglycaemia, lowered resistance to infection, muscle and joint pains, and muscle weakness.

The aim of functional mesotherapy is to replenish intracellular glutathione, prevent muscle weakness, and restore immunity. Glutathione preserves the mitochondrial power house (ATP production) and reverses the cytokine inhibition of muscle protein synthesis.

Glutathione

- Master antioxidant
- Tripeptide molecule
- Protects cells against ROS
- Detoxifies xenobiotics
- Regulates protein and DNA biosynthesis, and cell growth
- Improves endurance performance
- Prevents muscle lipid peroxidation and thiol oxidation in cardiomyocytes (mitochondrial ion channels).
- Tissue level decreases with aging, inflammation, physical activities, stress, and chronic degenerative diseases.

Glutathione Protocol 1: Oxidative Stress and Muscle Performance
- 10 ml syringe 1 containing:
    - lyophilized glutathione   600 mg
    - injectable water   4 ml
    - 1.4% sodium bicarbonate   3 ml
- 10 ml syringe 2 containing:
    - B-complex   2 ml
    - or vitamin C   1 g 2 ml
    - magnesium pidolate   1.2 g 2 ml
    - procaine   2% sulfite free 2 ml

Glutathione Protocol 2: Neuronal Fatigue and Chronic Pain:
- 10 ml syringe 1 containing:
    - lyophilized glutathione   600 mg
    - injectable water   4 ml
    - 1.4% sodium bicarbonate   3 ml
- 10 ml syringe 2 containing:
    - placenta extracts   2 ml
    - cobalamine   1 mg 2 ml
    - procaine 1% 2 ml

Glutathione Protocol 3: Joints Wear and Tear:
- 10 ml syringe 1 containing:
    - lyophilized glutathione 600 mg
    - injectable water 4 ml
    - 1.4% sodium bicarbonate 3 ml
- 10 ml syringe 2 containing:
    - non cross-linked hyaluronic acid 2.5 ml
    - placenta extracts 2 ml

Sites and Techniques
- On the skull **IED**
- On the neck **IED, IDS, IDP, DHD**
- Both sides of the spine **IED,IDS,IDP,DHD**
- Liver and kidneys: anterior & posterior dermatomes **IED, IDS, IDP,DHD**
- On limbs **IED, IDS, IDP, DHD**
- Pre-auricular area, over the tragus **IDP**
- Retro auricular papulas
- Mastoid Process tip **IDS, IDP, DHD**
- Around the Vertebrae (C1ªC4) of the neck **IDP,DHD**
- In the membranous external auditory canal through the retro auricular fold **DHD**
- Subcutaneous retro auricular infiltration: 2 ml in one injection
- Acute condition: twice a week or more
- During intensive training: once a week
- Maintenance: twice a month
- Day 1, Day 8, Day 15, Day 21

Mesotherapy Protocols for Overtraining
Protocol for Immunity Enhancement:
- Glutathione protocol 1
- Plus syringe 3 containing:
    - medium chain triglycerides (MCT) Vit. D3 2 ml
    - pentoxyfilline 2 ml
- Frontal & maxillary areas: **IED,IDS,IDP**
- Nape of Neck: **IED,IDS,IDP,DHD**
- Carotid triangle: **IED,IDS,IDP**
- T1→ T 7 anterior and posterior left and right dermatomes: **IED,IDS,IDP**
- Abdominal and inguinal plexi: **IED,IDS,IDP,DHD**
- D 1, D 8, D 15
- The month before cold or damp seasons

Protocol for Pain Management:
On the insertion of the tendons **IDP**
- lidocaine WP 1% 2 ml
- piroxicam 1 ml
- thiocolchicoside 3 ml
- etamsylate 2 ml
- (**IED, IDS, IDP, DHD**) 0.1ml-0.5ml /Pt and on irradiations
- depending on the site **IED IDS IDP DHD**
- On knees, elbows and muscle areas
- Eventually amitryptilline 1 ml on all sensitive areas **IED, IDS** only if suspicion of painful chronic fatigue syndrome (CFIDS)
- It is advisable to plan mesotherapy injections before the time when pains occur
- 1 per week four weeks in the first phases

- 1 per month for maintenance

Protocol for Fatigue:
- Glutathione protocol 3
- On the skull: **IED**
- On the back: **IED,IDS,IDP,DHD**
- On the thorax: **IED,IDS,IDP**
- On the medial side of limbs: **IED,IDS,IDP**
- 1 per week four weeks in the first phases
- 1 per month for maintenance

Respiratory Capacity Protocol – VO2 Max Improvement
- Glutathione protocol 1
- Plus syringe 3 containing:
  - pentoxyfilline   3 ml
  - N-acetylcysteine   2 ml
  - or ambroxol   2 ml
- T1 → T 7 anterior and posterior left and right dermatomes
- **IED IDS IDP**

Protocol for Tissues Protection:
- Glutathione protocol 3
- Plus Syringe 3 for bones, containing:
  - salmon calcitonin   100 UI 1 ml
  - MCT vitamin D3   2 ml

- Plus Syringe 3 for joints, containing:
  - salmon calcitonin   100 UI 1 ml
- Plus inflammation→ piroxicam   1 ml
- Plus stiffness→ thiocolchicoside 2 ml
- Plus calcifications→ EDTA   0.5 ml
- Neck: **IED,IDS,IDP,DHD**
- Spine and 1.5 cm, 3 cm, 5 cm on both sides of the spine: **IED,IDS,IDP**
- Pathologic bones and joints: **IED,IDS,IDP,DHD**
- Muscles: **IED,IDS,IDP,DHD**

CONCLUDING REMARKS
Mesotherapy is the treatment of choice for many sports related conditions. This is because it is safe and effective at alleviating pain, promoting fast and optimal tissue healing, promoting organ reserve, and increasing performance. The major advantages of mesotherapy are that it uses very low doses of drugs, is virtually side effect free (side effects are rare), and that it is a relatively cheap treatment. It is important to note that mesotherapy is a medical specialty requiring training and knowledge of pharmacology. Proper training is required in order to achieve optimal results.

REFERENCES
1. Pistor M Mésothérapie pratique ed.Masson Paris 1998
2. Conférences de consensus en mésothérapie 2000 Ed. SFM
3. Laurens D, Mrejen D. ENATOME I, ENATOME 11. 1989-1990. (National study on tolerance of mesotherapy).
4. Burnham EL, Moss M, Ziegler TR. Myopathies in critical illness: characterization and nutritional aspects. *J Nutr.* 2005;135:1818S-1823S.

5. Kim HJ, Nel AE. The role of phase II antioxidant enzymes in protecting memory T cells from spontaneous apoptosis in young and old mice. *J Immunol.* 2005;175:2948-2959.
6. Balog T, Sobocanec S, Sverko V, Krolo I, Rocić B, Marotti M, Marotti T.The influence of season on oxidant-antioxidant status in trained and sedentary subjects. *Life Sci.* 2006;78:1441-1447.
7. Castagné V, Rougemont M, Cuenod M, Do KQ. Low brain glutathione and ascorbic acid associated with dopamine uptake inhibition during rat's development induce long-term cognitive deficit: relevance to schizophrenia. *Neurobiol Dis.* 2004;15:93-105.
8. Dröge W. Oxidative stress and ageing: is ageing a cysteine deficiency syndrome? *Philos Trans R Soc Lond B Biol Sci.* 2005;360:2355-2372.

ABOUT THE AUTHOR

Dr. Janine Gaston Nhan graduated from Paris Medical School 1973. She is a Board Certified by the American Board of Anti-Aging & Regenerative Medicine (ABAARM) and a Fellow of the European Society of Anti-Aging Medicine (ESAAM). Dr. Gaston Nhan is a Certified Mesotherapist, AFMCP Graduate in Functional Medicine, Chronobiology, Neurodegeneration, Prevention of pathological aging, and Certified in Aesthetic & Laser Medicine. She is is the translator in French of the *Textbook of Functional Medicine*, author of the textbook *Mesotherapy in Anti-Aging Medicine*, and frequent lecturer at both the A4M's Annual Congresses and the Meetings of the French Mesotherapy Societies.

Chapter 14
Post Traumatic Brain Injury Hormonal Deficiency Syndrome

Mark Gordon, M.D.
Medical Director, Millennium Health Centers

ABSTRACT

Traumatic brain injury (TBI), typically resulting from vehicle accidents or acts of violence, is a major public health concern. Survivors often face lifelong impairments affecting functional status, memory, cognition, language, and mood, as well as physical functioning and metabolism. Within the past three years, a clear cause and effect has been established – post TBI hormonal deficiency syndrome. Prior to this new knowledge patients have been treated with symptomatic protocols that simply did not work. There is an increasing amount of evidence to suggest that post TBI hormonal deficiency syndrome affects many people who have sustained TBI and mild TBI, and research is now beginning to show that replacement of deficient hormones can lead to significant improvements. This paper will consider the incidence, clinical course, diagnosis, and treatment of post TBI hormonal deficiency syndrome.

INTRODUCTION

Traumatic brain injury (TBI), typically resulting from vehicle accidents or acts of violence, is a major public health concern. Survivors often face lifelong impairments affecting functional status, memory, cognition, language, and mood, as well as physical functioning and metabolism. Within the past three years, a clear cause and effect has been established – post TBI hormonal deficiency syndrome. Prior to this new knowledge patients have been treated with symptomatic protocols that simply did not work. There is an increasing amount of evidence to suggest that post TBI hormonal deficiency syndrome affects many people who have sustained TBI and mild TBI, and research is now beginning to show that replacement of deficient hormones can lead to significant improvements.

POST TRAUMATIC BRAIN INJURY HORMONAL DEFICIENCY SYNDROME
Incidence

An estimated 1.9 million Americans sustain a TBI each year. Approximately half of these cases result in at least short-term disability, and approximately 52,000 of those people die from their injuries. Of those that survive, many will develop progressive hormonal deficiencies, which lead to post concussion syndrome or post TBI hormonal deficiency syndrome, a cascade of deficiencies of hormones that will affect every aspect of functioning and will have a dramatic effect upon the patient's quality of life. Merriam *et al* found that just 20% of adults with growth hormone (GH) deficiency have a history of childhood-onset GH deficiency. Therefore, the remaining 80% are acquired in adult life, usually through acquired damage to the pituitary-hypothalamic region caused by TBI.

Post TBI hormonal deficiency syndrome is typically associated with severe head traumas with a Glasgow Coma Score of less than 7 or 8 with loss of consciousness and coma. Survivors of such head trauma often suffer from impairment of cognition, language, and mood, as well as physical functioning. However, more recent research suggests that relatively mild trauma can be enough to cause a TBI and post TBI hormonal deficiency.

Motor vehicle accidents and sports, such as boxing, martial arts, wresting, football, are common causes of TBI. As are slips and falls, blunt trauma, and shaken trauma. Even seemingly innocuous rides at amusement parks can be violent enough to cause jarring of the stock of the pituitary that can predispose us to TBI.

Kelly *et al* found that chronic GH deficiency develops in approximately 18% of patients with complicated mild, moderate, or severe TBI, and is associated with depression and diminished quality of life. Whilst Powner *et al* found that chronic hormone deficiency occurs in 30-40% of patients after TBI, with 10-15% of patients having more than one deficiency. Like Kelly, Powner found that 15-20% of TBI patients go on to develop GH deficiency. Results of the study by Powner *et al* also showed that 15% of TBI patients develop gonadal hormone deficiencies and 10-30% develop hypothyroidism. The researchers found that chronic adrenal failure is widespread amongst TBI patients and that nearly a third have elevated prolactin levels.

Aimaretti *et al* found that GH deficiency and secondary hypogonadism were the most common acquired pituitary defects induced by TBI in the transition phase (pediatric to adolescent). The results of this study suggest that it is extremely important to give all prepubescent children who have sustained a head injury a total hormone assessment, because that head injury may cause post TBI hormonal deficiency syndrome, which could cause a whole range of problems, including short stature, personality changes, functional disability, and problems with language skills and school skills. The most recent literature suggests that hormone levels should be determined immediately after the injury and then again a few weeks later.

Thomson *et al* found that post-traumatic hypogonadism is very common in the acute post-TBI phase, although most cases resolve themselves within six to twelve months. However, results of this study also showed that hypogonadism persists in 10 to 17% of long-term survivors. So, it can be seen that there is plenty of evidence in the medical literature to show that there is a clear relationship between head trauma and the development of one or multiple hormone deficiencies.

Symptomatology

Any brain function can be disrupted by TBI. Symptoms of post TBI hormonal deficiency syndrome include: excessive sleepiness, inattention, difficulty concentrating, impaired memory, an inability to learn new things, faulty judgment, depression, irritability, emotional outbursts, disturbed sleep, diminished libido, difficulty switching between two tasks, and slowed thinking.

Neuropathology

What effect do diminished hormone levels have on the brain? Firstly, the presence of adequate amounts of GH is crucial if the brain is to function correctly. This is because GH plays an important role in microtubular regeneration, lipid metabolism, and dendritic growth and regrowth. What about insulin-like growth factor (IGF-1)? IGF-1 deals with the functional use of glucose in the brain. Furthermore, Cheng *et al* found evidence indicating that IGF-1 depletion causes disruption in lipid and microtubule metabolism, leading to impaired neuronal, somatic, and dendritic growth.

The hippocampus is very important for memory. Research suggests that the functions mediated by GH receptors in the hippocampal area may be involved in the hormone's action on memory and cognitive function. Furthermore, beneficial effects of GH on certain functions, including memory, mental alertness, motivation, and working capacity have been reported.

Cranston *et al* conducted an interesting study using PET scans to investigate the effects of GH replacement on cerebral metabolism in adults with GH deficiency. The results showed that the resting cerebral metabolic rate in adults with GH deficiency is low. However, GH replacement to physiological levels increased resting cerebral metabolism towards normal levels, thus suggesting that GH has a direct effect upon the central nervous system and cellular metabolism.

Clinical Course

There are three phases to post TBI hormonal deficiency syndrome: the acute phase, the recovery phase, and the chronic phase. Schneider *et al* studied the prevalence of anterior pituitary insufficiency 3 and 12-months after TBI. Results showed that found that 56% of TBI patients had anterior pituitary insufficiency at 3 months. By 12-months this had dropped to 36%. However, GH deficiency actually increased over that period from 9% to 10%. Leal-Cerro *et al* conducted a similar study investigating the prevalence of TBI-mediated hypopituitarism in patients who had sustained a severe TBI within the last five years. Results showed that 17% were suffering from gonadotrophin deficiency, 6.4% were suffering from adrenocortiocotrophic (ACTH) deficiency, 5.8% were suffering from thyroid stimulating hormone (TSH) deficiency, and 1.7% developed diabetes insipidus. Overall, 24.7% of participants developed some type of pituitary hormone deficiency.

Koponen *et al* conducted a 30-year follow-up study on patients who had suffered TBI to determine the occurrence of psychiatric disorders. Their results showed that 48.3% of study participants had had an axis I disorder that began after TBI. The most common disorders after TBI were: major depression (26.7%), alcohol abuse or dependence (11.7%), panic disorder (8.3%), specific phobia (8.3%), and psychotic disorders. Nearly a quarter (23.3%) developed at least one personality disorder. These findings led the researchers to conclude: *"The results suggest that traumatic brain injury may cause decades-lasting vulnerability to psychiatric illness in some individuals. Traumatic brain injury seems to make patients particularly susceptible to depressive episodes, delusional disorder, and personality disturbances. The high rate of psychiatric disorders found in this study emphasizes the importance of psychiatric follow-up after traumatic brain injury.*"

The ER doctors and the neurologists, the very people who are responsible for the care of people with TBI, are seemingly doing nothing about the problems associated with TBI. The real key to treating these problems is hormone replacement. Aimaretti and Ghigo suggested that patients with TBI-induced hypopituitarism might benefit from appropriate hormone replacement therapy, such as anti-diuretic hormone (ADH), glucocorticoid, and thyroid hormones. They also wrote that gonadal and recombinant human GH (rhGH) replacement therapy should be given if deficiencies are found.

Diagnosis and Treatment of Post TBI Hormonal Deficiency Syndrome

The first and foremost thing to do in order to diagnose, or rule out, post TBI hormonal deficiency syndrome is evaluate the patient – regardless of their age. Many of the patients that I see cannot even remember sustaining a head injury, because they were two or three when they were dropped on their head or when they accidentally banged their head on the wall and ended up in the emergency room. Remember, even very mild head injuries can have their consequences – they may be subtle but they are also long-term consequences.

To evaluate patients you should perform a full hormonal assessment via a spot or 24-hour urine test for hormones and their metabolites, or serum testing. These are the most accurate and reliable testing formats for TBI. Salivary testing is not recommended for TBI. It is also important to test for neuro-endocrine markers. This can be done with either spot or 24-hour urine testing. It is important to use a laboratory with neurotransmitter expertise.

In order to treat post TBI hormonal deficiency syndrome it is necessary to identify the hormonal deficiencies present and then begin the process of replenishing the deficient hormones.
Important points to remember when you suspect that a patient may have post TBI hormonal deficiency syndrome include:

- It is vital not to use the intensity of the trauma to predict the onset of post TBI hormonal deficiency syndrome – even the most subtle injuries can sometimes be enough to cause a TBI.
- It is vital that you perform hormonal testing immediately after the precipitating event to establish a baseline.
- Do not use age as a predictor. Even in a 45-year-old patient it is vital to enquire about any historical head trauma – even head trauma that occurred in their childhood.
- Although GH cannot be used at present for the treatment of TBI, it can still be used to treat adult GH deficiency syndrome. However, being aware of the etiology of such a deficiency is extremely important because you may well need to adopt a totally different approach to a patient's treatment.
- Consider early hormonal supplementation to minimize the physical and psychological sequelae.
- Hormonal assessments can be done at three-month intervals from the date of injury, or more frequently based upon treatment.

CONCLUDING REMARKS

For 40 years researchers have been looking at what they can do to help people with TBI, each and every one of these studies was futile because nothing they came up with helped. They tried a whole gambit of drugs and nothing worked. Even now, few people are aware of the existence of post TBI hormonal deficiency syndrome, which means that it is down to anti-aging physicians to intervene and once again be at the cutting edge of medicine. It is up to us to educate our fellow physicians about post TBI hormonal deficiency syndrome and how to treat it.

REFERENCES

Agha A, Rogers B, Sherlock M, O'Kelly P, Tormey W, Phillips J, Thompson CJ. Anterior pituitary dysfunction in survivors of traumatic brain injury. *J Clin Endocrinol Metab*. 2004;89:4929-4936.

Aimaretti G, Ambrosio MR, Di Somma C, Gasperi M, Cannavo S, Scaroni C, *et al*. Hypopituitarism induced by traumatic brain injury in the transition phase. *J Endocrinol Invest*. 2005;28:984-989.

Aimaretti G, Ghigo E. Traumatic brain injury and hypopituitarism. *ScientificWorldJournal*. 2005;5:777-781.

Cheng CM, Mervis RF, Niu SL, Salem N, Witters LA, Tseng V, Reinhardt R, Bondy CA. Insulin-like growth factor 1 is essential for normal dendritic growth. *J Neurosci Res*. 2003;73:1-9.

Cranston IC, Marsden PK, Carroll P, Sonksen PH, Russell-Jones D. Effects of hGH replacement on cerebral metabolism in adults with growth hormone deficiency. *Growth Hormone & IGF Research*. 1998;8:317-318.

Estes SM, Urban RJ. Hormonal replacement in patients with brain injury-induced hypopituitarism: who, when and how to treat? *Pituitary*. 2005;8:267-270.

Kelly DF, McArthur DL, Levin H, Swimmer S, Dusick JR, Cohan P, Wang C, Swerdloff R.

Neurobehavioral and quality of life changes associated with growth hormone insufficiency after complicated mild, moderate, or severe traumatic brain injury. *J Neurotrauma*. 2006;23:928-942.

Koponen S, Taiminen T, Portin R, Himanen L, Isoniemi H, Heinonen H, Hinkka S, Tenovuo O.

Axis I and II psychiatric disorders after traumatic brain injury: a 30-year follow-up study. *Am J Psychiatry*. 2002;159:1315-1321.

Leal-Cerro A, Flores JM, Rincon M, Murillo F, Pujol M, Garcia-Pesquera F, Dieguez C, Casanueva FF. Prevalence of hypopituitarism and growth hormone deficiency in adults long-term after severe traumatic brain injury. *Clin Endocrinol (Oxf)*. 2005;62:525-532.

Merriam GR, Carney C, Smith LC, Kletke M. Adult growth hormone deficiency: current trends in diagnosis and dosing. *J Pediatr Endocrinol Metab*. 2004;17:1307-1320.

Nyberg F. Growth hormone in the brain: characteristics of specific brain targets for the hormone and their functional significance. *Front Neuroendocrinol*. 2000;21:330-348.

Powner DJ, Boccalandro C, Alp MS, Vollmer DG. Endocrine failure after traumatic brain injury in adults. *Neurocrit Care*. 2006;5:61-70.

Schneider HJ, Schneider M, Saller B, Petersenn S, Uhr M, Husemann B, von Rosen F, Stalla GK. Prevalence of anterior pituitary insufficiency 3 and 12 months after traumatic brain injury. *Eur J Endocrinol*. 2006;154:259-265.

ABOUT THE AUTHOR

After 14 years of clinical orthopedics and 20 years as a residency trained board certified family physician, Dr. Mark Gordon integrates anti-aging medical theories into a program of sports rehabilitation. Using nutrition, exercise and his knowledge of supplementation he has helped a number of injured patients return to their activities in a significantly reduced time. Pre-operative programs help surgical outcome and reduce the down time for both sports and non-sports related injuries. Many natural products are available to accomplish these goals. Dr. Mark Gordon has been recognized as a leader in the area of anti-aging medicine and holds associate clinical professorships at USC and UCLA. Dr. Gordon has recently been reappointed as Medical Director for CBS Studios, and Medical Consultant to HBO and FX. In these positions he is available for consultation on areas of preventive, anti-aging and alternative medicine. He writes articles on nutritional supplementation and hormonal replacement, some of which have been published in *Max Muscle* and *Planet Muscle*.

Chapter 15
New Minimally Invasive Laser Treatment for Prostate Disease

Mahmood Hai, M.D., F.I.C.S.
Senior Urology Consultant at Oakwood Hospital; Chief of Urology at Annapolis Hospital

ABSTRACT

Transurethral Resection of the Prostate (TURP) has in the past been referred to as 'the gold standard' for treatment of obstructive Benign Prostatic Hyperplasia (BPH) because of its exceptional affect on obstructive symptoms of BPH and speed of procedure; however, it is a procedure associated with significant limitations and risks. Over the last two decades, laser technology for the treatment of Benign Prostatic Hyperplasia (BPH) has undergone an evolution from theory to practical application. Recent generations of laser treatments now enable similar symptom improvements while providing advantages in morbidity associated with TURP.[1]

A significant step forward was made with the discovery of the KTP laser. The KTP laser works by selectively delivering energy to hemoglobin which consequently results in vaporizing thermal energy.[2] Recent studies[3] have confirmed that KTP (potassium titanyl phosphate) laser resection of the prostate – otherwise known as photoselective vaporization of the prostate (PVP) – provides equivalent or superior clinical outcomes, lesser morbidity and lower overall economic burden when compared to TURP. It also provides a means of treating BPH in patients with co-morbidities that precluded TURP in the past.[4-9] Furthermore, a comparison of common BPH treatments using typical diagnostic tests, such as AUA symptom score, IPSS and maximum flow rate (Qmax), shows remarkable superiority of PVP over other procedures.[10]

Initial research of a 60 watt KTP laser showed significant improvement in symptom and urologic measures immediately and at 2 and 5 years.[11, 12] Subsequently an 80W laser was created to address slow procedure times. Data on this system are similar to the earlier results at early and longer term time points.[13-16] Further development led to the release of a 120W KTP laser. Initial outcomes in 64 patients at our site show shorter operative time, decreased irritative bladder symptoms of frequency and urgency and less hematuria.[17] Long term evaluations are still needed to verify consistency of long term outcomes with this higher power system.

PVP has demonstrated improvements over TURP with respect to morbidity and has well established short and long-term symptomatic and urodynamic improvements consistent with TURP. KTP has evolved into a viable treatment that should affect our approach in the management of the obstructive BPH.

Keywords: BPH, PVP, Prostate, Laser

INTRODUCTION

Benign Prostatic Hyperplasia (BPH) with associated lower urinary tract symptoms (LUTS); including urgency, frequency, nocturia, incontinence, hesitancy, poor flow, intermittency, straining, dysuria, dribbling, and incomplete emptying; is a common medical condition in the aging male.[18] BPH by definition involves microscopic or palpable enlargement of the prostate with or without LUTS.[19] The incidence increases from 40% among males between the ages of 50 and 60 years to 90% among males older than 80 years of age.[20] BPH is often diagnosed using subjective patient questionnaires such as the International Prostate Symptom Score (IPSS) as well as more objective measures including digital rectal examination (DRE), serum prostate specific antigen (PSA), urinary flow, post void residual tests and cystoscopy, intended to diagnose obstruction.

TREATMENT OF BPH

Watchful waiting is often the first form of BPH treatment utilized, which includes adjustment of fluid intake, changes in diet, daily routines, and overall health as well as regular assessments for a careful differential diagnosis. A physical examination and medical history are necessary elements for a formal diagnosis. The DRE should include size estimation, shape, symmetry, and texture of the prostate. Measuring post-void residual volume of urine may be appropriate in patients to check the response to medical therapy. Laboratory tests may include glucose, electrolytes, urinalysis, and PSA assay. This option is appropriate management for patients who are asymptomatic, not bothered by their symptoms, or have not developed complications due to BPH such as bladder outlet obstruction, urinary tract infections, hydronephrosis, acute urinary retention, hydroureter, hematuria, bladder dysfunction, renal failure, etc. No specific treatment or intervention is done and this period can last from months to years depending on the rate of disease progression.

Once symptoms affect quality of life, both the European Association of Urology (EAU) and the American Urology Association (AUA) recommend escalation to medical therapy which consists of alpha-1-adrenergic blockers (alpha-blockers) and androgen hormone inhibitors (5 alpha-reductase inhibitors) both approved by the US Food and Drug Administration (FDA) for treatment of BPH. These drug classes diminish symptoms by either reducing the volume of glandular tissue or by reducing the prostatic muscle fiber response to stimulus. In particular, 5 alpha-reductase inhibitors, Dutasteride and Finasteride, are agents which by reducing the conversion of Testosterone to the active agent dihydrotestosterone (DHT) reduce prostate volume. Alpha blockers, including Alfuzosin, Doxazosin, Tamsulosin, and Terazosin, work essentially by relaxing the external sphincter and bladder neck, thereby allowing a better flow of urine. A combination of alpha-blocker and 5 alpha-reductase may be appropriate for men with larger prostates. Lastly, phytotherapeutic or herbal compounds have been used but their mechanism of action is currently unknown. Data suggests clinically meaningful outcomes in some patients.

Surgical intervention is considered the first line therapy for BPH when the disease results in further medical complications such as urinary retention or renal insufficiency. Additionally, the AUA and EAU recommend balancing patient choice and management of risk factors when selecting between medical therapy and minimally invasive surgical treatments. With the advancement of safer and less invasive surgical methods and with the desire of younger patients to skip pharmaceuticals, surgery is quickly becoming a potential first line treatment for BPH even in patients with no resultant complications.

SURGICAL TREATMENTS FOR BPH
Open Prostatectomy
Surgical removal of the prostatic adenoma is now rarely used except for very large BPH.

Transurethral Resection of the Prostate
The long standing gold standard surgical treatment for BPH, transurethral resection of the prostate (TURP), is currently undergoing intense scrutiny due to the high cost and significant morbidity associated with the procedure. TURP has exceptional clinical efficacy and well established long-term durability[21]; however, significant concerns remain regarding the relatively high incidence of postoperative morbidity and the major economic burden on world healthcare systems.[22, 23] As a result of these concerns, there have been continued efforts to introduce technology that could address these concerns without sacrificing clinical outcomes.

History of Surgical Lasers for BPH
Lasers were first introduced in urology as a coagulative device (Nd:YAG/VLAP) but failed to deliver sufficient outcomes. Initial forms of laser treatment were often either too slow or unable to generate adequate tissue resection in order to achieve clinical outcomes similar to that of TURP. Techniques such as VLAP and Interstitial Laser Coagulation (ILC) were replaced by newer more powerful technology and techniques. Technology has rapidly evolved to offer physicians a tissue vaporization tool able to achieve rapid and efficient debulking of the prostate while still maintaining desired hemostasis similar to that of the earlier coagulative lasers. These recent generations of laser treatments have overcome the limitations of early laser techniques demonstrating similar clinical improvements while providing advantages in morbidity associated with TURP.[24] Laser procedures for BPH have typically been performed with three primary lasers of differing wavelength and application techniques. While newer wavelengths have been introduced, there is little to no human clinical data to support their use for BPH.

Holmium Laser Techniques
The Ho:YAG laser (2140 nm) was the second laser wavelength introduced and has been utilized in several forms. The energy of holmium laser is strongly absorbed by water and because prostate debulking is done with irrigation, the technique requires close contact with tissue in order to achieve the

desired effect. This is coupled with a high absorption of energy in the tissue which limits the depth of penetration of energy.

The first technique introduced was Holmium Laser Resection or E-nucleation of the Prostate (HOLRP or HOLEP). This technique involves cutting out chunks of the prostatic lobes through an end-firing fiber with morcellation of the resected tissue.[25] Although some centers have produced good results, this technology has not gained popularity primarily because of a high learning curve, unexpected bleeding, difficulty in morcellating and removing tissue and long procedure duration. While still used, this technique is most appropriate for larger prostates.[26]

Holmium Laser Ablation of the Prostate (HOLAP) was first performed in 1994, using a side-firing fiber with a 60W machine that was aimed at vaporizing tissue rather than cutting tissue.[27] In a randomized study by Mottet et al, HOLAP demonstrated clinical outcomes similar to that of TURP.[28] Of the few patients available for long-term, seven year, follow-up in a study by Tan et al, the maximum flow (Qmax) improved by 83% and symptom score reduced by 47% with a reoperation rate of 15%.[29, 30] Recently, HOLAP has been marketed for small prostates with an increased laser power of 100 watts aimed at overcoming tissue vaporization speeds.[31] This procedure continues to be used, but long term data is unavailable.

Greenlight 532nm Laser Treatment

Development

Photoselective vaporization of the prostate (PVP) using a 532 nm wavelength is the most recent technological discovery that has generated favorable outcomes.[32-34] The 532 nm wavelength is in the visible spectrum as green light and is strongly absorbed by oxyhemoglobin. Energy absorption by oxyhemoglobin heats the tissue leading to formation of vapor bubbles inside the prostatic tissue which instantly disintegrates the collagen matrix, effectively vaporizing the tissue. Continued exposure leads to progressive vaporization of the newly exposed tissue layers. Converse to previous laser technologies, the diffusion of laser energy in the peripheral tissue planes is superficial and results in a relatively thin coagulation zone of 1-2 mm. This coagulation zone provides hemostasis without significant thermal damage.[35] As power increases the mechanism of action and the avascular layer remain, but the rate of tissue vaporization increases allowing faster treatment without affecting the hemostatic properties of the laser.

The use of a 532 nm laser in urology dates back to the late 1980's. In 1990 a laser console (Laserscope 800) was made available that had a combined energy source of 100W Nd:YAG and 38W KTP. The low power KTP laser provided slow and limited vaporization and was only useful for smaller glands. The clinical outcomes were first presented by Hai in 1995.[36, 37] Following Hai, Kuntzman et al established the scientific foundation of higher energy PVP with a prototype 60 watt KTP laser in cadavers and living canines.[38] In 1998, Malek, et al published their first live human clinical outcomes with the 60 watts KTP laser, which showed significant improvement in subjective and objective clinical measures of BPH.[39] Malek et al subsequently reported the long term outcomes of this cohort at 2 and 5 years. The long term results confirmed significant and sustained improvements in symptomatic and urodynamic outcomes (Figure 1).[40, 16] The 60W laser was still limited by the relatively low rate of tissue vaporization at that time, but had great interest due to the clinical outcomes and low incidence of complications reported. As a result, an 80W laser (Greenlight PV, AMS) was created.

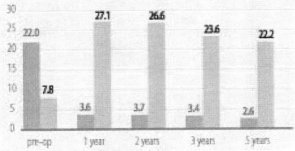

Figure 1. Long-term outcomes after PVP
(Results from Malek, Kuntzman and Barrett)

Greenlight PV 80W Laser
Prospective Single Arm Studies

The first clinical study of the 80W system was performed by Hai and Malek.[41] This study demonstrated the efficacy of Greenlight PVP with improvement in urinary flow (Qmax) of 198%, reduction of AUA symptom score by 89% and reduction of post void residual volume (PVR) of 98% at 12 months. Since the publication of the initial experience with the 80W KTP Greenlight laser, numerous articles and abstracts have been published in urologic literature. These results led investigators to expand the evaluation of PVP using the 80W KTP laser into a multi-institutional study with a larger cohort of patients. In 2004, Te *et al* published the first multi-center study (six medical institutions) of 139 patients evaluating PVP as a treatment of BPH through 1 year of follow-up.[42] This study again demonstrated all patient outcome parameters were significantly improved at twelve months by 82%, 77%, 190%, and 78% in AUASI, QoL, Qmax, and PVR, respectively. The degree of improvement was consistent with TURP and continued to support the original findings of the 60W laser. This group went on to publish their outcomes annually out to three years; each reinforced the durability of treatment with Greenlight.[23, 43-45]

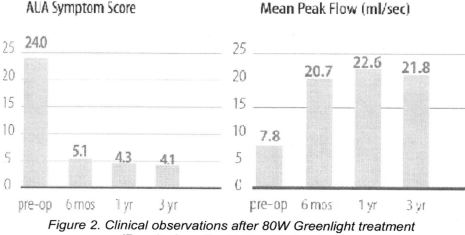

Figure 2. Clinical observations after 80W Greenlight treatment
(Results from Te, Malloy, Stein, et al.)

The major adverse events encountered have been prolonged dysuria 5-9.4%, delayed hematuria 3-8.6%, urinary retention requiring re-catheterization 1-5%, bladder neck contracture 1.4-2%, with no incidence of permanent urinary incontinence or impotence. Because of the preservation of the bladder neck fibers, retrograde ejaculation was seen only in 26-50% of patients.

Various centers including the New York Presbyterian Hospital,[46] University of Baseland, University of Munich,[47] King College Hospital, London[48] and urologists in private practice[49, 50] have all confirmed that the PVP technique is simple to learn and has a high degree of reproducibility with good outcomes as well as reduced morbidity, catheterization time and hospitalization.

My personal long-term experience with PVP using the Greenlight PV has shown promising results at 5-years with significant improvements overall. Compared to baseline values, 5-year outcomes showed improvements of 79%, 80%, 110%, 173% for AUA, QOL, voided volume (VV), Qmax, as well as 10%, 18%, and 77% reduction in PSA, TRUS, and PVR respectively. All results are statistically significant, p<0.05. Out of 242 patients followed for 5 years, 18 were treated with repeat PVP and 3 with transurethral incision of the bladder neck (TUIBN), for an overall retreatment rate of 8.7% which is much less than the reported retreatment following TURP.

Greenlight Comparisons to TURP

Transurethral Resection of the Prostate (TURP) has in the past been referred to as 'the gold standard' for treatment of obstructive BPH because of its exceptional effect on obstructive symptoms of BPH and speed of procedure. However, TURP has also been associated with significant clinical limitations and patient risks. Early studies on PVP spurred the development of further research focused on comparing outcomes of PVP to TURP[51-62] and other transurethral treatments.[63, 64] Many of the authors found PVP to be a superior procedure, particularly when compared to minimally invasive treatments.

124

Several groups of physicians have released series of prospective Greenlight PV studies comparing PVP to a TURP control group. Of the main clinical studies performed to date, the majority have been multi-center, non-randomized, controlled trials. Nearly all of these studies focused on the traditional measures of BPH including IPSS or AUA score for subjective symptom relief, Qmax, PVR, hospitalization time, and catheterization time. Qmax improvement was generally similar to TURP; although, a couple sources suggest some incremental change from TURP. Relative IPSS or AUASI score outcomes were similar to Qmax changes. Out of nine citations, post-operative clinical outcomes were significantly different in 1, non-significant in 7, and no conclusion in 1. These results are supported by single arm studies in that the degree of change was consistent among all studies.

Only a single study in Australia has taken on a multi-center, randomized, prospective study to compare PVP to TURP. All surgeons had performed less than 5 cases each prior to the start of the study but had extensive experience performing TURPs. Early results from 76 subjects showed non-significant differences in urinary outcomes and symptom scores for the two modalities but patients in the TURP arm did experience more significant adverse events including clot retention and bleeding. Additionally, care for the TURP cases cost 22% more when considering all factors. These early results support previously reported finding similar to single-arm studies.

Greenlight PVP's primary benefit over TURP comes in the degree and severity of the intervention. Two claims made in support of PVP are shorter hospitalization and catheterization times. In the seven studies with data reported on hospitalization times, differences between the mean hospitalization time for PVP and TURP ranged from 0.91 to 3.4 days, with PVP having significantly shorter hospitalization times in all studies. Of the eight studies reporting catheterization times, the range of differences in mean PVP and TURP catheterization time was 1.1 to 2.0 days. All studies showed significantly shorter catheterization times for PVP. Overall, study results clearly show that PVP is indeed associated with significantly reduced hospitalization and catheterization times when compared to TURP.

Finally, post-operative morbidity was recorded, but many of the studies were not powered to detect differences of events occurring at relatively low rates. The following is a summary of the results observed in these two-armed studies:

- **Capsular perforation:** Of the articles reporting complications, the range of reported capsular perforation rates were from 2.5-5% for TURP while none occurred for PVP. In addition, Park *et al* stated that more capsule perforations occurred in the TURP group than in the Greenlight PV group. These rates are slight elevated over historical reported rates for TURP, of 1-2%. This complication is rare but expected with TURP while this is considered very rare with PVP.

- **Clot retention requiring bladder washout:** Clot retention again was mentioned in several of the articles, including rates for TURP of 2.3%, 2.5%, 5.0%, and 26.2% while this was not reported in any of the PVP groups.

- **Urinary tract infection:** UTI incidence was reported in four articles, all with comparable occurrence rates between the two groups which would be expected.

- **Stricture:** Stricture rates were highly variable with rates between 2.7% and 21% for TURP, and 2.0%-13.2% for PVP. Three articles reported rates similar between groups, while two others showed some difference between groups, one favoring TURP and one favoring PVP. Outside of one outlier, all studies reported rates consistent with non-comparative study results.

- **TUR Syndrome, Hyponatremia:** TUR Syndrome was reported in only two studies, each with single occurrences (1%, 2.6%); these rates are consistent with other TURP specific literature.

- **Excessive bleeding:** Excessive bleeding is defined as bleeding that required active management or stoppage of the procedure, but without requiring transfusion. The incidence rates for TURP ranged from 10.5%-18%, while this was not reported in any PVP group. The decrease in bleeding for PVP is primarily driven by the way that green light interacts with tissue.

- **Impotence/Erectile Dysfunction:** Two studies reported the incidence of ED, at 0% and 2.7% for TURP, while no incidents or ED were reported for PVP.

- **Retention requiring indwelling catheter:** Of the four studies reporting on transient retention requiring placement of an indwelling catheter, all four reported rates higher in the PVP group. Rates for TURP ranged from 0%-3.4%, while PVP had a significantly higher rate, with ranges between 3.0%-8.2%.

- **Bleeding requiring transfusion:** In addition to the excessive bleeding, some cases are severe enough to require transfusion. Of the five papers, 2 reported no occurrence in either group, while the other three reported significantly greater rates in the TURP group with occurrences between 2.6%-3.4%. No blood transfusion was needed in any of the PVP patients.

All series made conclusions stating equivalent or reduced incidence of complications associated with PVP. Evaluating the complications above, it is clear that PVP does indeed have lower intra- and peri-operative risks. Long-term risks such as stricture appear to be equivalent between the groups. Dysuria, hematuria, and retrograde ejaculation surprisingly were not reported. All occur with both TURP and PVP and, based on occurrence rates, would have been expected. It is possible that these events were not included because they did not require additional medical intervention for resolution.

Alivizatos et al have taken the randomized trial one step further and recently published one year outcomes of PVP compared to open prostatectomy.[65] The study showed that while some differences were observed in volume removal measures (TRUS prostate volume, PSA) and the QOL question of the IPSS, in all other measures there were no statistical or clinical meaningful differences. Another paper by Stovsky et al comparing PVP, ILC, TUMT, TUNA, and TURP using an analytical model for estimating procedure and outcome costs, concluded that PVP was superior in both clinical efficacy and total healthcare cost in the long run.[66]

Greenlight Outcomes in Special Populations

Further studies with large prostates,[38, 48, 67, 68] high risk patients,[69-71] patients with hematologic impairments[72] and patients with acute[73] and chronic[74] retention have all confirmed the versatility of the PVP procedure showing advantages over TURP in the ability to deal with concomitant and high risk patients. Due to the risk of bleeding and TUR Syndrome, traditionally TURP has not been used in glands greater than 80g or in patients who require anticoagulation or are ASA category 4. PVP can be performed safely in all these patients.

Greenlight HPS 120W Laser

Despite positive clinical outcomes and inconclusive data on speed of surgery, the Greenlight procedure was considered to be a bit slower than TURP and occasionally technically challenging because the laser fiber needed to be within 1 mm of the tissue for optimal vaporization. The Greenlight HPS (HPS) was developed to continue the improvements in procedural efficiency that were observed with previous increases in power. The higher powered laser allows the user to address both of the above issues. By introducing greater power, faster vaporization is possible when held near 1mm from the tissue. As well, the greater power and more collimated beam allow the user to be within 3 mm of the tissue and still maintain efficient vaporization of tissue. These two options allow greater flexibility in technique for physicians treating BPH. The HPS system also allows for programmable energy allowing the user to decrease output power if the physician is working near a critical structure and wants to use less power and go more slowly. The consistency of results observed with power increases from the 38W to 60W and then to 80W suggests that another incremental change in power will result in similar results to the outcomes of the 80W laser. Early results suggest that this will be true.[75] Initial outcomes in 300 patients at our site show shorter operative time, decreased irritative bladder symptoms of frequency and urgency and less hematuria compared to the 80W Greenlight PV system. Long term evaluations are still needed to verify consistency of long term outcomes with this higher power system.

CONCLUDING REMARKS

Early successful results with the 60W and 80W laser drove further research that consistently showed significant improvements in all objective and subjective measures of BPH. These studies demonstrated outcomes comparable to previous series of TURP and thus further research comparing the two methodologies were started.

These comparative studies continued to show consistent Greenlight results with respect to Qmax, IPSS, catheterization, and hospitalization times as well as morbidity. The cumulative evidence of these trials has demonstrated comparable results between the two therapies, with an edge in morbidity, catheterization and hospitalization times for Greenlight. While no tests for equivalence were performed, it is clear that PVP outcomes are comparable if not better than TURP and the degree of symptomatic and functional improvements are similar with much decreased operative and post-operative morbidity.

In summary, physician research has reported the advantages of PVP to include: (a) fewer intra-operative bleeding events than TURP; (b) no absorption of irrigant fluid, thus reducing the risk of diluted hyponatremia;[76] (c) it can be used in high-risk special patient populations, for instance, patients on anticoagulation;[77, 78] or patients with other co-morbidities, for example, severe cardiac or pulmonary disease[79] (d) a broader range of potential anesthesia could be used; and (e) catheterization and/or hospital-stay time is shorter. Additionally the added economic benefits derived from the device could have an enormous positive impact on healthcare world-wide.

REFERENCES

1. Anson K. Could the latest generation potassium titanyl phosphate lasers be the ones to make transurethral resection of the prostate an operation of historical interest only? *Curr Opin Urol.* 2004;14:27-29. Review.
2. Malek RS, Nahen K. Photoselective Vaporization of the Prostate (PVP): KTP Laser Therapy of obstructive Benign Prostatic Hyperplasia. *AUA Update, Lesson 20.* 2004;23:153-160.
3. Stovsky MD, Griffiths RI, Duffs SB. A Clinical Outcomes And Cost Analysis Comparing Photoselective Vaporization Of The Prostate To Alternative Minimally Invasive Therapies And Transurethral Prostate Resection For The Treatment Of Benign Prostatic Hyperplasia. *J Urol.* 2006;176:1500-1506.
4. Reich O, Bachmann A, Zaak D, Hofstetter A, Sulser T, Steif CG. Photoselective Vaporization of the Prostate (PVP): Prospective Evaluation in 85 High Risk Patients. *J Urol.* 2005;173:422. Supplement.
5. Sandhu JS, Nb CK, Gonzalez RR, Kaplan SA, Te AE. Photoselective laser vaporization prostatectomy in men receiving anticoagulants. *J Endourol.* 2005;19:1196–1198.
6. Fu WJ, Hong BF, Wang XX, Yang Y, Cai W, Gao JP, Chen YF, Zhang CE. Evaluation of greenlight photoselective vaporization of the prostate for the treatment of high-risk patients with benign prostatic hyperplasia. *Asian J Androl.* 2006;8:367-371.
7. Malloy TR, Harryhill JF, Smith AL. Potassium-Titanyl-Phosphate (KTP) *Laser Vaporization of the Prostate in Hematologically Impaired Patients with Benign Prostatic Hypertrophy.* Amer Society for Las Medicin Surg. April 2005 Annual Meeting.
8. Mueller EJ. *Photoselective Vaporization of the Prostate (PVP): a Case Report of a Hematologically Impaired High Risk Patient with Acute Urinary Retention Secondary to Bladder Outlet Obstruction.* Amer Society for Las Medicin Surg April 2005 Annual Meeting.
9. Bachmann A, Ruszat R, Siefert HH, Casella R, Wyler S, Sulser T. Photoselective Vaporization of the Prostate (PVP) in Men with Preoperative Catheterization Due to Chronic Urinary Retention. *J Urol.* 2005;173:424. Supplement.
10. Malek RS, Hai MA, Nseyo UO, Lapeyrolerie J. Photoselective Vaporization of the Prostate: Breakthrough Treatment for BPH.
11. Malek RS, Kuntzman RS, Barrett DM. High Power Potassium-Titanyl-Phosphate Laser Vaporization Prostatectomy. *J Urol.* 2000;163:1730-1733.
12. Malek RS, Kuntzman RS. Photoselective Vaporization of the Prostate: 5-Year Experience with High Power KTP Laser. *J Urol.* 2003;169(4)supl:390.
13. Te AE, Malloy TR, Stein BS, Ulchaker JC, Nseyo UO, Hai MA, Malek RS. Photoselective Vaporization of the Prostate for the Treatment of Benign Prostatic Hyperplasia: 12-Month Results from the First United States Multi-Center Prospective Trial. *J Urol.* 2004;172: Part 1:1404-1408.
14. Malloy TR, Stein BS, Ulchaker JC, Nseyo UO, Hai MA, Malek RS, Te AE. Photoselective Vaporization of the Prostate (PVP) for the Treatment of Benign Prostatic Hyperplasia (BPH): 24-Month Results from a Prospective Multi-Center Clinical Trial. *J Urol.* 2004;171:399. Supplement.
15. Te AE, Malloy TR, Stein BS, Ulchaker JC, Nseyo UO, Hai MA. Impact of Prostate-Specific Antigen and Prostate Volume as Predictors of Efficacy Outcomes in Photoselective Vaporization Prostatectomy (PVP):Analysis and Results of Ongoing Prospective Multi-Center Study at 3 Years. *J Urol.* 2005;173:421. Supplement.
16. Te AE, Malloy TR, Stein BS, Ulchaker JC, Nseyo UO, Hai MA, Malek RS. Photoselective Laser Vaporization of the Prostate (PVP) for the Treatment of Benign Prostatic Hyperplasia (BPH): The First Multi-Center Prospective Trial. *J Urol.* 2003;169:465. Supplement.
17. Hai MA. *Initial Experience with Greenlight HPS Laser in the Treatment of Obstructive Benign Prostatic Hyperplasia.* June 2007, 40th Congress of the International College of Surgeons.

18. Abrams P, Cardozo L, Fall M *et al*. The standardization of terminology of lower urinary tract function: report from the Standardization Sub-committee of the International Continence Society. *Neurourol Urodyn.* 2002;21:167-178.

19. Levy A, Samraj GP. Benign prostatic hyperplasia: when to 'watch and wait,' when and how to treat. *Cleveland Clinic Journal of Medicine.* 2007;74:S15-S20.

20. Ackerman SJ, Rein AL, Blute M, Beusterien K, Sullivan EM, Tanio CP, Manyak MJ, Strauss MJ. Cost Effectiveness of Microwave Thermotherapy in Patients with BPH: Part I – Methods. *Urology* 2000;56:972-980.

21. Lepor H, Rigaud G. The Efficacy of Transurethral Resection of the Prostate in Men with Moderate Symptoms of Prostatism. *J Urol.* 1990;143:533-537.

22. Mebust WK, Holtgrewe HL, Cockett AT, Peters PC. Transurethral Prostatectomy: Immediate and Postoperative Complications. A Cooperative Study of 13 Participating Institutions Evaluating 3,885 Patients. *J Urol.* 2002;167:999-1003.

23. Madersbacher S, Marberger M. Is Transurethral Resection of the Prostate still Justified? *BJU International.* 1999;83:227-237.

24. Anson K. Could the latest generation potassium titanyl phosphate lasers be the ones to make transurethral resection of the prostate an operation of historical interest only? *Curr Opin Urol.* 2004;14:27-29. Review.

25. Gilling PJ, Kennett KM, Fraundorfer MR. Holmium laser resection v transurethral resection of the prostate: results of a randomized trial with 2 years of follow-up. *J Endourol.* 2000;14:757-760.

26. Shah HN, Mahajan AP, Sodha HS, Hedge S, Mohile PD, Bansal MB. Prospective Evaluation of the Learning Curve for Holmium Laser Enucleation of the Prostate. *J Urol.* 2007;177:1468-1474.

27. Gilling PJ, Cass CB, Malcolm AR, Fraundorfer MR. Combination holmium and Nd:YAG laser ablation of the prostate: initial clinical experience. *J Endourol.* 1995;9:151-153.

28. Mottet N, Anidjar M, Bourdon O, Louis JF, Teillac P, Costa P, Le Duc A. Randomized comparison of transurethral electroresection and holmium: YAG laser vaporization for symptomatic benign prostatic hyperplasia. *J Endourol.* 1999;13:127-130.

29. Tan AH, Gilling PJ, Kennett KM, Fletcher H, Fraundorfer MR. Long-term results of high-power holmium laser vaporization (ablation) of the prostate. *BJU Int.* 2003;92:707-709.

30. Tan AH, Gilling PJ. Holmium laser prostatectomy. *BJU Int.* 2003;92:527-530. Review.

31. Wilson LC, Gilling PJ. Lasers for Prostate Surgery – An Update. Business Briefing: *European Kidney and Urologic Disease.* 2006:44-47. Review.

32. Malek RS. Photoselective KTP laser vaporization of obstructive BPH. In: Baba S, Ono Y (Eds). *Recent Advances in Endourology 8: Interventional Management of Urological Diseases.* Tokyo: Springer Verlag; 2006: 103-122.

33. Malek R, Kuntzman RS, Barrett DM. Photoselective potassium-titanyl-phosphate laser vaporization of the benign obstructive prostate: observations on long-term outcomes. *J Urol.* 2005;174:1344-1348.

34. Te AE. The Development of Laser Prostatectomy. *BJU Intl.* 2004;93:262-265.

35. Malek RS, Nahen K. Photoselective Vaporization of the Prostate (PVP): KTP Laser Therapy of obstructive Benign Prostatic Hyperplasia. *AUA Update, Lesson 20.* 2004;23:153-160.

36. Hai MA. *Laser Ablation of the Prostate Using Only KTP Energy.* 13th World Congress of Endourol and ESWL 1995. Poster.

37. Hai MA. *Current Experiences with KTP as the Sole Energy Source for Laser Prostatectomy.* Society for Laparo. Surg. Annual Meeting 1995. Poster.

38. Kuntzmann RS, Malek RS, Barrett DM, Bostwick DG. High Power (60W) Potassium-Titanyl-Phosphate Laser Vaporization Prostatectomy in Living Canines and in Human and Canine Cadavers. *Urology* 1997;49:703-708.

39. Malek RS, Barrett DM, Kuntzman RS. High Power Potassium-Titanyl-Phosphate (KTP/532) Laser Vaporization Prostatectomy: 24 hours later. *Urology* 1998;51:254-256.

40. Malek RS, Kuntzman RS, Barrett DM. High Power Potassium-Titanyl-Phosphate Laser Vaporization Prostatectomy. J Urol. 2000;163:1730-1733.

41. Hai MA, Malek RS. Photoselective vaporization of the prostate: initial experience with a new 80 W KTP laser for the treatment of benign prostatic hyperplasia. *J Endourol.* 2003;17:93-96.

42. Te AE, Malloy TR, Stein BS, Ulchaker JC, Nseyo UO, Hai MA, Malek RS. Photoselective Vaporization of the Prostate for the Treatment of BPH: 12 Month results from the first United States Multicenter Prospective Trial. *J Urol.* 2004;172:1404-1408.

43. Malloy TR, Stein BS, Ulchaker JC, Nseyo UO, Hai MA, Malek RS, Te AE. Photoselective Vaporization of the Prostate (PVP) for the Treatment of Benign Prostatic Hyperplasia (BPH): 24-Month Results from a Prospective Multi-Center Clinical Trial. *J Urol.* 2004;171:399. Supplement.

44. Te AE, Malloy TR, Stein BS, Ulchaker JC, Nseyo UO, Hai MA. Impact of Prostate Specific Antigen Level and Prostate Volume as Predictors of Efficacy in Photoselective Vaporization Prostatectomy: Analysis and Results of an Ongoing Prospective Multicenter Study at 3 years. *BJU Intl.* 2006;97:1229-1233.

45. Te AE, Malloy TR, Stein BS, Ulchaker JC, Nseyo UO, Hai MA, Malek RS. Photoselective Laser Vaporization of the Prostate (PVP) for the Treatment of Benign Prostatic Hyperplasia (BPH): The First Multi-Center Prospective Trial. *J Urol.* 2003;169:465. Supplement.

46. Sandhu JS, Ng CK, Gonzalez R, Kaplan SA, Te AE. High-Power Photoselective Laser Vaporization Prostatectomy (PVP) in Men with Large Prostates: The New York Presbyterian Series of 64 Patients. *J Urol.* 2004;171:400. Supplement.

47. Bachmann A, Ruszat R, Wyler S, Reich O, Seifert H, Muller A, Sulser T. Photoselective Vaporization of the Prostate: The Basel Experience after 108 Procedures. *Eur Urol.* 2005;47:798-804.

48. Muir G. Advances in Laser Treatment for Benign Prostatic Hyperplasia. *Eur Kidney and Urol Dis.* 2005;44-47.

49. Mueller E. *Photoselective Vaporization of the Prostate (PVP) for Treatment of Benign Prostatic Hyperplasia (BPH): The Methodist Experience.* Presented at the James C Kimbrough Urological Meeting January 2005.

50. Jung G, Ok Y, Choi E. High-Power KTP Photoselective Laser Vaporization Prostatectomy for Treatment of Benign Prostatic Hyperplasia (BPH). *Eur Urol.* 2005;4:151. Supplement.

51. Reiter R. *Photoselective Vaporization of the Prostate (PVP): Is This a Safer & Less Costly Alternative to TUR? The UCLA Experience.* James C Kimbrough Urological Meeting, Jan 2005.

52. Bouchier-Hayes DM, Anderson P, Van Appledorn S, Bugeja P, Costello AJ. KTP laser versus transurethral resection: early results of a randomized trial. *J Endourol.* 2006;20:580-585.

53. Bachmann A, Schurch L, Ruszat R, Wyler S, Seifert H, Muller A, Lehmann K, Sulser T. Photoselective vaporization of the prostate versus transurethral resection of the prostate: a prospective bi-center study of perioperative morbidity and early functional outcome. *Eur Urol.* 2005;48:965–972.

54. Bouchier-Hayes DM. Photoselective vaporization of the prostate—towards a new standard. *Prostate Cancer Prostat Dis.* 2007;10:S10-S14.

55. Sarica K, Altay B. Photoselective vaporization (PVP) versus transurethral resection of the prostate (TURP) for prostates >80 G: a prospective randomized trial. *Eur Urol Suppl.* 2007;6:163.

56. Bachmann A, Ruszat R, Straumann U, Wyler A, Schurch L, Forster T, Reich O, Lehmann K, Sulser T. Photoselective Vaporization of the Prostate (PVP) Versus Transurethral Resection of the Prostate (TURP). *Eur Urol Suppl.* 2006;5:236.

57. Ruszat R, Sulser T, Seifert HH, Wyler S, Forster T, Leippold T, Bachmann A. Photoselective Vaporization (PVP) vs. Transurethral Electroresection of the Prostate (TURP): A Comparing Cost Analysis. *Eur Urol Suppl.* 2006;5:271.

58. Han DH, Chung JW, Kim JY, Jung BJ, Hong JH, Lee SW. Impact of 80 watt KTP photoselective laser vaporization prostatectomy versus transurethral resection of the prostate on prostate volume and severity of obstruction: 6-month results of a prospective trial. *J Urol.* 2007;177(4 suppl).

59. Park J, Song SH, Lee SB, Hong B, Ahn TY. Photoselective vaporization of the prostate for benign prostatic hypertrophy: comparison of short-term treatment outcomes with TURP. *Eur Urol Suppl.* 2006;5:235.

60. Tugcu V, Tasci AI, Sahin S, Karakas F, Zorluoglu F. Photoselective vaporization of the prostate (PVP) versus transurethral resection of the prostate (TURP): a prospedtive nonrandomized bi-centre trial, 2-year follow-up. *Eur Urol Suppl.* 2007;6:191.

61. Sulser T, Schurch L, Ruszat R, Reich O, Lehmann K, Bachmann A. Prospective comparison of photoselective laser vaporization (PVP) and transurethral resection of the prostate (TURP). *J Urol.* 2005;173(4 Supplement):422.

62. Park J, You CH, Hong B, Choo MS, Kim CS, Ahn H, Ahn TY. Comparison of treatment outcomes between photoselective vaporization and transurethral resection of the prostate depending on experiences of surgery. *Eur Urol Suppl.* 2007;6:193.

63. Te AE, Sandhu JS, Gonzalez RR, Egan C, Kaplan SA. High Power KTP Photoselective Vaporization Prostatectomy (PVP) versus Trans-Urethral Electrovaporization of the Prostate (TVP) for the Treatment of Benign Prostatic Hyperplasia (BPH): A Prospective Comparative Trial. *J Urol.* 2004; 171:402.

64. Malek RS, Hai MA, Nseyo UO, Lapeyrolerie J. Photoselective Vaporization of the Prostate: Breakthrough Treatment for BPH.

65. Alivizatos G, Skolarikos A, Chalikopoulos D, Papachristou C, Sopilidis O, Dellis A, Kastriotis I, Deliveliotis C. Transurethral Photoselective Vaporization versus Transvesical Open Enucleation for Prostatic Adenomas >80 ml: 12-mo Results of a Randomized Prospective Study. *Eur Urol.* 2007 Nov 29; [Epub ahead of print]

66. Stovsky MD, Griffiths RI, Duff SB. A Clinical Outcomes and Cost Analysis Comparing Photoselective Vaporization of the Prostate to Alternative Minimally Invasive Therapies and Trans-Urethral Prostate Resection for the Treatment of Benign Prostatic Hyperplasia. *J Urol.* 2006;176:1500-1506.

67. Sandhu JS, Ng C, Vanderbrink BA, Egan C, Kaplan S, Te AE. High Powered Potassium-Titanyl-Phosphate Photoselective Vaporization of Prostate for Treatment of Benign Prostatic Hyperplasia in Men with Large Prostates. *J Urol.* 2004;64:1155-9.

68. Chandrasekera SK, Barber NJ, Walsh K, Thompson PM, Muir GH. Greenlight PVP: Safety and Efficacy in Large Prostates > 100 cm3. *J Urol.* 2004;173:425. Supplement.

69. Reich O, Bachmann A, Zaak D, Hofstetter A, Sulser T, Steif CG. Photoselective Vaporization of the Prostate (PVP): Prospective Evaluation in 85 High Risk Patients. *J Urol.* 2005;173:422. Supplement.

70. Sandhu JS, Ng CK, Gonzalez RR, Kaplan SA, Te AE. Photoselective laser vaporization prostatectomy in men receiving anticoagulants. *J Endourol.* 2005;19:1196–1198.

71. Fu WJ, Hong BF, Wang XX, Yang Y, Cai W, Gao JP, Chen YF, Zhang CE. Evaluation of greenlight photoselective vaporization of the prostate for the treatment of high-risk patients with benign prostatic hyperplasia. *Asian J Androl.* 2006;8:367-371.

72. Malloy TR, Harryhill JF, Smith AL. *Potassium-Titanyl-Phosphate (KTP) Laser Vaporization of the Prostate in Hematologically Impaired Patients with Benign Prostatic Hypertrophy.* Amer Society for Las Medicin Surg April 2005 Annual Meeting.

73. Mueller EJ. *Photoselective Vaporization of the Prostate (PVP): a Case Report of a Hematologically Impaired High Risk Patient with Acute Urinary Retention Secondary to Bladder Outlet Obstruction.* Amer Society for Las Medicin Surg April 2005 Annual Meeting.

74. Bachmann A, Ruszat R, Siefert HH, Casella R, Wyler S, Sulser T. Photoselective Vaporization of the Prostate (PVP) in Men with Preoperative Catheterization Due to Chronic Urinary Retention. *J Urol.* 2005;173:424. Supplement.

75. Wong C, Araki M, Tonkin JB. High-Power Potassium-Titanyl-Phosphate or Lithium Triboride Laser Photoselective Vaporization Prostatectomy for Benign Prostatic Hyperplasia: A Systematic Approach. *J Endourol.* 2007;21:1141-1144.

76. Barber NJ, Zhu G, Donohue JF, Thompson PM, Walsh K, Muir GH. Use of Expired Breath Ethanol Measurements in Evaluation of Irrigant Absorption During High-Power Potassium Titanyl Phosphate Laser Vaporization of Prostate. *Urology.* 2006;67:80-83.

77. Sandhu JS, Ng CK, Gonzalez RR *et al.* Photoselective laser vaporization prostatectomy in men receiving anticoagulants. *J Endourol.* 2005;19:1196-1198.

78. Reich O, Bachmann A, Siebels M, Hofstetter A, Stief CG, Sulser T. High Power (80W) Potassium-Titanyl-Phosphate Laser Vaporization of the Prostate in 66 High Risk Patients. *J Urol.* 2005;173:158-160.

79. Chepurou AK. Holmium laser treatment of benign prostatic hyperplasia *Urologiia.* 1999;4:39-41.

ABOUT THE AUTHOR

Dr. Mahmood Hai is a Senior Urology Consultant at Oakwood Hospital, Chief of Urology at Annapolis Hospital, and the Medical Director of Cherry Hill Medical Center. He is a Fellow of the International College of Surgeons, and a member of many urology associations. Dr. Hai has used lasers in urology for nearly twenty years.

Chapter 16
Personalizing Hormone Treatment: The Whole Picture
Patrick Hanaway, M.D.
Chief Medical Officer, Genova Diagnostics

ABSTRACT

Many physicians and their female patients are facing difficult questions regarding the decision to use hormone replacement therapy (HRT). The current confusion surrounding HRT highlights the peril of applying a "one size fits all" approach. An individualized approach includes phenotypic and genotypic testing. The first questions that many physicians ask are:

- Should a women entering menopause begin HRT?
- Who needs it and who doesn't?

Once the decision to begin HRT is determined, the delivery system and dosage are required. We have learned a great deal about the various delivery systems for bioidentical HRT, as well as other hormones. Now the questions become:

- How does one determine the unique and individual needs of the patient?
- How does one personalize the treatment?

Determining the specific, individualized needs of each patient allows us to personalize our treatment. Hormonal assessments, based upon the 3-dimensional perspective of urine, serum, and saliva, will help to generate the best answers in meeting the needs of each individual patient. This will enable the physician to determine the best combination of hormonal therapies that will provide the maximum benefits and minimum risks.

The aim of this paper is to answer these questions, and therefore provide the anti-aging physician with the knowledge necessary to personalize a patient's hormone treatment program.

INTRODUCTION

Many physicians and their female patients are facing difficult questions regarding the decision to use hormone replacement therapy (HRT). The current confusion surrounding HRT highlights the peril of applying a "one size fits all" approach.

When considering prescribing HRT, it is very important that the physician has a good understanding of:

- The interrelationships between hormones,
- The hormonal metabolic pathways (i.e. how the hormones are transformed when they circulate and move into the cell), and
- The intracellular and intranuclear effects of hormones and their metabolites.

Of course, the first thing that the physician needs to determine is whether or not the patient would actually benefit from HRT, or whether they may benefit more from nutritional support and/or lifestyle changes. Then, if it is decided that HRT is the best course of action, it is necessary to determine what hormones need replacing, which form of delivery is most suitable, and what dosage is required. The thing to focus on when deciding on these factors is balance – the goal of the anti-aging physician is to determine the best combination of hormonal therapies that will provide the maximum benefits and the minimum risks.

This is where we need to think about the concept of biochemical individuality or genomic predisposition. Remember; one size does not fit all! By looking at biochemical individuality we can begin to modify and personalize treatment recommendations in order to maximize the benefits of health and wellbeing for the patient.

The concept of biochemical individuality in Western medicine began to develop at the turn of the century when we started to gain an understanding of genetics. The term "biochemical individuality" was first coined by Roger Williams in 1956 to explain genetic variance in disease susceptibility, nutrient needs, and drug responsiveness among otherwise seemingly healthy people. But, if we look at Ayurvedic medicine, Traditional Chinese Medicine (TCM), and ancient Greek medicine, we will find the common belief that we are all inherently different, and that it is important to work with those differences.

Unfortunately, mainstream Western medicine is, at present, standing firmly by the 'medicine for the masses' approach and is keen to apply the same therapeutics to every person who comes in. This approach does not work very well, and what sets anti-aging physicians apart from the majority is that we have the wisdom and foresight to be able to see that this approach is not working for everybody. Our aim is to understand and highlight the differences between individuals; to personalize our care.

In my practice, I have found that I need to individualize and target specific therapies for each person. But when I recognized the importance of this, I did not have the tools to help me understand the role, relationship, and interaction of specific hormones. The aim of this paper is to provide you with these tools.

THE IMPORTANCE OF THE STEROIDOGENIC PATHWAYS

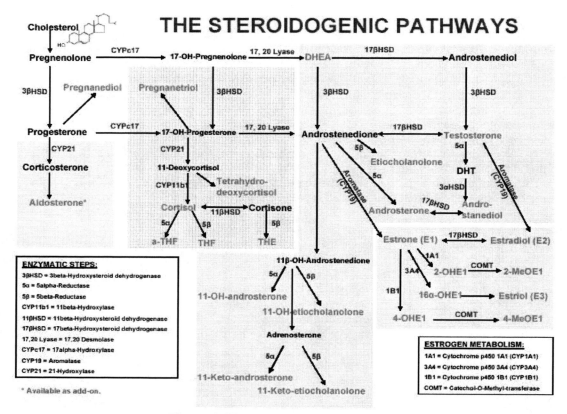

Figure 1. The steroidogenic pathways.

It is very important to be aware of the steroidogenic pathways when prescribing HRT. As can be seen in Figure 1, cholesterol is a precursor for all the steroid hormones, and all the hormones are interrelated. Another important point that is apparent when we look at Figure 1 is that pregnenolone, progesterone, and DHEA are prohormones, and it is vital that everyone has sufficient amounts of these prohormones in order to be able to drive the other pathways. So, whenever we are thinking about prescribing a patient HRT, it is vital that we determine their pregnenolone, progesterone, and DHEA levels, and ensure that their levels are adequate.

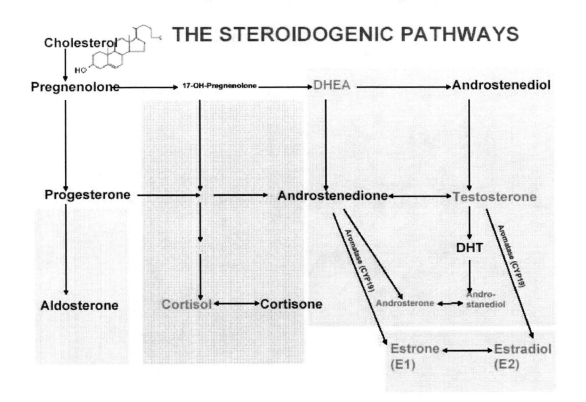

Figure 2. A simplified version of the steroidogenic pathways.

If we look at Figure 2, which is a simplified version of the steroidogenic pathways, the importance of pregnenolone, progesterone, and DHEA, and their role in the production of testosterone and (via aromatase) the production of estrone and estradiol, is clearly obvious.

An interesting thing happens to the steroidogenic pathway when we have a lot of stress in our lives. When we are stressed, we have a preferential drive towards the synthesis of cortisol and cortisone, and the precursors that are necessary for the production of DHEA and sex hormones are blocked. Thus, stress impedes the production of DHEA and the sex hormones. We need to keep this in mind. If we are driving everything through the stress reaction to synthesize cortisol and cortisone, then we are going to end up with imbalances between anabolic and catabolic hormones.

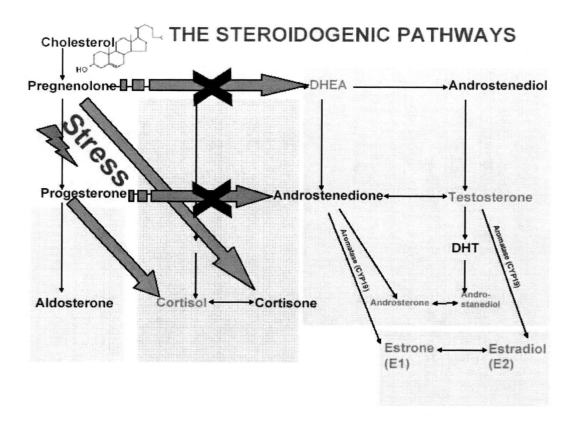

Figure 3. The impact of stress upon the steroidogenic pathways.

For optimum health we need to ensure that we maintain the correct balance between anabolic hormones, which aid rest and recovery, and catabolic hormones, which are the breakdown or "wear and tear" hormones. Androgens, such as DHEA and androsterone, are anabolic steroids, and they are often referred to as 17-ketosteroids (17-KS). On the other side of the balance are hormones such as cortisol and cortisone, which are catabolic steroids, and these are referred to as 17-hydroxysteroids (17-OHCS). We can actually look at the ratio of 17-KS to 17-OHCS in urine and use it to see whether or not HRT is benefiting the patient.

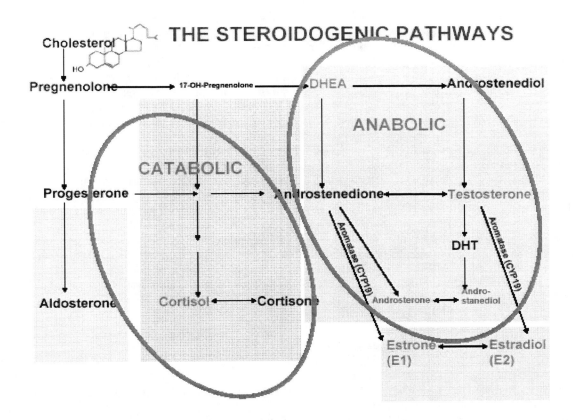

Figure 4. The steroidogenic pathways lead to the production of both anabolic and catabolic steroids.

So, we can see the importance of the interrelationship between these hormones and we can use and understand that interrelationship in clinical practice. The ratio or balance of various metabolic groups (e.g. anabolic and catabolic steroids) reflects the relationship between the hormones and metabolic pathways, whereas levels of individual hormones and metabolites do not.

PERSONALIZING HORMONE TREATMENT
Which is the Best Method for Measuring Hormone Levels?

When thinking about measuring hormone levels most doctors automatically think about blood tests. However, it is very important to think about what a circulating hormone actually is. The majority of circulating hormone is bound and is not bioavailable, and therefore using blood samples to determine a patients hormone levels is not going to tell you anything about the patient's free or bioavailable hormone levels. One effective way to find out about bioavailable hormone levels is to use saliva samples. At the same time, neither serum nor saliva sampling are going to tell us you how that hormone is taken into the cell and metabolized, to find out about that you need to be looking at urine. Thus, we have three sample types, and each has their own benefits and disadvantages.

For example, when we measure estradiol in the serum, we measure all of the estradiol, both bound and unbound. However, only 1% to 3% of the total estradiol is actually free to bind to estrogen receptors. The rest of it is bound. Some of it is loosely bound to albumin, but much of it is tightly bound to sex hormone binding globulin (SHBG). Therefore, the free fraction of a circulating hormone, which is the part that we are interested in, makes up a very small amount of the total hormone level. While estradiol does not have a diurnal variation, serum levels of certain hormones (cortisol, growth hormone, insulin, and others) fluctuate significantly throughout the day.

In reviewing the hormonal physiology, we return to estradiol, which is produced as 17-beta estradiol in the ovary. It then travels through the body, via the blood, where the vast majority (97-99%) of it is bound to SHBG or albumin. When estradiol reaches the tissues, the free fraction of the hormone passes through the estrogen receptor and moves into the cell and is metabolized. There are two different effects that occur here. There are immediate effects caused by the estradiol binding to the membrane-bound estrogen receptor, and there are long-term effects that occur when the estradiol has passed into the cell and moved into the nucleus. So, there are non-genomic signaling mechanisms that are caused by the binding of estradiol to the estrogen receptor on the cell membrane, and genomic signaling mechanisms that are triggered when estradiol moves into the nucleus of the cell. Urinary measures of the estrogen metabolites are the best way to evaluate the genomic effects of hormones, while saliva and serum are probably the best way of looking at the non-genomic effects of hormones. So, with urine, we can begin to understand the estrogenic effect on gene expression.

The classic clinical example of this membrane-bound signaling effect versus the nuclear effect of genomic expression for a circulating hormone is with progesterone. For example, transdermal progesterone is the best form of progesterone for managing the symptoms of menopause in the majority of patients, however there is a subset of patients who suffer from agitation, restlessness, and sleeping difficulties, and these patients respond better when given oral micronized progesterone. This is because with oral micronized progesterone there is an increase in serum progesterone levels that you do not get with transdermal progesterone, and that helps with the symptoms. That is an immediate, non-genomic effect, which is due to the progesterone binding to the progesterone receptor. That effect is different from the other beneficial effects of the progesterone, which occur at the genomic level.

Therefore, when thinking about how you should measure a patient's hormone levels, your need to consider:

- The physiology of the specific hormone
- The clinical question begin asked
- The therapeutic modalities being used

Growth Hormone

Growth hormone (GH) levels fluctuate wildly in the serum, so, measuring serum GH is not clinically useful. Salivary levels of GH are not measurable. However, urinary levels can be measured via a 24-hour or first morning void (FMV) urine collection, to give an average, or a spot urine sample can be used before and after a stimulation test incorporating insulin or anaerobic exercise.

Typically, we see that there is about 14% drop in GH every decade, and so by the time a person reaches their 70s or 80s they only have about 5% of the GH that they had in youth. GH acts as an anti-inflammatory hormone. While supplementing with growth hormone can be of benefit, you should only prescribe it to those people who have a recognized adult GH deficiency. Thus, you need to determine who really meets the definition of GH deficiency and will benefit from supplementation with GH. There are other therapeutic interventions than can also help to increase GH levels, such as dietary changes and exercise.

DHEA

DHEA can be measure in lots of different ways. Serum levels of DHEA-sulfate (DHEA-S) provide a useful measurement of total body stores, because they are much more stable than serum DHEA levels. Conversely, salivary levels of DHEA provide a useful measure of free hormone availability, while much lower levels of DHEA-S are found in saliva.. Urinary levels of DHEA are sensitive and reproducible. In addition, DHEA downstream metabolites and the 17-KS/17-OHCS ratio can also be evaluated.

If we look at Figure 5, we will see that DHEA levels decline with age. Now, some endocrinologists will say, "This is normal, DHEA levels are supposed to decline over time," but if you have a loss of DHEA, you also lose your ability to rest and recover. DHEA is one of the principle anabolic steroids. So, one very important way of supporting our patients is by ensuring that they have an adequate amount of DHEA.

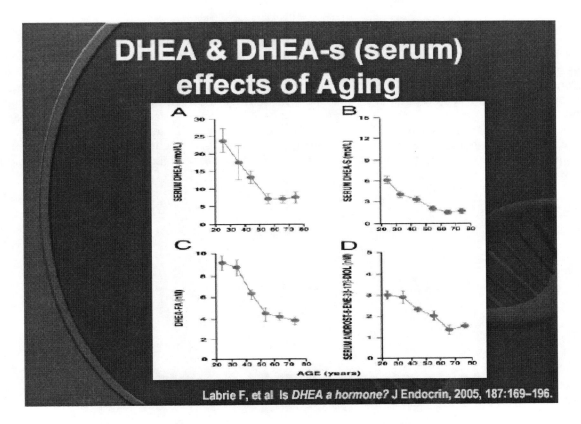

Labrie F, et al Is *DHEA a hormone?* J Endocrin, 2005, 187:169–196.

Figure 5. The effect of aging on DHEA levels.

What can we do to support patients with depleted DHEA levels? There are a number of things that will help to increase DHEA levels, one of which is DHEA supplementation. However, there are many other things that can help to increase DHEA levels, including: meditation, good nutrition, adequate and good quality sleep, and supplementary magnesium.

Cortisol

What about addressing adrenal stress and measuring cortisol levels? In order to measure serum levels it is necessary to conduct a corticotrophin-releasing hormone (CRH) stimulation test. This has been considered the 'gold standard' from endocrinologists, but the difficulty in performing this test in most offices makes it functionally prohibitive. The best way to look at cortisol clinically is to use salivary samples to look at the diurnal variation of cortisol. Cortisol levels reach a peak between 6 and 8am and then decline throughout the day. Patients in whom this diurnal variation is not present are often candidates for adrenal support and therapies. Urinary levels of cortisol help determine the total cortisol throughput within the body, and help to identify those who will benefit from bioidentical cortisone treatment. The evaluation can be done as a 24-hour collection or as a first morning void (FMV) sample. The anabolic-catabolic balance can also be used to determine if a patient is going to respond well to cortisol therapy.

CONCLUDING REMARKS

The goal of the anti-aging physician is to help patients become and remain healthy for as long as possible. One way that we can do this is by evaluating the specific, individualized needs of each patient in order to personalize their treatment. Hormonal assessments, based upon this 3-dimensional perspective of urine, serum, and saliva, will help to generate the best answers in meeting the needs of each individual patient. This approach will enable us to determine the best combination of hormonal therapies that will provide the patient with the maximum benefit and the minimum risks.

ABOUT THE AUTHOR

Dr. Patrick Hanaway is a board-certified family physician with a Medical Degree from Washington University and residency training at the University of New Mexico. Dr. Hanaway received his Bachelors degree from the University of Wisconsin in Molecular Biology and has done research in muscle biology, neurochemistry, lipid metabolism, public health, preventive medicine, immunology, digestion, and nutrition. In addition to being a family physician, Dr. Hanaway is a board-certified holistic physician and currently is on the American Board of Holistic Medicine. Dr. Hanaway founded Family to Family: Your Home for Whole Family Health in Asheville, NC, and is currently Chief Medical Officer for Genova Diagnostics. Dr. Hanaway has lectured extensively on the clinical application of nutrition and genomics; particularly in the areas of endocrinology, digestion, oxidative stress, inflammation, and achieving long-term wellness.

Chapter 17
Stress and Steroid Synthesis
Patrick Hanaway, M.D.
Chief Medical Officer, Genova Diagnostics

ABSTRACT

In normal circumstances, the body produces a fine balance of both DHEA and cortisol; however an interesting thing happens to the steroidogenic pathway when we have a lot of stress in our lives. When we are stressed, we have a preferential drive towards the synthesis of cortisol and cortisone, and the precursors that are necessary for the production of DHEA and sex hormones are blocked. This process is called "cortisol steal". The aim of this paper is to examine the effects of stress upon steroid hormone synthesis.

INTRODUCTION

When there is a sympathetic response in the body a stress signal is sent to the hypothalamus and to the anterior pituitary gland. The stress signal then stimulates the release of adrenocorticotrophic hormone (ACTH), which, in the adrenal cortex, produces cortisol (a catabolic and anti-inflammatory hormone) and DHEA (an anabolic hormone).

CORTISOL

If we look at the overall actions of cortisol it can be seen that it is actually a counter-regulatory hormone. Cortisol maintains blood glucose levels during stress reactions and provides additional glucose to the brain, heart, lungs, and skeletal muscle. It also promotes hepatic protein synthesis and gluconeogenesis, however it stimulates protein catabolism elsewhere in the body.

What this means, if we think in terms of the normal fight or flight stress response, is that cortisol helps to provide us with the extra glucose required by the skeletal muscles if we need to make a quick getaway. However, it does this at a price and will sacrifice some things in the process. One of the things that cortisol will sacrifice is the immune system. Cortisol works with the liver to aid the process of gluconeogenesis, however in order to support the liver it will promote the breakdown of fat elsewhere in the body in order to help provide extra energy.

Cortisol is also an anti-inflammatory hormone, as it downregulates inflammatory cytokines. When enough cortisol has been produced as a result of the stress signal it provides inhibitory feedback to the hypothalamus and the pituitary promoting the downregulation of both corticotrophin-releasing hormone (CRH) and ATCH.

Cortisol levels are usually at their highest first thing in the morning when you get up. Levels then gradually decline over the course of the day. This normal diurnal variation, which can be shown by salivary sampling, is an indication of a healthy adaptation to stress. Acute stress will lead to excess levels of cortisol first thing in the morning, whilst long periods of stress will result in deficient levels of cortisol first thing in the morning.

DHEA

The anabolic hormone DHEA is a prohormone for sex steroids. Whereas cortisol slows down or inactivates the immune system, DHEA stimulates the immune system. It also improves insulin sensitivity. Thus meaning that insulin works better when there are sufficient amounts of DHEA present. When there is insufficient DHEA, there is a decrease in insulin sensitivity and a corresponding increase in insulin resistance. DHEA also maintains tissue strength and repair, supports bone density, is anti-atherogenic, neuroprotective, and promotes a sense of well-being.

DHEA-sulfate (DHEA-S) is the primary storage form of DHEA in the body. When we measure DHEA in serum, we are really measuring DHEA-S. DHEA-S constitutes the largest concentration of steroids in the body. There is approximately 100-500 times more DHEA-S in the body than testosterone and over a 1000 times more DHEA-S than there is estrogen.

DHEA and DHEA-S levels peak somewhere between 20 and 30 years of age (some studies say between 20 and 40 years of age), and thereafter both DHEA and DHEA-S levels decrease markedly. So, as we get older our DHEA levels decline, thus depleting our ability to manufacture sufficient amounts of both anabolic or so-called "rest and recovery" hormones and sex hormones. Results of a study of 2500 aging African-American women by Haren *et al* showed that participants DHEA-S and estradiol (E2) levels declined in parallel.[1] The study also found that lower DHEA-S levels were independently associated with increased problems of physical disability and depression.

THE EFFECT OF STRESS ON STEROID HORMONE SYNTHESIS

One of the great pioneers of modern medicine who has been largely forgotten is Hans Selye. Selye discovered that all the mammals he studied reacted to stress in a certain way. He called this response General Adaptation Syndrome (GAS). Stress can be caused by a vast number of things, from "fight or flight" responses, fear, anxiety, worry, depression, feelings of defeat or helplessness, to infection, inflammation, illness, pain syndromes, and hypoglycemia. Our environment is also a great source of stress – we are under constant bombardment from both physical and mental stressors in the form of light pollution, air pollution, and noise pollution. All of these factors, plus inadequate sleep, poor nutrition, and other hallmarks of our modern lifestyle mean that we are now exposed to approximately 1000 times more stressors in our lives than we were one hundred years ago.

The body responds to stress by secreting cortisol. As soon as the body is exposed to a stressor cortisol levels rise, they then plateau, and finally they begin to drop. Cortisol levels fall again much quicker in younger, more resilient, people than in older people. However, when we are placed under chronic stress we do not respond to cortisol as well, and therefore cortisol production is upregulated. The end result is permanently elevated cortisol levels. We learnt earlier that cortisol is a catabolic hormone. It breaks things down. Therefore permanently raised cortisol levels are far from desirable.

If we think about the steroidogenic pathway shown in Figure 1, we can see that cholesterol is a precursor for all the steroid hormones, and that all the hormones are interrelated. Cortisol and DHEA are derived from the same precursors. So, the body has to determine whether it will produce cortisol, DHEA, or both. In normal circumstances, the body produces a fine balance of both DHEA and cortisol; however an interesting thing happens to the steroidogenic pathway when we have a lot of stress in our lives. When we are stressed, we have a preferential drive towards the synthesis of cortisol and cortisone, and the precursors that are necessary for the production of DHEA and sex hormones are blocked. This process is called "cortisol steal". The net result of cortisol steal is that the person will have higher cortisol levels and lower levels of DHEA and all of the other hormones that are downstream from DHEA.

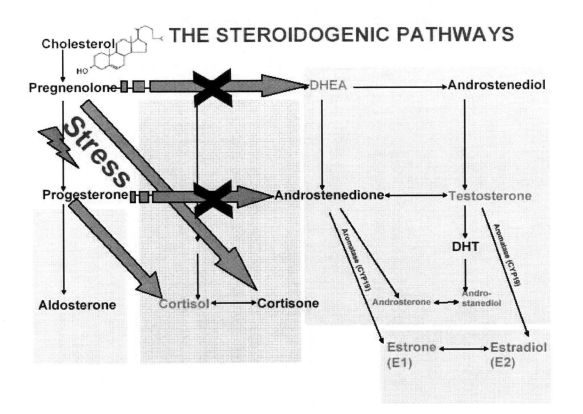

Figure 1. The impact of stress upon the steroidogenic pathways.

Cortisol steal is not uncommon. Many of us are continuously exposed to different types of stressors. The day-to-day difficulties involved with trying to balance both work and family life is enough to cause adrenocorticol hyperactivity and adrenal upregulation. Of course, adrenocorticol hyperactivity is life-saving in the short-term, as catabolism frees up energy reserves. However, over the long-term, persistent cortisol production is associated with immune suppression, hyperglycemia, insulin resistance, central adiposity, hypertension, memory impairment due to hippocampal damage, hyperlipidemia, and impaired hepatic T4 to T3 conversion.

Persistently high cortisol output also leads to cortisol receptor desensitization in the hippocampus, which, in turn, leads to a chronically high CRH output. CRH is an independent neurotransmitter and persistently high levels of CRH can cause a number of unpleasant gastrointestinal symptoms (reduced gastric emptying and colonic contractility, diarrhea, and bowel inflammation) and depression.

If adrenocorticol hyperactivity is allowed to continue it will come to a point where the adrenal glands simply cannot keep on producing such high levels of cortisol. Some people refer to this point as phase III adrenal fatigue. Phase I is where the adrenal glands are functioning normally, phase II is characterized by the upregulation of cortisol and the depletion of DHEA, and phase III is where you have not only a depletion of the DHEA, but also a complete depletion in cortisol levels. It is important to note that phase III adrenal fatigue is not the same as Addison's disease - if you give people with phase III adrenal fatigue a large dose of cosyntropin and you checked their cortisol levels 15, 30, and 60 minutes later, you would see that they do have some response. So, phase III adrenal fatigue is not as serious as Addison's disease, but it still has consequences. Low cortisol levels are associated with fatigue, hypotension, hypocglycemia, sugar cravings, heightened inflammatory responses, and greater conversion of T4 to T3.

The Anabolic-Catabolic Balance

The idea of the anabolic-catabolic balance has been around for the past 30 years, yet it is still a relatively new idea to most physicians. A lot of the early literature about the anabolic-catabolic balance came from Eastern Bloc countries where they were working with their Olympic athletes to try to optimize their anabolic capabilities. The scientists found that a fine balance exists between anabolic and catabolic hormones, and shifting that balance too far in either direction leads to problems.

Of course, chronic stress and the cortisol steal effect is going to disrupt the fine balance that exists between anabolic and catabolic hormones. For optimum health we need to ensure that we maintain the correct balance between anabolic hormones, which aid rest and recovery, and catabolic hormones, which are the breakdown or "wear and tear" hormones. Androgens, such as DHEA and androsterone, are anabolic steroids, and they are often referred to as 17-ketosteroids (17-KS). On the other side of the balance are hormones such as cortisol and cortisone, which are catabolic steroids, and these are referred to as 17-hydroxysteroids (17-OHCS).

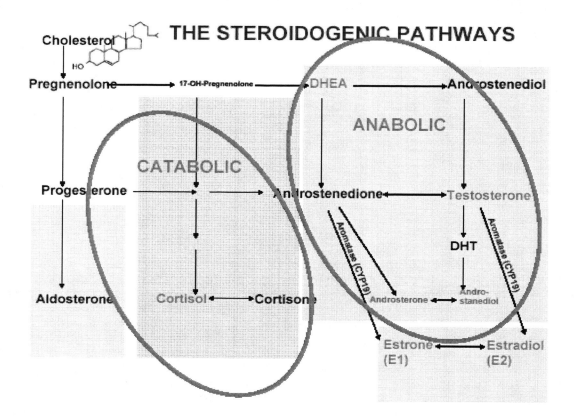

Figure 2. The steroidogenic pathways lead to the production of both anabolic and catabolic steroids.

It is now possible determine the ratio of 17-KS to 17-OHCS in the urine and use it to provide you with a valuable insight into the anabolic or catabolic state of your patient. Nishkaze[2] wrote about this test: *"The measurement of 17-KS, which decreases with failing health, when combined with 17-OHCS, may make it possible to evaluate distortions in the organism (disturbance of adaptability), which bring the presence of illness or the susceptibility to illness in each person to our notice. Further adding a new dimension to clinical diagnostic acumen in an objective evaluation of psychosocial stress...where results of clinical routine tests are often within normal limits."*

The ratio of 17-KS-S/17-OHCS is altered by both mental and physical stress. Results of a study by Furuya *et al* showed: *"In subjects with severe mental stress the ratio of 17-KS-S/17-OHCS showed markedly reduced values with a transient marked increase in 17-OHCS. There was a decrease in the levels of 17-KS-S in depressives, which was more pronounced during severe depression...These results suggest that measurement of 17-KS-S is indispensable for current research on psychosocial stress."[3]*

142

Whilst results of a study by Kano *et al* of children with atopic dermatitis or renal disease show that stress also has profound effects upon the anabolic-catabolic balance in children.[4]

IDENTIFYING PROBLEMS WITHIN THE STEROIDOGENIC PATHWAYS

It is important not to jump to conclusions when treating a patient that you suspect of having a hormone imbalance. A good example of this is a 56-year-old postmenopausal patient of mine who came to my office complaining of fatigue and hot flashes. Now, the first thing the vast majority of doctors would think about in this scenario is estrogen. They would think about the hot flashes and prescribe estrogen and maybe check her serum estrogen levels. I would do things a little differently, I would give her some estrogen to help her with her climacteric symptoms, and then I would run a whole series of lab tests, including taking a look at the diurnal variation of her cortisol levels.

The results of the lab tests showed that this woman had a very low level of DHEA, and very low levels of progesterone metabolites. She also had relatively low estrogen levels, which we could tell from her symptoms, but she also had low levels of her anabolic hormones and androgens. Her anabolic/catabolic ratio was also very low at 0.44 (should be at least 1, but ideally around 1.2). So, we can determine that this patient is suffering from the cortisol steal effect. Her body is driving everything towards the production of cortisol, to the point that she does not have enough DHEA to be able to manufacture the estrogen, testosterone, and other androgens that her body needs. Therefore she has developed multiple hormone deficiencies and is starting to develop symptoms of those deficiencies.

Thus, we can see that this lady had several major issues going on, which all needed addressing. If we simply address her problems symptomatically by giving her estrogen, we are going to miss the point. If a patient has low levels of both estrogens and androgens we need to think about the steroidogenic pathways and the enzymes involved in those pathways. Do they have adequate amounts of DHEA and DHEA-S to be able to produce those hormones? What should you do?

Well, the obvious answer to this problem is that we should simply replenish the patient's DHEA levels. However, it is not quite that simple. If you give someone DHEA, and they have a genomic predisposition to drive everything to make 4-hydroxyestrone or 16-alpha-hydroxyestrone, and they are not able to make the proper methyl derivatives, you are actually increasing that person's risk of breast cancer by giving them DHEA. Similarly, if you have got a patient who has problems with aromatase activity, and they are not converting testosterone into the estrogens, and you give them DHEA, you are ultimately increasing the problem of androgenic drive, which will only serve to worsen any problems the patient may have, for example polycystic ovary syndrome (PCOS). Therefore it is important to understand all of the pathways involved in steroid synthesis. [See Fig. 3.]

The Importance of Aromatase Activity Pathways

DHEA and DHEA-S are converted to androstenedione by 3-beta-HSD. Androstenedione is converted to estrone and testosterone, and testosterone is also converted to estradiol. The conversion of androstenedione to estrone and testosterone to estradiol both involve aromatase activity pathways. There are many factors that upregulate and downregulate aromatase activity. Upregulated aromatase activity will lead to high estrogen levels and low androgen levels, whilst donwregulated aromatase activity will lead to high androgen levels and low estrogen levels.

Factors that upregulate aromatase activity include: abdominal obesity, elevated cortisol and glucocorticoid levels, hyperinsulinemia, zinc deficiency, inflammatory cytokines, alcohol, the herb Coleus forskohlii, and the asthma drug Isoproterenol. Therefore several issues that contribute to cortisol steal also upregulate aromatase activity. So, if a patient has problems that put them at high risk of cortisol steal, it is likely that they are also going to be aromatizing androgens into estrogen. This can cause issues, ranging from concerns about strength and libido, to very serious issues concerning increased risk for prostate and breast cancer as well.

So, what should we do if the patient has upregulated aromatase activity? The pharmaceutical companies have invested a lot of money into developing aromatase inhibitors, should we be giving those to our patients? No, we should be dealing with the causes of upregulated aromatase activity (and cortisol steal) in the first instance; medication should be the last resort. Decreasing abdominal obesity, combating inflammation, eating a well-balanced diet, and managing stress could be of significant help to many problems with the steroidogenic pathways.

Many factors that inhibit aromatase activity can be found in food, these include: flavonoids (e.g., chrysin, naringenin, and hesperitin), phytoestrogens (e.g., flaxseed), procyanidins in grape seed and red wine, and vitamin c. This demonstrates how nutrition and the right kind of nutritional supplements can be used to balance hormones. When I see a patient who has an abundance of estrogen, but virtually no 17-ketosteroids because they are driving everything through the aromatase pathway, I will treat them nutritionally. Giving them DHEA is not the answer. DHEA can be useful but it is vital that you know what is going to happen to it. The bottom line is that lowering stress levels, getting plenty of sleep, eating lots of fruit and vegetables and less animal products, losing weight if necessary, and taking regular exercise can do wonders.

Dihydrotestosterone

Another example of why it is vital that we know everything about the steroidogenic pathways is that of a 39-year-old male who was medicating himself with large amounts of AndroGel. Unsurprisingly, his testosterone levels were really high. His free testosterone levels were higher than we could even measure with our assays, his estradiol levels were very high, and his dihydrotestosterone (DHT) level was really low. Thus, he was driving everything right down through aromatase and increasing his overall estradiol levels. So, this is an indication of increased aromatase activity resulting in estrogen excess.

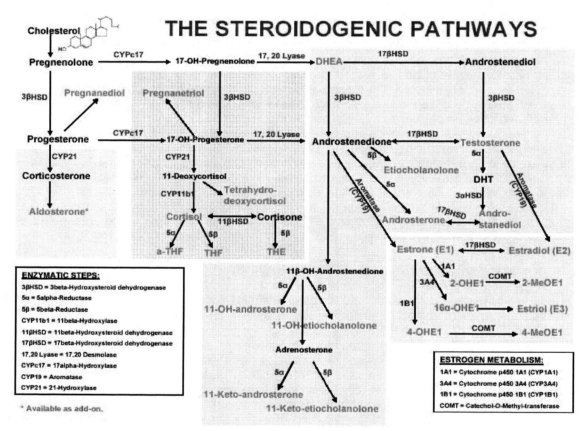

Figure 3. The steroidogenic pathways.

If we look at the steroidogenic pathways (Fig. 3) we can see that testosterone is converted into DHT by an enzyme called 5-alpha reductase (5α). A number of factors will upregulate 5-alpha-reductase activity, including: insulin resistance, obesity, high protein diet, sodium restriction, licorice, DHEA, and hyperthyroidism. Whilst factors that will downregulate 5-alpha-reductase activity include: vegetarian diet, herbal 5-alpha-reductase inhibitors (e.g., Saw palmetto, pygeum, and stinging nettles), pharmaceutical 5-alpha-reductase inhibitors (e.g., Proscar), flaxseed lignans, epigallocatechin gallate (EGCG) – an antioxidant found in green tea, and progesterone. All of these things will help to decrease DHT production.

Cortisol and Cortisone

What is the difference between cortisol and cortisone? Cortisol is the active form and cortisone is the inactive form. An enzyme called 11-beta hydroxysteroid dehydrogenase (11βHSD) catalyzes the conversion of inactive cortisone to active cortisol. Therefore the amount of active cortisol circulating around the body is dependent upon the activity of 11βHSD. When 11βHSD is highly expressed there is an increase in adipose tissue and an increase in the metabolism of sex steroids. Thus, we want to try to inhibit this process. Factors that drive 11βHSD expression include obesity (especially abdominal obesity), metabolic syndrome, hyperinsulinemia, hypothyroidism, hypertension, and inflammation.

CONCLUDING REMARKS

We have learnt that stress has a profound effect upon steroid synthesis. Elevated cortisol levels are undesirable, and the phenomena of cortisol steal compounds the problem by depleting the body of DHEA and it downstream hormones.

It is very important to be aware of the pathways involved in steroid hormone synthesis and also to ensure that you are aware of exactly what a patient's problem is. Simply prescribing DHEA for a patient with elevated cortisol levels is not the answer!

Abdominal obesity is a major problem. It makes people make more DHT and estrogens, and it keeps cortisol active. Addressing the problem of abdominal obesity, will also help to reduce the insulin resistance, metabolic syndrome, and inflammation, and will be of major benefit to your patient. Other steps that can help to resolve many of the problems that occur within the steroidogenic pathways include: eating a well-balanced diet containing lots of fruit and vegetables and few animal products, lowering stress levels, getting plenty of sleep, and taking regular exercise. Specific nutritional and herbal supplements can also be of help to specific problems, for example EGCG will help to lower DHT production and phytoestrogens can help to downregulate aromatase activity.

REFERENCES

1. Haren MT, Malmstrom TK, Banks WA, Patrick P, Miller DK, Morley JE. Lower serum DHEAS levels are associated with a higher degree of physical disability and depressive symptoms in middle-aged to older African American women. *Maturitas*. 2007;57:347-360.
2. Nishikaze O. [Distortion of adaptation--wear & tear and repair & recovery--17-KS-sulfates and stress in humans.] *J UOEH*. 1993;15:183-208. [Japanese]
3. Furuya E, Maezawa M, Nishikaze O. [17-KS sulfate as a biomarker in psychosocial stress] *Rinsho Byori*. 1998;46:529-537. [Japanese]
4. Kano K, Yamada Y, Arisaka O. Urinary 17-hydroxycorticosteroids and 17-ketosteroid sulfates in normal children and in children with atopic dermatitis or renal disease. *Rinsho Byori*. 2001;49:807-812.

ABOUT THE AUTHOR

Dr. Patrick Hanaway is a board-certified family physician with a Medical Degree from Washington University and residency training at the University of New Mexico. Dr. Hanaway received his Bachelors degree from the University of Wisconsin in Molecular Biology and has done research in muscle biology, neurochemistry, lipid metabolism, public health, preventive medicine, immunology, digestion, and nutrition. In addition to being a family physician, Dr. Hanaway is a board-certified holistic physician and currently is on the American Board of Holistic Medicine. Dr. Hanaway founded Family to Family: Your Home for Whole Family Health in Asheville, NC, and is currently Chief Medical Officer for Genova Diagnostics. Dr. Hanaway has lectured extensively on the clinical application of nutrition and genomics; particularly in the areas of endocrinology, digestion, oxidative stress, inflammation, and achieving long-term wellness.

Chapter 18
Treatment of Osteoarthritis with Horizontal Therapy

Achim Hansjürgens, Ph.D.
Researcher, Hako-Med Group

ABSTRACT

Horizontal Therapy is based on the fact that bioelectric changes in living tissues are strictly combined with biochemical changes and vice versa. Cells are electrical and chemical in nature and act by combining these two fields to produce an effect. Horizontal Therapy imitates the natural cell functions. In other words, Horizontal Therapy is able to create biochemical and bioelectrical therapeutic effects simultaneously in cells in the treatment area. This paper will discuss the use of Horizontal Therapy in the treatment of osteoarthritis.

Keywords: pain management, osteoarthritis, physical therapy, horizontal therapy, metabolism, regeneration

INTRODUCTION

Horizontal Therapy is based on the fact that bioelectric changes in living tissues are strictly combined with biochemical changes and vice versa. Cells are electrical and chemical in nature and act by combining these two fields to produce an effect. Horizontal Therapy imitates the natural cell functions. In other words, Horizontal Therapy is able to create biochemical and bioelectrical therapeutic effects simultaneously in cells in the treatment area. Traditional Electrotherapy can only create bioelectrical effects; it cannot create bioelectrical and biochemical effects simultaneously in the treated area.

HORIZONTAL THERAPY

The new Medical Concept (MC) for Horizontal Therapy: The MC contains 2 classes of therapeutic effects: Class A: bioelectrical effects, Class B: Biochemical effects.

Class A: Bioelectrical effects

Bioelectrical effects are induced by action potentials in excitable cells. Different effects are created according to the following two principles:

- Function imitation principle uses the normal range of the physiological discharge frequencies for the stimulation of nerves and/or muscles.
- Function fatigue principle uses higher stimulating frequencies above the normal discharge frequency range of the stimulated excitable cells. Therefore the opposite effects of the imitation principle are achieved by the fatigue principle.

The frequency boundaries between the imitation principle and the fatigue principle are: 10 Hz for the sympatic nerves, 20 Hz for the striped musculature, and approximatley 100 Hz for the majority of the sensory nerves.

Class B: Biochemical Effects

Biochemical effects are caused by a biophysical mechanism and electrophysiological effects are caused by sustained depolarization in nerves (blockade) and muscles (contractures)

New Medical Concept of Horizontal-Therapy

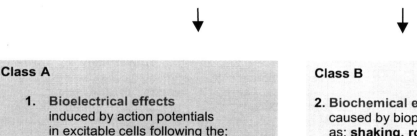

Class A

1. **Bioelectrical effects**
   induced by action potentials
   in excitable cells following the:

   • **principle of imitating functions**

   and the

   • **principle of fatiguing functions**

Class B

2. **Biochemical effects**
   caused by biophysical mechanism
   as: **shaking, rotary, oscillation or oscillating** processes on ions and molecules

3. **Electrophysiological effects**
   caused by sustained depolarization in nerves (blockade) and muscles (contractures)

Horizontal-Therapy
Simultaneous application of class A and class B effects

TREATMENT OF OSTEOARTHRITIS WITH HORIZONTAL THERAPY

The electrical alternating field of some thousand waves per second created by Horizontal Therapy increases the probability that enzymes and their substrates will meet, while also increasing the chance that they will bind at the enzymes optimal active "docking" sites. These effects, which support metabolism and also have regenerative functions, mainly happen intracellularly in the chondrocytes and in cells involved in the inflammatory process.

Horizontal Therapy promotes the metabolism, circulation, lymph transport, and the diffusion processes in the treated area. The function of the chondrocytes is improved by Horizontal Therapy as is the production of hyaluronic acid.

HORIZONTAL THERAPY AND PAIN MANAGEMENT

There are seven features of Horizontal Therapy that make it useful for pain management:
1. Counter irritation – Gate Control Theory
2. Release of endorphins in the central nervous system – longer lasting pain relief
3. Distribution of pain mediators - longer lasting pain relief
4. Pain fibre block – longer lasting pain relief due to the post hyperactivity depression (PHD) effect
5. Transient excitatory activity (TEA), a very intensive counter irritation, which leads to central pain relief.
6. Reduction of pain causing factors – longer lasting pain relief
7. Acupuncture whole body pre-treatment

REFERENCES

1. Carniel R, Saggini R. **Critical Review of the use of Electrotherapy.** XXII Congresso Nazionle, Anno 2006, Associazione Nazionale Specialisti in Medicina Dello Sport, Iniversita "G. DÁnnunzio" Chair of Physical and Rehabilitative Medicine, "G. D'Annunzio" University, Chieti, Pescara.
2. Felicetti G, *et al*. Use of Horizontal-Therapy in chronic Backache: Evaluation of therapeutic Efficacy. *Eur Med Phys*. 2004; 40 (Suppl. 1-3):421-424.
3. Saggini R, *et al*. Gonarthrosis: Treatment with Horizontal-Therapy, Multicenter study. Eur Med Phys. 2004;40 (Suppl. 1-3):594-598.
4. Chiappano G, Felicetti G, Brignoli E, Sciarra T, Maini M, Giustini A. Evaluation of Functional Recovery and Pain Progress in Patients Subjected to Total Knee Replacement Surgery and Subsequent Electro analgesia Cycles. *Eur Med Phys*. 2005;41 (Suppl. 1-4):603-606.
5. Jokic A, Hansjürgens K, Sremcevic N, Hansjürgens A, Pekmezovic T, Vasic S, Markovic S. **Gonarthrosis: Treatment by Horizontal Therapy, a comparative study.** 4th World Congress of the International Society of Physical and Rehabilitation Medicine Seoul, Korea, June 2007.
6. Zambito A, Bianchini D, Gatti D, Rossini M, Adami S, Viapiana O. Interferential and horizontal therapies in chronic low back pain due to multiple vertebral fractures: a randomized, double blind, clinical study. *Osteoporos Int*. 2007;18:1541-1545. Epub 2007 Jul 4.
7. Singh BB, Zarow FM, Traina A, Scaringe J. A specific electrotherapy technique in the treatment of osteoarthritis of the knee: three case reports. Altern Ther Health Med. 2000;6:110-112.
8. Hansjürgens A, Klotzbücher M. *Summary of Clinical Case Studies Utilizing Horizontal Therapy for the Treatment of 496 Patients Suffering from Osteoarthritis, Lumbar Pain and other Pain Conditions*. Annual Congress 2002, The Korean Pain Society.

ABOUT THE AUTHOR

Dr. Hansjuergens graduated from the Universities Berlin and Karlsruhe 1967. He received his Ph.D. in electrophysiology concerning Dynamic Interferential Currents (DIC) and field distribution in living tissue 1982 from Strasbourg, France. He developed both DIC and Horizontal Therapy, and suggested the medical concept of Electrical Differential Treatment (EDT) in cooperation with the university hospitals Muenster, Munich and Heidelberg. He introduced these medical therapies in Europe, America, and Asia. DIC has been standard in Physiotherapy for many decades.

Chapter 19
Signaling Pathways Targeted by Curcumin:
Basis for Anti-Photoaging and Anti-Carcinogenic Therapy

Madalene C.Y. Heng, M.D., FRACP, FACD
Clinical Professor of Medicine/Dermatology at UCLA School of Medicine

ABSTRACT

Increasing interest has been focused on certain dietary botanicals and their potential use in the treatment of photoaging skin and prevention of photocarcinogenesis. In this review, the biochemical mechanisms and injury pathways involved in photoaging and photocarcinogenesis are summarized, with specific focus on potential targets for the preventive use of curcumin in these conditions.

INTRODUCTION

Photoaging of the skin has assumed increasing importance particularly in the context of an increasingly aging population. Chronic solar exposure not only produces photoaging, characterized by skin fragility, scaling, and pigmentary changes, but is also associated with the development of premalignant and malignant non-melanoma and melanoma skin cancers (Runger 1999; Bachelor 2003).

Photocarcinogenesis is initiated by DNA damage, most commonly induced by UVB (280-320 nm) and UVA (320-400 nm) solar radiation. It has since been observed that although the UVB wavelengths causes burning of the skin, these rays have low penetrating properties, and are not capable of penetrating tissue much below the surface of the epidermis. More recently, the role of UVA (320-400 nm) in photocarcinogenesis has been increasingly recognized (Runger 1999; Bachelor 2004). Unlike UVB, which, because of its limited penetrating properties predominantly affects the epidermal keratinocytes, UVA damages basal cells and melanocytes and easily penetrates into the mid-dermis, where it interacts with dermal fibroblasts, stromal tissue, and blood vessels. It is now believed that the changes of photoaging, including loss of elastic tissue, dryness, scaling, and patchy hyperpigmentation, result mainly from chronic UVA exposure. In comparison with UVB rays, it has been observed that although wavelengths in the UVA spectrum do not produce burning, the UVA rays are capable of penetrating far below the epidermis, and the effects of prolonged UVA exposure have been observed to affect the mid and even the lower dermis. The inadequacy of sunscreens to protect against UVA-induced free radical formation has been recently reported and has important implications both in photoaging and in melanoma and non-melanoma photo-induced tumorigenesis (Haywood 2003; Bachelor 2004).

Epidemiologic studies have implicated sunlight exposure as a risk factor in the development of basal cell and squamous cell carcinomas, although correlation is better for squamous cell carcinomas than for basal cell carcinomas and melanomas. Point mutations and mutagenic bipyrimidine dimers have been observed with combined UVB and UVA exposure. Point mutations of the type seen in UVB exposure have been observed in the p53 gene on chromosome 17p in 40-56% of basal cell carcinomas. However, limited association between basal cell carcinomas and sites of UVB (280-320 nm) exposure suggests that additional factors must be involved It is possible that the mutagenic effects of UVA may add to the genotoxic effects of UVB in initiation of melanomas and non-melanoma skin cancers.

Increasing interest has been focused on certain dietary botanicals and their potential use in the treatment of photoaging skin and prevention of photocarcinogenesis. In this review, the biochemical mechanisms and injury pathways involved in photoaging and photocarcinogenesis are summarized, with specific focus on potential targets for the preventive use of curcumin in these conditions.

STEPS INVOLVED IN PHOTOCARCINOGENESIS

Specifically, photocarcinogenesis involves three steps: (A) tumor initiation with DNA damage induced in a single cell as a result of the genotoxic effects of the mutagenic photoproducts; (B) tumor promotion, with clonal expansion of the clone of DNA-damaged cells, and (C) tumor transformation of the damaged clone by further DNA and stromal changes, leading to disregulated growth and acquisition of metastatic potential.

A. Tumor Initiation (DNA Damage)

It has been shown that although oxidative lesions are the main type of DNA damage involved with UVB exposure, other genotoxic products are generated with solar UVA exposure that may be even more mutagenic. In particular, unlike UVB-generated [6-4]-photoproducts, which are quickly repaired, UVA-generated bipyrimidine photoproducts are poorly repaired and isomerize into Dewar products that are highly mutagenic (Douki 2003). In addition, the induction of singlet oxygen formation by UVA is the basic event leading to signal transcription-factor-mediated gene expression in UVA-damaged skin.

B. Tumor Promotion with Clonal Expansion

1. Induction of Gene Transcription: Activation of Transcription Factors

(a) Nuclear Factor-kappa B (NF-κB) – Nuclear factor-kappa B (NF-B) is a family of related protein dimers that bind to a common sequence on the DNA, the κB site. In the quiescent state, the NF-κB dimers are located in the cytoplasm. When activated by free radicals generated by ultraviolet light exposure, as well as by other injurious stimuli such as radiation, endotoxins, carcinogens, tumor promoters, and inflammatory cytokines, the activated NF-κB dimers, a complex made of p50/p65 subunits, are translocated to the nucleus. NF-κB then goes on to induce transcription of over 200 genes involved in cell proliferation, cell transformation, inhibition of apoptosis, and metastases.

Curcumin, the active ingredient in turmeric, is an indirect but potent inhibitor of NF-κB activation. The process of activating NF-κB dimers involves the removal of the inhibitory protein, IκBα, by phosphorylation of its kinase (IκBα kinase, a serine/threonine kinase), which in turn is activated by phosphorylase kinase. Curcumin, a selective phosphorylase kinase inhibitor, blocks NFκB activation by blocking its IκBά kinase Blocking NF-κB activation is an important mechanism for the anti-inflammatory and anticarcinogenic effect of curcumin.

(b) Activator protein-1 (AP-1) – AP-1 is a transcription activator which bears similarity to a DNA-binding protein encoded by the tumor transforming viral oncogene. The complex consists of members of the JUN and FOS family of proteins. The inducers of AP-1 include environmental stresses such as ultraviolet light, various growth factors, and inflammatory cytokines. AP-1 has been implicated in growth regulation and cell transformation by activating the cyclin D1 gene, which promotes the initiation of cells into the G1 phase of the cell cycle. AP-1, by suppressing the p53 tumor suppressor gene, causes uncontrollable growth and cell transformation. Curcumin has been shown to also suppress the activation of AP-1.

2. Cell Proliferation

(a) Mitogen Activated Protein (MAP) Kinases – The mitogen activated protein kinase pathway which results in cell proliferation of epidermal cells involves activation of MAP kinase kinase kinase (MAP 3Kinase), which then activates MAP kinase kinase (MAP 2Kinase). These kinases are serine threonine kinases, which when activated go on to activate MAP kinase (MAPK), a growth factor-dependent receptor tyrosine kinase (see below under Growth Factor Signaling Pathways). Activation of the tyrosine kinase at the cell membrane level is responsible for triggering intracellular pathways resulting in cell growth and cell proliferation.

The MAP kinases are responsible for activating NK-κB-induced proliferative pathways, including the extracellular signal regulated protein kinases (ERK), c-jun N-terminal kinases (JUN), stress-activated protein kinases (SAPK), and p38 protein kinases. In skin cancers, stress activated pathways are particularly important, since stress activated promoters, such as ultraviolet light, activate NF-κB through phosphorylation of ERK, JNK, SAPK and p38 kinases. All these kinases are serine/threonine kinases believed to be activated by phosphorylase kinase and blocked by curcumin.

(b) Growth Factor Signaling Pathways – Growth factors are proteins that bind to receptors on the cell surface, with resultant activation of cell proliferation and/or differentiation. Growth factors that are implicated in carcinogenesis include: epidermal growth factor (EGF), platelet-derived growth factor, fibroblast growth factors (FGFs), insulin-like growth factor (IGF), transforming growth factors (TGFα and TGFβ) as well as cytokine growth factors such as TNFα (tumor necrosis factor-ά) and IL-1 (interleukin-1). These growth factor-induced signaling pathways are involved in non-malignant proliferation, e.g. psoriasis, as well as in proliferation of transformed cells.

The binding of growth factors to its tyrosine-kinase based receptor results in phosphorylation of the receptor, activation of the receptor, and triggering of serine-threonine based signaling pathways resulting in cell growth and proliferation. Curcumin has been shown to inhibit the tyrosine-kinase activity of this receptor, and also inhibits serine/threonine-dependent pathways, furthermore, it is probable that the effect of curcumin may be achieved through its inhibition of phosphorylase kinase. Phosphorylase kinase, which is involved in tyrosine-kinase dependent phosphorylation reactions, is also involved in serine/threonine kinase-dependent phosphorylation (see MAP kinases). In addition, since inhibition of phosphorylase kinase depletes ATP levels, the curcumin treated ATP-depleted cell may also have difficulty maintaining the growth factor receptor in its folded state.

3. Apoptosis-Cell Survival Balance

The balance between cell survival and cell death determines the number of existing cells. In cancer, the balance is tipped towards cell survival of UV-damaged cells. Cell death (apoptosis) helps to remove excess, damaged, or abnormal cells. It has been observed that activation of NF-κB promotes cell survival, and downregulation of NF-κB sensitizes the cells to apoptosis induction. Inhibition of NF-κB by curcumin promotes apoptosis of photodamaged cells and retards photoaging as well as the development of skin malignancies.

(a) Apoptotic Proteins – Apoptotic proteins include the caspase family, in particular caspase 8, caspase 9, and caspase 3, which trigger DNA fragmentation when activated, leading to loss of membrane potential, and leakage of cytochrome c into the cytoplasm. Other apoptotic proteins include PARP and Bax proteins, which are also involved in the apoptotic process. It has been observed that NF-κB-dependent expression of cell survival genes block apoptosis, thus promoting survival of photodamaged cells. On the other hand, curcumin, which inhibit NF-kB activation, sensitizes cells to apoptosis induction (Aggarwal B, 2003), thus killing off photodamaged cells. Curcumin has been observed to cause p53-dependent apoptosis in human basal cell carcinoma cells. (Jee et al,1998).

(b) Antiapoptotic proteins – Anti-apoptotic proteins such as Bcl-2 and Bcl-xL inhibit apoptosis and increase cell survival. On the other hand, downregulation of apoptosis suppressor proteins such as Bcl-2 or Bcl-xL by curcumin has been shown to induce apoptosis in cancer cell lines. This leads to activation of nuclear DNA fragmentation through mitochondrial disruption and cytochrome c release through activation of the caspase-dependent apoptotic pathways. NF-κB-dependent expression of cell survival genes, including survivin, TRAF1, and TRAF2, block apoptosis of photodamaged cells. By downregulating anti-apoptotic proteins, curcumin promotes apoptosis of photodamaged cells, thus improving photoaging skin and reduce the development of premalignant and malignant skin lesions.

(c) Cell Survival Kinase (Akt) – The cell survival kinase, Akt, is a serine/threonine protein kinase activated by growth and survival factors. Akt is activated by phosphorylation at the Thr308 and Ser473. Activated Akt promotes cell survival by activating NF-kB signaling pathway, and by inhibiting apoptosis of photodamaged cells. Since the activation of NF-κB is dependent on removal of its inhibitory IkBά protein achieved by activation of the serine threonine IkBά kinase, inhibition of IkBα kinase would result in inhibition NF-κB. Both IkBά kinase (NFkB activator) and Akt (survival kinase) are serine/threonine kinases activated by phosphorylase kinase and inhibited by curcumin. Thus, curcumin promotes apoptosis of photodamaged cells both by promoting NFκB-dependent apoptosis and by Akt-dependent cell survival.

C. Cell Transformation and Metastatic Potential

1. Dysregulated Cell Cycle and Tumor Transformation

Proteins that regulate the cell cycle, in particular the timing of cell cycling events are important in tumor transformation since loss of this regulation is the hallmark of the cancerous cell. These proteins are known as the cyclins, which are in turn, regulated by cyclin-dependent kinases.

Cyclin D1, a subunit of cyclin dependent kinase, cdk-4, and cdk-6, is the rate-limiting factor regulating the G1 phase of the cell cycle. Overexpression of cyclin D1, and other cyclin-dependent kinases, causes excessive growth promotion and dysregulation of the cell cycle associated with tumorigenesis, with increased expression related to proliferating cell nuclear antigen expression. Curcumin has been known to block the dysregulated cell cycle in cancers. Cyclin D1 expression is regulated by NF-κB, and suppression of NF-κB by curcumin leads to downregulation of cyclin D1. Curcumin also induces AF-1/p-21-mediated G1 phase arrest of the cell cycle (Aggarwal B, 2003), thus retarding proliferation of premalignant and malignant cells.

2. p53 Transcription Factor and Tumor Transformation

p53 is a transcription factor which functions as a tumor suppressor. It regulates many cellular processes including signal transduction and cell cycle control. It is also responsible for cellular response to DNA damage and subsequent cellular genomic stability. It activates the transcription of genes such as p21WAF1 and Bax to induce apoptosis of DNA damaged cells, resulting in the inhibition of growth of DNA damaged cells, including cancer cells. Mutant p53 loses its ability to bind DNA effectively. Consequently, the p21WAF1 protein is not formed to regulate cell division, with resultant uncontrollable growth and tumor formation. In one study, over 90% of squamous cell carcinomas and more than 50% of basal cell carcinomas were linked to deletion of p53 suppressor gene expression. The antitumorigenic effect of curcumin may lie in its ability to upregulate p53 and p21WAF-1/CIP1, perhaps by apototic removal of damaged cells with mutated p53 and low P21 WAF-1 expression. It has been observed that curcumin, selectively induces apoptosis in deregulated cyclin D1-expressed cycling G2 phase tumor cells in a p53-dependent manner.

3. Proteins in Tumor Invasion and Metastases: Cell Adhesion Molecules and Matrix Metalloproteinases

The penetrating properties of UVA into the dermis allow ultraviolet radiation of this wavelength band to affect dermal fibroblasts and mesenchymal tissue, inducing the production of tissue metalloproteinases seen in photoaging skin. Tissue injury and resultant inflammatory response result in generation of cytokines and growth factors, which activate transcription factors, such as AP-1 and NF-kB. These synergize to activate metalloproteinase promoter genes, inducing gene transcription. In the case of UVA exposure, it has been shown that singlet oxygen generated as a result of UVA exposure may mediate transcription factor-induced expression of cell adhesion molecules. The upegulation of matrix metalloproteinases promote invasiveness of the tumor into the dermis and deeper tissues. The expression of cell adhesion molecules, such as intercellular adhesion molecule-1 (ICAM-1), which allows tumor anchorage and vascular invasion, is also intimately involved in tumor metastases. Two metalloproteinases, MMP-2 and MMP-9, have been observed to be closely involved in promoting tumor metastases. Specifically, MMP-2 and MMP-9 are responsible for digestion of collagen IV in basement membranes, and collagen V in the subendothelial fibrillary component of epithelial and endothelial cells, thus enabling the tumor cells to invade into the dermis, as well as penetrate blood vessels. Metalloproteinase-2 (MMP-2) expression, in particular, has been shown to correlate with aggressiveness of cutaneous squamous cell carcinomas. Curcumin downregulates the expression of both matrix metalloproteinase-2 (MMP-2) and matrix metalloproteinase-9 (MMP-9), and may reduce the potential for tumor metastases, which rely on these proteins for tissue invasion.

CURCUMIN: A SELECTIVE INHIBITOR OF PHOSPHORYLASE KINASE

Curcumin (diferuloylmethane) is a dietary phytochemical found in the rhizome of the plant (*Curcuma longa*) from which turmeric is derived. Its anticarcinogenic properties have been extensively reviewed by Aggarwal *et al* (2003). The pathways targeted by curcumin are summarized in Fig 1. As detailed above, curcumin appears to block carcinogenesis in a multi-targeted fashion, which at first glance appears confusing because its many reported effects are difficult to reconcile from the viewpoint of an underlying fundamental mechanism. We propose a unifying concept which may explain the multifaceted inhibitory effects of curcumin in inflammation, anti-aging, and photocarcinogenesis through its selective inhibitory activity on phosphorylase kinase, a protein kinase with unique properties and multiple specificities.

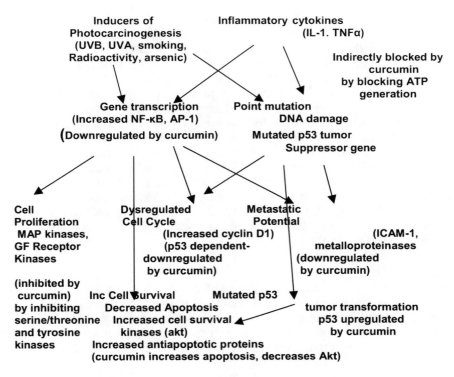

Figure 1. Pathways in photocarcinogenesis: targets for curcumin.

Phosphorylase Kinase: a Protein Kinase with Multiple Specificities

Protein kinases usually catalyze phosphotransfer reactions from ATP to either serine/threonine or tyrosine residues. This is because protein kinases, with the exception of phosphorylase kinase, allow only one configuration at its substrate binding site. In the case of phosphorylase kinase, however, the substrate binding site may be altered by utilizing a hinge joint between the subunits of the phosphorylase kinase molecule, thus altering the size of the substrate binding site. In addition, the substrate binding site can be made to alter its shape by causing it to swivel first in one plane (by binding to magnesium) and in another plane (by binding to manganese). In this way, phosphorylase kinase is able to phosphorylate substrates of multiple specificities, including protein kinases with serine/threonine, tyrosine, phosphatidylinositol, troponin etc... as specific moieties.

In support of the above mode of action of phosphorylase kinase, Graves *et al* (1999) provided evidence that in the phosphorylase kinase molecule, the spatial arrangement of specificity determinants can be manipulated so that phosphorylase kinase can utilize other substrates. It is possible that this flexibility may be the result of both the presence of the hinge joint between the subunits of phosphorylase kinase, a flexibility further enhanced by the ability of the molecule to alter the substrate binding site by metal ion (magnesium or manganese) specificity. This flexibility enables phosphorylase kinase to take part in a multiplicity of phosphorylation reactions.

Moreover, Yuan *et al* (1991) provided evidence of dual specificity depending on ion binding (magnesium, manganese). The ability of phosphorylase kinase subunits to adapt to different enzyme configurations, allow for one enzyme to accept many substrates, including serine/threonine kinases, tyrosine kinase, and phosphatidylinositol kinase

Phosphorylase Kinase: an ATP Generator

In addition, phosphorylase kinase is the only known enzyme which catalyzes the phosphorylation of glycogen phosphorylase b to glycogen phosphorylase a, since no other kinase has yet been observed to be able to duplicate this reaction. In doing so, phosphorylase kinase breaks down glycogen to produce ATP. Also known as ATP-phosphorylase b phosphotransferase, phosphorylase kinase, therefore, integrates multiple calcium-calmodulin-dependent signaling pathways while coupling these reactions to glycogenolysis and ATP-dependent phosphorylation.

Curcumin: a Selective Phosphorylase Kinase Inhibitor

We have previously reported that curcumin gel inhibits phosphorylase kinase activity in the skin (Heng *et al*, 2000). In addition, we have also demonstrated that inhibition of phosphorylase kinase activity by curcumin correlates with apoptosis of cells expressing proliferating cell nuclear antigen (PCNA) as shown by the Ki-67 immunocytochemical marker (Heng *et al*, 2000). Proliferating cell nuclear antigen (PCNA) is expressed in both premalignant (actinic keratoses, solar lentigenes) and malignant (basal cell carcinoma, squamous cell carcinoma and malignant melanoma), as well as in non-malignant cell proliferation (psoriasis, eczema). By inhibiting phosphorylase kinase, curcumin thus benefits photodamaged cells by inhibiting serine/threonine kinases (e.g. IκBά kinase, a kinase responsible for NFκB activation; MAP kinases responsible for cell proliferation; and Akt responsible for increased cell survival of photodamaged cells. Curcumin also inhibits cyclin kinases involved in cell cycling. By its action on tyrosine kinase inhibition, it inhibits growth factor dependent proliferation. By upregulating the p53 suppressor gene, it promotes apoptosis of photodamaged cells, and promotes p53-dependent cell regulation, and inhibits cell transformation.

CLINICAL IMPLICATIONS

Unfortunately, curcumin does not seem to be well absorbed when taken orally, and high doses of curcumin have failed to produce detectable blood levels. Curcumin in a topically gel, however, has been effective in many skin problems, particularly in skin lesions induced by injury. The injury pathway induced by ultraviolet light which results in photoaging and photocarcinogenesis are summarized in Fig 2, which also illustrates the potential role of curcumin gel in the treatment of a variety of skin conditions.

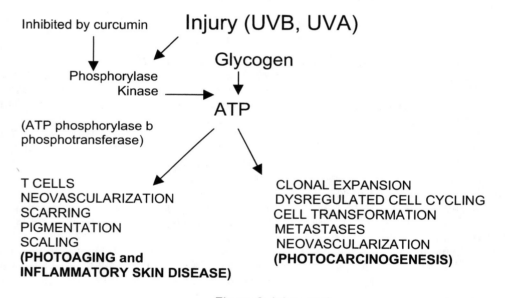

Figure 2. Injury pathway

Inflammatory Skin Disease and Scars

We have shown that inhibition of phosphorylase kinase activity by topical curcumin gel results in resolution of increased T lymphocyte population in inflammatory skin disease (psoriasis, eczema, burns, acne) thus accounting for the anti-inflammatory activity of curcumin gel (Heng *et al*, 2000). Clinically, curcumin in the form of a topical gel has been observed to have anti-inflammatory properties and to decrease redness and inflammation in sun-damaged skin. It has been observed to produce healing of superficial burns with minimal or no scar formation. Our observations also include a decrease in scarring in acne and pseudofolliculitis with curcumin gel. We had previously reported that curcumin gel produced resolution of psoriasis, correlating with suppression of phosphorylase kinase activity (Heng *et al*, 2000).

Photodamaged Skin

In photodamaged skin, topical curcumin in a gel base has been observed to improve the texture of photodamaged skin resulting in decreased appearance of wrinkle formation. It has also been effective in decreasing solar induced hyperpigmentation, and improving solar-induced telangiectasia. In photodamaged skin with actinic keratoses and solar lentigenes, curcumin gel has been observed to reverse these changes. These observations are consistent with reports that curcumin is capable of inducing apoptosis of damaged cells (Aggarwal 2003, Jee 1998), and shown in the following series of photographs.

We present clinical photographs (before and after curcumin gel application) taken from patients with various types of photodamaged skin as clinical evidence of the efficacy of curcumin gel in improving patients with these conditions.

In Figure 3, the patient had confluent actinic keratoses over most of her exposed areas, with scars from multiple surgeries for non-melanoma skin cancers. A large keratotic lesion was observed in the lower presternal chest (Fig. 3a, magnified in Fig. 3c) which partially resolved after 6 months with curcumin gel and sunscreen (Fig. 3b, magnified in Fig. 3d). Resolution was observed after 12 months with curcumin gel (Fig. 3e). Note the residual loss of pigmentation in the presumed apoptotic area after resolution of the keratotic lesion (Fig. 3e) and the general improvement in the remaining skin (Fig. 3e).

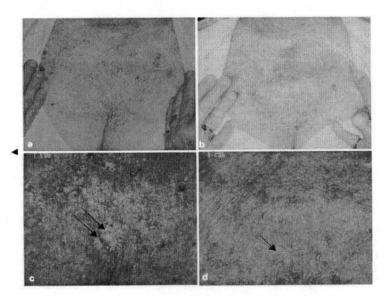

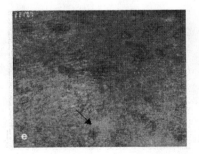

Figure 3: (a and c) severely photodamaged skin anterior chest, with large actinic keratosis before treatment with curcumin gel and sunscreen; (b and d) marked improvement 6 months after curcumin gel and sunscreen therapy; (e) resolution of actinic keratosis with apoptotic changes (unequal arrows) 12 months after curcumin and sunscreen treatment.

We have also observed that the more advanced the premalignant lesion, the more dramatic the resolution. For example, in Fig. 4a-c, the large biopsy proven prelentigo maligna on the left was mostly resolved after 10 months of curcumin gel (with sunscreen on top). However, the less involved smaller pigmented lesion to the right of the prelentigo maligna (Fig. 4a-c) was less improved after 10 months of curcumin gel (also with sunscreen on top) sunscreen).

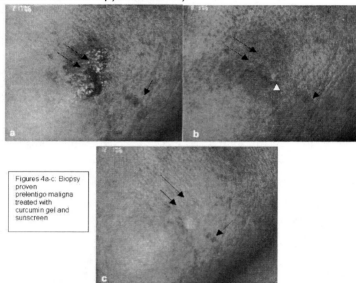

Figures 4a-c: Biopsy proven prelentigo maligna treated with curcumin gel and sunscreen

Figure 4: (a) Biopsy proven prelentigo maligna on cheek of patient before treatment by curcumin gel and sunscreen; (b) improvement noted after 6 months of treatment with curcumin gel and sunscreen; (c) further improvement (unequal arrows) was noted 10 months after initiation of therapy. Observe marked improvement in the lesion on the left (double arrows), and much less improvement in the lesion on the right (single arrow).   Arrowhead indicates the scar resulting from the punch biopsy

Curcumin gel decreases pigmentation induced by solar damage, particularly if used together with a good sunscreen (SPF 45-70). In such patients, wrinkles secondary to photoaging were observed to improve with increasing use.   In Fig. 5a-c, there is resolution of pigmentary solar lentigenes over 12 months, with gradual decrease in wrinkles over this period (Figs. 5a-c).

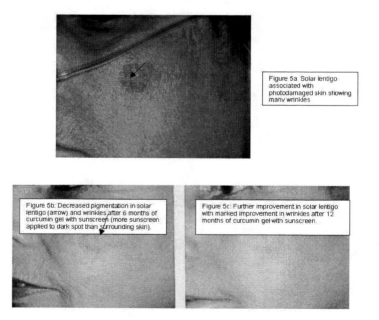

Figure 5a Solar lentigo associated with photodamaged skin showing many wrinkles

Figure 5b: Decreased pigmentation in solar lentigo (arrow) and wrinkles after 6 months of curcumin gel with sunscreen (more sunscreen applied to dark spot than surrounding skin).

Figure 5c: Further improvement in solar lentigo with marked improvement in wrinkles after 12 months of curcumin gel with sunscreen.

We have also observed improvement in skin quality of photodamaged skin, with decreased atrophy, and improvement in telangiectasia resulting in decreased erythema after 6 months or more of curcumin gel application (Fig. 6a, b).

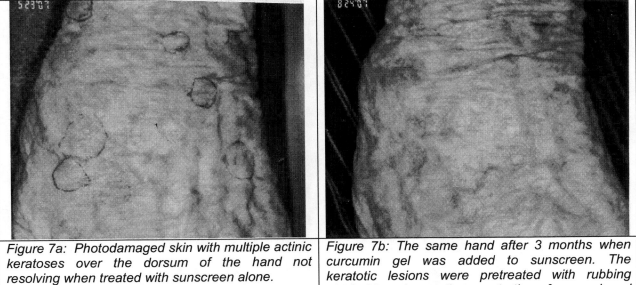

| Figure 6a: Photodamaged skin with atrophy, telangiectasia and pigmentary changes treated with sunscreen alone. | Figure 6b: Photodamaged skin 6 months after curcumin gel applied under sunscreens. Note improvement in skin atrophy, telangiectasia, and pigmentation. |

In severely photodamaged skin with increased skin roughness from multiple actinic keratoses, curcumin gel therapy used together with sunscreens result in improvement of the skin quality and smoothness. Many actinic keratoses are seen to resolve with curcumin gel together with sunscreen without surgery (Figs. 7a, b).

| Figure 7a: Photodamaged skin with multiple actinic keratoses over the dorsum of the hand not resolving when treated with sunscreen alone. | Figure 7b: The same hand after 3 months when curcumin gel was added to sunscreen. The keratotic lesions were pretreated with rubbing alcohol to enhance the penetration of curcumin gel under the keratotic scale. Sunscreen was applied before sun exposure. Note the resolution of many of the keratotic lesions. |

REFERENCES

1. Bachelor MA, Bowden GT. UVA-mediated activation of signaling pathways involved in skin tumor promotion and progression. *Semin Cancer Biol.* 2004;14:131-138.
2. Runger TM. Role of UVA in the pathogenesis of melanoma and non-melanoma skin cancer. A short review. *Photodermatol Photoimmunol Photomed.* 1999;15:212-216.
3. Haywood R. Sunscreens inadequately protect against ultraviolet A-induced free radicals in skin: implications for skin aging and melanoma. *J Invest Dermatol.* 2003;121:862-868.
4. Douki T, Reynaud-Angelin A, Cadet J, Sage E. Bipymidine photoproducts rather than oxidative lesions are the main type of DNA damage involved in the genotoxic effect of solar UVA radiation. *Biochemistry* 2003;42:9221-9226.
5. Aggarwal B, Kumar A, Bharti AC. Anticancer potential of curcumin: preclinical and clinical studies. *Anticancer Research.* 2003;23:363-398.
6. Jee SH, Shen SC, Tseng CR, Chiu HC, Kuo ML. Curcumin induces a p53-dependent apoptosis in human basal cell carcinoma cells. *J Invest Dermatol.* 1998;111:656-661.
7. Graves D, Bartleson C, Bjorn A, Pete M. Substrate and inhibitor recognition of protein kinases: what is known about the catalytic subunit of phosphorylase kinase? *Pharmacology and Therapeutics.* 1999;82:143-155.
8. Yuan CJ, Huang CYE, Graves DJ. Phosphorylase kinase: a metal ion dual specificity kinase. *J Biol Chem.* 1991;268:17683-17686.
9. Heng MCY, Song MK, Harker J, Heng MK. Drug induced suppression of phosphorylase kinase activity correlates with resolution of psoriasis as assessed by clinical, histological and immunohistochemical parameters. *Br J Dermatol.* 2000;143:937-949.

ABOUT THE AUTHOR

Dr. Madalene Heng is Clinical Professor of Medicine/Dermatology at UCLA School of Medicine. From 1979 to 2003, she was Chief, Division of Dermatology, UCLA San Fernando Valley Medicine Program. She is currently practicing at the Centers for Family Health, Community Memorial Hospital, Ventura, California. Dr. Heng is a reviewer for the Journal of the American Academy of Dermatology, American Journal of Geriatric Medicine, British Journal of Dermatology, Lancet, London, and International Journal of Angiology. With more than 130 scientific publications, including 71 published peer-reviewed articles on topics such as phosphorylase kinase activity and psoriasis, pathophysiology of disease, and wound healing, Dr. Heng is able to link treatment of diseases to their etiology at the basic science level. Dr. Heng is the developer of curcumin gel (Psoria-Gold).

Chapter 20
Metabolic Syndrome X: The Most Important Anti-Aging Initiative

Stephen Holt MD, LLD (Hon.), ChB, PhD, DNM, FRCP (C),
MRCP (UK), FACP, FACG, FACN, FACAM, OSJ
Distinguished Professor of Medicine, NYCPM (New York USA);
Scientific Advisor to Natural Clinician LLC

ABSTRACT

The global epidemic of obesity threatens longevity. Considerable evidence supports the notion that a physically active person of normal bodyweight lives longer than the overweight, inactive individual. Obesity causes premature morbidity and mortality as a consequence of obesity-related diseases. Furthermore, an overweight status is often associated with metabolic problems, such as the Metabolic Syndrome X. The association between being overweight and the occurrence of the Metabolic Syndrome X presents a unifying concept of premature aging, because of its attendant morbidity and mortality. This paper will discuss the role of Integrative Medicine in the management of both Metabolic Syndrome X.

INTRODUCTION

We have "super-sized" America, yet we still exude complacency about our overweight status. Globally, based upon body mass index (BMI) measurements, there are nearly 2 billion people who are overweight and 400-500 million people who are obese. Approximately one-third of US adults fall within the category of obesity and almost 20% of teenagers are overweight. Unfortunately, we have the fattest and most idle children in the world.

The global epidemic of obesity threatens longevity. Considerable evidence supports the notion that a physically active person of normal body weight lives longer than the overweight, inactive individual. Obesity causes premature morbidity and mortality as a consequence of obesity-related diseases. Furthermore, an overweight status is often associated with metabolic problems, such as the Metabolic Syndrome X. The association between being overweight and the occurrence of the Metabolic Syndrome X presents a unifying concept of premature aging, because of its attendant morbidity and mortality.

Data in the late 1980's showed that more than 40 million Americans have Metabolic Syndrome X, yet people still continue to deny that this syndrome even exists. Today, approximately 70 million Americans, and as many as 65% of African-American or Hispanic females between the age of 50 and 65 have Metabolic Syndrome X. So, what is Metabolic Syndrome X? Metabolic Syndrome X is characterized by the variable combination of obesity, hypertension, and abnormal blood lipids, linked by resistance to the hormone insulin. The variable constellation of problems encountered in Syndrome X has been associated with many other diseases (Syndrome X, Y, Z...)[1] Metabolic Syndrome X is under-diagnosed and often mistreated by both conventional and alternative medicine.

We know that Metabolic Syndrome X is causally linked with the development of cardiovascular disease, female endocrine disorders, polycystic ovary syndrome (PCOS), non-alcoholic fatty liver disease, gestational diabetes, cancer, compromise of immune function, and changes in eicosanoid status (Syndrome X, Y, and Z...). Furthermore, it also increases the risk of death from all common causes. The fact that Metabolic Syndrome X impairs the immune system and promotes inflammation means that it is also linked to all diseases in which inflammation is now known to play a major role, for example Alzheimer's disease.

To reiterate, the pathophysiology of Metabolic Syndrome X creates a platform for the development of many diseases, [1, 2, 3] and this is why I coined the terms Syndrome X, Y, and Z...[1] This conglomeration of syndromes results in the commonest cause of premature death and disability in Western society, and is now emerging in many urbanized areas of third world nations. The legacy and increasing prevalence of Metabolic Syndrome X has not been fully experienced in modern society. Some credible opinions imply that we may have a current generation of adults who may outlive their children.

Prevalence data about Metabolic Syndrome X from the National Health Nutritional Survey led the Centers for Disease Control and Prevention (CDC) to conclude: *"While proper management of the individual abnormalities of this syndrome can reduce morbidity and mortality, it seems unlikely that management of the individual abnormalities of this syndrome provides better outcomes than a more integrated strategy."* This is an unusual statement to be made by the government, as they are actually saying in a covert manner that this issue is not amenable to conventional medical treatment. I believe that this statement implies that if we are to combat Metabolic Syndrome X we need to adopt an integrative approach, not a standard allopathic approach.

One must conclude that the effective prevention and treatment of Metabolic Syndrome X requires a multifaceted approach to impact all cardinal components of the disorder. Current allopathic treatments have been too focused on individual components of Metabolic Syndrome X, and their focus on drug treatments tends to form a "back-up plan" for management.[1, 4, 5] In contrast, natural approaches with lifestyle modification and nutritional and/or nutraceutical interventions may provide versatile and powerful, first-line management options for Metabolic Syndrome X.[1] In summary, Syndrome X and obesity often "go hand-in-hand" and managing one without the other is "mismanagement."

LOOKING AT OBESITY FROM NEW SCIENTIFIC PERSPECTIVES

It is time to start looking at obesity and its related diseases with thoughts from outside the "conventional medical box". In the last year we have gained a greater understanding of the epidemiology of obesity and of how fat cells themselves regulate energy metabolism, and of neurohormonal control. We have discovered the incretins GLP-1 and GLP in recent years, and we know much more about the workings of the central nervous system as a fuel-sensing system. We also have new information on how positive lifestyle changes can control or prevent further weight gain. And, we have some new, rather innovative, drug and nutriceutical approaches. Unfortunately, we also have the potential over-utilization of bariatric surgery.

The Relationship between Gut Hormones, Sleep, and Obesity

Sleep deprivation, overweight status, and Metabolic Syndrome X appear to be inextricably linked in many people. The mechanisms of this association are not yet fully understood. Reduction in sleep duration in healthy young men is associated with major changes in the levels of the hormones ghrelin and leptin, which control hunger and appetite, and these changes promote weight gain.[6] An established association between short sleep duration and obesity has led to the proposition that some individuals may need more sleep in order to prevent or treat obesity.[6-8] I conclude that if you do not get obese patients to sleep, they will not lose weight, with any efficiency.

Ghrelin, which is sometimes known as "the hunger hormone", is an orexigenic, or appetite-promoting, hormone. Ghrelin is unusual because all of the other gut hormones that we have studied in detail tend to regulate energy balance by giving signals of satiety. What is clear now is that ghrelin secretion is elevated during episodes of insomnia, and perhaps even further elevated with the use of non-benzodiazepine sleeping drugs. Furthermore, insomnia causes blood levels of the satiety hormone leptin to fall. Together, the decrease in leptin levels and the increase in ghrelin levels form the fundamental basis of nocturnal eating disorder, otherwise known as nocturnal fridge raiding syndrome.

The incretins glucose-dependent insulinotropic polypeptide (GIP) and glucagon-like peptide-1 (GLP-1) are gut hormones, which are secreted within minutes of oral nutrient intake. Incretin receptor activation leads to glucose-dependent insulin secretion. They also slow the rate of absorption of nutrients into the bloodstream, and play a role in reducing food intake. GLP-1 is secreted by the intestines. It has direct effects on the brain (increases progenitor cell formation), bone (increases bone formation and decreases resorption of bone), pancreas (increases insulin secretion, insulin biosynthesis, and β-cell proliferation, and decreases β-cell apoptosis), and adipose tissue (increases lipogenesis). The effects of GLP-1 on pancreatic function suggest that dysregulation of this hormonal axis could be related to insulin resistance. GIP and GLP-1 are attracting a lot of attention as their actions suggest that they may provide us with new therapeutic targets for the treatment of Metabolic Syndrome X and type-II diabetes.

Hoodia Gordonii

Research into fuel sensing by the central nervous system (CHS) has been ongoing for many years. The neurohormonal control of hunger, appetite, satiety, and eating behavior are extremely complex. This control is altered by socio-behavioral factors, which can probably overcome any regulatory mechanisms that we have to control our eating behavior. There are lipostatic, glucostatic, and aminostatic theories of appetite control. However, the hypothalamus, which is the main regulatory organ for human appetite, plays a central role in all of these hypotheses of appetite regulation.

Hoodia Gordonii is a plant from South Africa, which seemingly acts directly on the hypothalamus and suppresses the appetite. A number of very interesting articles have been published about this plant; however it has proved very difficult to identify and isolate its appetite-suppressing constituents. Despite these unresolved problems Hoodia Gordonii (and perhaps Carralluma Fimbriata from East India) could prove to be among the most significant ethnobotanical discoveries of the last century.

Obesitis: A Concept that Further Unifies Modern Disease Theories?

Obesity and excess body fat can be classified as pro-inflammatory conditions and inflammation is a key factor in the pathophysiology of Metabolic Syndrome X. Not only does obesity raise the level of pro-inflammatory messenger molecules in the body, it also precipitates or contributes to several disorders of inflammation, including cardiovascular disease, cancer, arthritis, liver disease, and asthma.[3] This inflammatory disease "link" compounds the undesirable effects of insulin resistance.

The hallmarks of Metabolic Syndrome X and many cases of pre-Type II, or early Type II diabetes mellitus involves the presence of insulin resistance.[9] Insulin acts by specific receptor binding which precipitates many intracellular events.[9] Current evidence suggests that insulin resistance is determined partially by chemical mediators that are released from immune competent cells or fat cells.[9, 10] For example, elevated levels of the inflammatory cytokine tumor necrosis factor-alpha (TNF-alpha) are associated with overnutrition, and reduction of TNF-alpha activity is associated with weight loss or improvements in insulin resistance.[11] An understanding of many factors that link inflammation and tissue damage have come from recent studies of non-alcoholic fatty liver disease, which is a common component of Metabolic Syndrome X [1, 12], as well as the association of Alzheimer's disease with the syndrome.[1, 11, 13, 14]

Up to one third of blood levels of the inflammatory cytokine, IL-6 may emanate from adipose tissue and weight loss is often associated with reduction in blood markers of inflammation e.g. C-reactive protein (CRP) and IL-18.[14] Popular healthcare authors have attempted to link inflammation with many common diseases, but their interpretation of this important association is limited or naive because only changes in eicosanoid status are emphasized (e.g. The Zone).[15] While correcting eicosanoid precursor pathways with Omega 3 fatty acids is an important anti-inflammatory and insulin-sensitizing maneuver, it is not a comprehensive treatment strategy.[1, 3-4, 9, 12, 16-18]

Recent studies have confirmed the anti-inflammatory actions of certain substances found in fat tissue.[11] These substances have been referred to as adipocytokines, and include: leptin, adiponectin, and visfatin.[11] Adiponectin is manufactured by fat cells and blood levels of this protein are reduced in states of obesity, insulin resistance, type II diabetes mellitus, and atheroma.[16, 18] Adiponectin exhibits potent anti-inflammatory effects by suppressing TNF-alpha synthesis and promoting the availability of anti-inflammatory cytokines, e.g. interleukin-10 or interleukin-1-receptor antagonist.[19-20] The metabolic "plot" thickens in "obesitis" where imbalances of pro-inflammatory and anti-inflammatory cytokines exist.

The final common pathway of tissue damage often involves oxidative damage to the tissues due to the generation of free radicals, which is perhaps exacerbated by a reduction in antioxidant defenses in the body.[19] Of course, the progression of the complications of obesity, Metabolic Syndrome X, and diabetes mellitus is often related to oxidative tissue stress, with the development of advanced glycation end products (AGES).[1] Therefore, the treatment of obesity-related disease seems quite incomplete without supporting antioxidant activity in the clinical management of the obese or overweight person.

THE INTEGRATIVE APPROACH TO MANAGING OBESITY

Integrative Medicine can offer the optimal pathway to the management of an overweight status, especially if the modern approach of allopathic medicine is complemented by holistic care. (Table 1.) Many people can shed a few pounds of bodyweight in the short term, but sustained weight control involves many management principles, other than diet alone.

The last thing that we need is another diet promise for weight loss. That said, carbohydrate restriction, or the Atkins diet, in the short-term can result in apparently safe and effective, accelerated weight loss.[21] The Atkins diet is a re-description of the William Banting diet, which was first described in 1863. Since inception, low carbohydrate diets have been popularized every two decades in the last century, most notably by Yudkin and Atkins and copycat variations such as the South Beach Diet or Zone Diets. However, long-term restriction of carbohydrate intake, with increased fat and protein consumption, is probably neither safe nor effective and compliance is a problem.[21] Low carbohydrate diets result in rebound weight gain, largely because of lack of compliance and the frequent failure of carbohydrate restriction alone to overcome insulin resistance.[21]

Research shows that patients are approximately 50% more likely to comply with face-to-face lifestyle advice programs than with internet-based programs and diet books. So, regular face-to-face contact with your patients is important if you want them to succeed with sustained weight control. It is also important that you manage patient expectations. The majority of patients have unrealistic weight loss expectations. A realistic goal for most patients is to lose approximately 10% of their body weight.

The keys to sustained weight control are continued practitioner contact and the long-term use of supplements – and drugs if absolutely necessary – together with positive life style change. Without positive lifestyle change, there cannot be a health benefit from any weight control program. It is vital that you manage Metabolic Syndrome X as well as weight loss. This was the shortfall of the Atkins and other similar diets – carbohydrate restriction alone does not overcome insulin resistance.

There is no miracle weight-loss diet or supplement, weight management is about dietary calorie-control, behavior modification, aerobic exercise, the management of the underlying metabolic disorder, and the clear preemptive management of obesity-related disease and "obesitis."

Table 1. A Holistic Weight Management Program for Natural Clinicians (As proposed by the Author)

FACTORS TO ADDRESS	ACTIONS
Mutual acceptance of weight status by doctor and client. Required commitments and targets for weight and health management must be set	Weight assessment BMI measurement Fat distribution Definition of realistic weight loss targets with health focus. Avoid unrealistic weight loss expectations. Assess psychological well being and behavior
Identify and exclude specific secondary causes of obesity	Congenital disorder, thyroid disease, Cushing's Syndrome, psychiatric disease, drugs, surgery, metabolism and insulin resistance syndrome, Metabolic Syndrome X, etc.
Is Metabolic Syndrome X present?	The overweight person with Syndrome X has increased risk of many diseases (Syndrome X, Y, Z…) Failure to address insulin resistance syndrome in the presence of obesity is incomplete medical management. (medical malpractice)
Diet	Tailored to specific weight control targets and objectives. Short-term accelerated weight loss with low carbohydrate approach. Long term maintenance with balanced diets includes: restricted simple sugar, trans-fatty acids and saturated fats, moderate protein intake (1g/Kg) with vegetable protein inclusion (soy), moderate salt intake. Planning required for special circumstances of liver disease, diabetes mellitus, hypertension and, again, beware of Syndrome X.
"Obesitis": Obesity is an inflammatory disorder	All factors that may suppress inflammation are worthy interventions. The common pathway of inflammation often involves oxidative stress. Various nutraceuticals may suppress inflammation and/or independently or simultaneously sensitize the actions of insulin, e.g. alpha-lipoic acid, hydrophilic and lipophilic antioxidants, and eicosapentanoic acid (EPA), given in enteric coated capsules for compliance and enhanced bioavailability of active constituents.
Correct Biorhythm	Reductions in sleep duration and quality promote weight gain, abnormal glucose metabolism, and insulin resistance. Without healthy sleep, weight loss cannot be sustained and eating disorders emerge, especially nocturnal "fridge-raiding"
Behavior Modification	Many approaches, but must alter attitudes to food and remove positive reinforcements to overeating. Frequent social gluttony
Exercise	Movement is an absolute prerequisite for weight control. Energy into the body must be balanced by energy expenditure. Aerobic exercise must be matched to physical fitness levels. Panacea benefits from exercise are apparent.

Adjunctive Approach	Dietary supplements for weight control are often associated with illegal treatment claims for obesity and many have a poor scientific basis for their use. Stimulant weight loss supplements should be avoided in the mature, obese person. Reductions in net calorie intake are the goal, but modern nutraceutical technology has combined appetite suppression with attempts to alter metabolic changes associated with obesity e.g. dysglycemia and insulin resistance syndrome, the hallmark of Metabolic Syndrome X. Drugs used in weight control have onerous side effects. Hoodia gordonii shows promise for non-stimulant appetite suppression and it can be combined with natural substances that alter dysglycemia e.g. green tea and chlorogenic acid (found in green coffee bean) etc.
Surgical Intervention?	A variety of approaches. Contemporary interests, focus on non-invasive surgery e.g. gastric banding. Surgery for obesity results in a circumstance of forced malnutrition. The clinical course and natural history of the post-obesity surgery patient has not been evaluated in the long-term. The nutritional status of the post-surgical obese individual is often mismanaged. A big question mark exists with obesity surgery in children and teenagers. Careful selection required for surgery, but holistic care of these patients must occur to decrease post-surgical morbidity and mortality. Surgery is "the last ditch".

CONCLUDING REMARKS

There is no successful, sustainable, stand-alone intervention for weight control. Please do not look for it or encourage your patients to seek it out because it does not exist! Integrative Medicine can offer the optimal pathway to the management of an overweight status, if the modern science of allopathic medicine is complemented by holistic care (a loose definition of integrative medicine Sleep, diet, exercise, nutrition, and inflammation must be addressed. Nutraceuticals and, if necessary, pharmaceutical intervention, should be considered. Physicians need to ensure that they are abreast of all new scientific developments and perspectives. If you fail to manage Metabolic Syndrome X and its complex pathophysiology in many overweight people, you are on the edge of poor practice. The integrative approach is clearly the only approach to such a complex disorder as obesity.

REFERENCES

1. Holt S. *Combat Syndrome X, Y and Z*...Wellness Publishing; 2002.
2. Reaven GM, Banting Lecture, 1988. Role of insulin resistance in human diabetes. *Diabetes.* 1998;37:1595.
3. Handelsman Y. Guest Editorial. *Metabolic Syndrome and Related Disorders.* Mary Ann Liebert Inc. 2005;3(4):281-283.
4. Bloomgarden ZT. Approaching treatment of the insulin resistance syndrome. *Metabolic Syndrome and Related Disorders.* Mary Ann Liebert Inc. 2005;3(4):328-331.
5. Fonseca VA., Bratcher C., Thethi T. Pharmacological treatment of the insulin resistance syndrome in people without diabetes. Metabolic Syndrome X and Related Disorders. Mary Ann Liebert Inc. 2005;3(4):332-338.
6. Spiegel K, Tasali E, Penev P, Van Cauter E. Sleep curtailment in healthy young men is associated with decreased leptin levels, elevated ghrelin levels, and increased hunger and appetite. *Ann Intern Med.* 2004;141:846-850.
7. Taheri S. The link between short sleep duration and obesity: we should recommend more sleep to prevent obesity? *Arch Dis Child.* 2006;91:881-884.
8. Kohatsu ND, Tsai R, Young T, VanGilder LF, Burmeister, Stromquist AM, Merchant JA. Sleep Duration and Body Mass Index in a Rural Population. *Archives of Internal Medicine.* 2006;166:1701-1705.

9. Bloomgarden ZT. Concepts of insulin resistance. *Metabolic Syndrome and Related Disorders.* Mary Ann Liebert Inc. 2005;3(4):284-293.
10. Pirola L, Johnston AM, Van Obberghen E. Modulation of insulin action. *Diabetologia.* 2004;47:170-184.
11. Wellen KE, Hotamisligil GS. Inflammation, stress, and diabetes. *J Clin Invest.* 2005;115:1111-1119.
12. Fonseca VA., Bratcher C., Thethi T. Pharmacological treatment of the insulin resistance syndrome in people without diabetes. Metabolic Syndrome X and Related Disorders. Mary Ann Liebert Inc. 2005;3(4):332-338
13. Meggs JL, Svec C. *The Inflammation Cure.* Contemporary Books, McGraw-Hill: New York, NY; 2004.
14. Grimble RF. Inflammatory status and insulin resistance. *Curr Opin Clin Nutr Metab Care.* 2002;5:551-559.
15. Sears B. *The Anti-Inflammation Zone.* Regan Books; 2005.
16. Bloomgarden ZT. Cardiovascular complications of insulin resistance. *Metabolic Syndrome and Related Disorders.* Mary Ann Liebert Inc. 2005;3(4):305-315.
17. Bloomgarden ZT. Approaching treatment of the insulin resistance syndrome. *Metabolic Syndrome and Related Disorders.* Mary Ann Liebert Inc. 2005;3(4):328-331.
18. Fonseca VA., Bratcher C., Thethi T. Pharmacological treatment of the insulin resistance syndrome in people without diabetes. Metabolic Syndrome X and Related Disorders. Mary Ann Liebert Inc. 2005;3(4):332-338
19. Matsuzawa Y, Funahashi T, Nakamura T. Molecular mechanism of Metabolic Syndrome X: contribution of adipocytokines adipocyte-derived bioactive substances. *Ann NY Acad Sci.* 1999;892:146-154.
20. Angulo P. Nonalcoholic fatty liver disease. *N Engl J Med.* 2002;346:1221-1231.
21. Holt S. *Enhancing Low Carb Diets.* Wellness Publishing; 2004.

ABOUT THE AUTHOR

Dr. Stephen Holt is a Distinguished Professor of Medicine and a medical practitioner in New York State. He has published many peer-review papers in medicine and he is a best-selling author with twenty books in national and international distribution. He has received several awards for teaching and research. As a full professor of medicine for 20 years and an adjunct professor of Bioengineering for 10 years, Dr. Holt is a frequent lecturer at scientific meetings and healthcare facilities throughout the world.

Chapter 21
Medical License Defense and Medical Liability Insurance Issues

Edward J. Kuhn, MBA*; Algis Augustine, Esq.
*Agent, Professional Liability Solutions, LLC

ABSTRACT

There are specific risks and liability issues associated with being a healthcare practitioner of anti-aging and alternative medicine. New liability insurance products are emerging to address these exposures, since standard insurance carriers and state-specific physician-owned mutual insurance companies are not covering these procedures.

Major carriers have created a new underwriting class for medical spas and practitioners of anti-aging medicine. Specialty insurance agents take a customized approach in procuring a comprehensive insurance policy that combines professional liability, general liability, and legal defense of your medical license in cases of state medical board investigations or disciplinary proceedings.

The importance of adequately considering these issues cannot be overemphasized. In many cases, a provider can be spared the expense, stress, and adverse publicity of a disciplinary proceeding by implementing preventative strategies in his or her everyday practice, for example by responding properly to informal board requests and, when necessary, retaining counsel to wage an effective settlement campaign.

The aims of this paper are to provide an overview of the risk and liability associated with practicing anti-aging and alternative medicine, illustrate solutions to risk management and avoiding medical liability claims, and to describe specific insurance products currently available on the market.

INTRODUCTION

There are specific risks and liability issues associated with being a healthcare practitioner of anti-aging and alternative medicine. New liability insurance products are emerging to address these exposures, since standard insurance carriers and state-specific physician-owned mutual insurance companies are not covering these procedures.

Major carriers have created a new underwriting class for medical spas and practitioners of anti-aging medicine. Specialty insurance agents take a customized approach in procuring a comprehensive insurance policy that combines professional liability, general liability and legal defense of your medical license in cases of state medical board investigations or disciplinary proceedings.

The importance of adequately considering these issues cannot be overemphasized. In many cases, a provider can be spared the expense, stress, and adverse publicity of a disciplinary proceeding by implementing preventative strategies in his or her everyday practice, for example by responding properly to informal board requests and, when necessary, retaining counsel to wage an effective settlement campaign.

The aims of this paper are to provide an overview of the risk and liability associated with practicing anti-aging and alternative medicine, illustrate solutions to risk management and avoiding medical liability claims, and to describe specific insurance products currently available on the market.

HOW DOES INSURANCE WORK?

There are three types of insurance companies: physician-owned mutual insurance companies, stock companies, and Risk Retention Groups (RRGs). The most predominant are the physician-owned mutuals. Each state has a mutual insurance company that is owned and operated by the doctors in that state. Physician-owned mutual insurance companies probably insure 75% to 80% of the physicians in the United States. Their purpose is to provide good quality insurance to their members at the lowest price possible. Unlike the stock companies, mutual insurance companies do not have to satisfy and answer to shareholders. RRGs function as a captive insurance company and are organized for the primary purpose of assuming and spreading the liability risk exposures of its member-owners. RRGs tend to be focused on specialties, especially high-risk specialties (a good example is that of the obstetricians in Pennsylvania who did not have any other alternative than to form their own insurance company).

So, how does insurance work? Basically, the money has to come in faster than it goes out, that is absolutely vital if an insurance company is to keep running. In order to do this insurance companies focus on something called underwriting profit, this is the amount of money that is left after from the premiums paid after all claims have been paid out and administrative expenses have been deducted. However, insurance companies make the majority of their money from investments, with 80 to 90% of premiums being invested in low-risk securities like bonds. At the moment, interest rates are going up and the price of bonds is going down, therefore market is starting to turn into what is referred to as a soft market. Because of this insurance companies are on the look out for business in order to make up the difference that they are losing on their investments, therefore they are cutting the prices of their premiums.

WHY DO YOU NEED LIABILITY INSURANCE?

Why do anti-aging physicians need liability insurance? There are a number of reasons as to why all anti-aging physicians need liability insurance. One of the most important is to gain hospital privileges. If you are an independent contractor a hospital would not let you walk through the door without some type of malpractice insurance. Secondly, if you are practicing alone, liability insurance protects your assets from lawsuits, and protects your reputation. It is important to be aware that personal injury attorneys follow trends. Probably the biggest growth area in anti-aging medicine is esthetic medicine, and as this industry grows economically the attorneys will start to take notice. So, at the moment the insurance companies are trying to build up their surplus, so that when claims start being made they will be ready to pay them out. Another reason why it is absolutely vital that every anti-aging physician has some type of liability insurance is that new procedures and techniques increase the need for insurance protection.

It is very important to be aware that underwriters take the view that risk exists because of what you do, and not necessarily how well you perform. So, if your specialty is seen as being high-risk, for example orthopedic surgery or obstetrics, your insurance company will rate you as a normal specialist of a high-risk specialty, even if you are renowned as being the top physician in the country in that specialty. The thing that it is important to remember with anti-aging medicine is that it is a new specialty. There are currently four or five underwriting companies that cover anti-aging medicine; however the market is now becoming more comfortable with anti-aging medicine, so it is likely that the number of companies offering cover will soon grow. A good example of the change in attitude towards anti-aging medicine is Botox. Five or six years ago it was simply not possible to insure anyone for Botox unless they were a dermatologist, but today, with millions of procedures having been done, the insurance companies can see that it is safe and they are starting to feel comfortable about underwriting it. So, as time goes on, more and more companies will start to feel comfortable with anti-aging medicine, and more and more companies will offer insurance for anti-aging physicians. Of course, more competition means stable prices.

What procedures are deemed as risky right now? It is funny how the insurance companies feel comfortable with a surgeon taking out a gallbladder, but they have a problem with someone giving a Botox injection. That is because that they know what the inherent risk with the surgery is as they have a lot of data, and they can therefore price it effectively. One particularly risky area of anti-aging medicine is bariatrics. Another area of high-risk is any non-FDA approved procedure or any treatment using a non-FDA approved compound.

It is important to note that the majority of claims and lawsuits are dismissed or settled out of court. Only a very few claims or lawsuits actually go all the way through the court system, and when they do it is more likely than not that the insurance company that is defending you will win – just 27% of claimants win.

As mentioned earlier, there are currently four to five companies that have broad enough coverage terms to cover anti-aging clinics and MedSpas – everything from prolotherapy to chelation. As agents, we look for the broadest coverage possible. The strong, financially stable companies that we currently work with are Berkshire Hathaway, Markel Corporation, General Star, and EDNA. The rates are very much determined by the overall profile of your practice, the size and scope of the practice, the type of procedures you offer, how many patient's are coming in, how many people are working under you, the practice history, and your overall education, experience, and training.

ORE INSURANCE PRODUCTS FOR YOUR PRACTICE

The type of liability policy that you buy is important, that is why you have to work very closely with your independent agent – tell him exactly what your insurance needs are so that he can formulate a good policy for you, customized for your clinic. What anti-aging physicians offer tends to vary significantly, some just want to do hormones, some want to focus entirely on esthetics, and some would like to do both. That is why it is important to have a customized policy.

What products are on the market right now? Firstly, there is professional liability insurance, which is commonly known as medical malpractice, and sometimes known as medical liability. Professional liability insurance provides comprehensive insurance coverage for your practice, including all procedures and employees/independent contractors. The vast majority of physicians will have some type of professional liability cover, however if you are starting to move into the anti-aging arena it is important to be aware that your old insurance policy may not cover you. Do not assume that the practice policy you have had for years will cover new procedures.

Another product is general liability insurance. General liability adds coverage for premises, products, and etcetera. Basically, general liability covers everything that professional liability does not cover, for example accidents on your premises. It is possible to buy stand-alone general liability insurance and combined professional and general liability insurance. It is probably best to buy a combined policy if you have a spa or a clinic, whereas if you are a medical director working at someone else's spa or clinic you would just need to buy a professional liability policy because the general liability would be the responsibility of the facility that employs you.

Finally, a very important new product that our agency has just come up with as a result of working closely with the American Academy of Anti-Aging Medicine is legal defense of license insurance. This policy will pay for legal defense in the event of any state medical license board investigations or disciplinary proceedings.

ADMINISTRATIVE PROTECTION

This section of the paper will discuss why administrative protection is important. Ways of protecting yourself and your practice, and what to expect when faced with administrative action will be covered.

Alternative medical providers are not looked upon in the same way traditional medical doctors are. If you are practicing traditional medicine, you do not need to consider many of the things discussed in this paper because you do not really need to have as many informed consents or be as cautious about the things you tell your patients because medical boards are mainly composed of people who are operating in the area of traditional medicine. As a rule, the people who sit on medical boards are not representing the people who are involved in anti-aging medicine or alternative medicine. They are representing those who practice traditional medicine. So, if you intend to do anything that veers even remotely off the road of traditional medicine you need to be aware that you are much more likely to face scrutiny from medical boards and licensing authorities.

Because of the misconceptions surrounding anti-aging medicine and alternative medicine the States have recently passed a number of rules that look on the surface to be like Medical Freedom Acts, which were designed to enable physicians to practice medicine in any way which they see fit as long as you do not hurt a patient and as long as no patient complains. However, what has happened is that the States have taken those laws and revamped them to make it more difficult to practice that way. If you are practicing anti-aging medicine, or you offer any type of complimentary and alternative medicine in your practice, it is vital that you make sure that you know the laws of your State.

RISK MANAGEMENT – PROTECTING YOURSELF AND YOUR PRACTICE

Risk management is extremely important if you want to avoid claims and/or medical board disciplinary actions. The first thing every physician should do to protect themselves is to keep exceptionally good records. In non-traditional medicine, record keeping is the most important thing you can possibly do, because if you keep really good thorough records and somebody has a problem, your records are your best defense. If your patient is improving don't just write down that they are improving, write how and why they are improving. For example, if your patient could not walk before you starting treating them and is now able to walk two blocks, write it down. The importance of detailed, thorough records cannot be overemphasized. If the medical board can see exactly how you have been treating your patients and that they are actually getting better, they will know that you are not some sort of charlatan. It is very hard for a board or any governmental entity to cause real problems for a doctor when they are succeeding.

It is also important to have systems in place just in case someone from the medical board pays you a visit. A good example of why it is important to know how and how not to act if someone from the board shows up at your practice comes from a doctor in Tennessee who had a State Investigator show up at his door about a particular issue involving a drug therapy. The doctor in question let the investigator in, invited him to have a look around his whole practice, let him meet his patients, and allowed him to take photographs of the different intravenous therapies he was giving at the time. Six months later he got a complaint for the initial issue involving the drug therapy that the State Investigator had questioned him about, as well as a whole bunch of complaints about other intravenous drug therapies he was involved in. The important point here is that none of the extra complaints would have been made if the doctor had not given the State Investigator free reign throughout his practice. Therefore, having systems in place should somebody show up with a subpoena, write you a letter, telephone you, or show up and say they want to ask you questions, is very important.

The number one thing to do if someone turns up at your practice is do not give them anything. If they hand you a subpoena, say thank you very much and tell them that you will get back to them in a couple of days when you have had time to talk to your lawyer. The next thing to do is to get in touch with your lawyer and check that all the relevant records are complete, then and only then you can give the records to the investigator if they have the right to receive them – some state laws do not allow the State to receive records without the patient's consent. You should, of course, be cooperative with the State Investigator, but do not give them free access to your practice and your files. Unfortunately, that is what most doctors do. They become afraid, panic sets in, and they give them the records, which are almost always incomplete, to the investigator, and then they get into more trouble.

Another essential form of protection is informed consent. A doctor should ensure that he has informed consent for any treatment or procedure he is going to carry out in his practice, just like he would if he were carrying out surgery in a hospital. The most important thing with informed consent forms is to make sure the patient understands exactly what treatment you are going to give them and what it involves, that there may well be forms of treatment available other than the one you are going to give them, and that you cannot promise them anything. For example, if you intend to give a patient chelation therapy, you might want to say that there may be other things that they could do such as going to see a cardiologist or other relevant specialist. If, once you have said that, the person says, "I understand that I have options, I understand that there are no promises, and I understand that may be some people consider this experimental or some people consider this worthless. I am making a decision on my own to undergo this therapy." If you are offering esthetic procedures, it is also crucial that you manage patient expectation. It is vital that a patient knows the limitations of the treatment you are offering. Once you have that informed consent you are protected. For extra protection, it is a good idea to have the patient sign every page of the form, and if you intend to give them an ongoing series of treatment it is wise to get the patient to sign a new informed consent every six months at a minimum so that you can demonstrate that your patient has been kept fully informed and that you have been entirely open and honest with them.

If you are unfortunate enough to have to attend a hearing it is important to be aware that they are not fair. Hearings at the administrative level are not fair. If you get before a board, try your best to get them to understand that you would very much like to get things resolved before the hearing. Is it possible to win at a hearing before a board? Yes, it is possible, but it is not probable. People have spent $300,000 - $500,000 fighting cases before boards. Therefore, if you are a doctor and you get a request from the board, ensure that you handle it immediately. Do not wait. This is when insurance products like legal defense of license come to the fore, as they will enable you to get someone knowledgeable working on your case without delay.

CONCLUDING REMARKS

If you practice anti-aging medicine, or are thinking of practicing anti-aging medicine, at this point in time you need to be cautious. Insurance companies are slowly coming around to the idea of anti-aging medicine and are developing products specifically designed for those who practice it. Make sure you go to a knowledgeable agent who will formulate a policy for you that is customized for your clinic. Ensure that you keep thorough and up-to-date records, have your patients sign informed consents on a regular basis, and make sure both you and your staff know exactly what to do and what not to do if you are paid a visit from the medical board.

ABOUT THE AUTHOR

Edward Kuhn is a licensed independent insurance agent for Liability Insurance Solutions/Professional Liability Solutions in Chicago, Illinois. He specializes in finding insurance solutions for healthcare practitioners. He has over twenty-five years of experience in the insurance and commercial finance industry. Prior to becoming an insurance broker in 1998, Mr. Kuhn was an underwriter and premium collection manager for a major insurance carrier.

Chapter 11
Conquering Diabetes with Gender-Specific Bioidentical Testostosterone
Edward M. Lichten, M.D., FACS, FACOG, FABAAM

ABSTRACT

Diabetes has reached full-blown epidemic proportions. In 1950, an estimated five million individuals in the US had diabetes. Today, there are an estimated 30 million people suffering from this condition. Furthermore, for every person with diabetes, there are another two people with pre-diabetes. Diabetes is not just about amputations, ulcers, macular degeneration, and kidney dialysis. We now know that diabetes is a cause of heart disease and that it also significantly increases the risk of developing cancer. This paper will demonstrate that diabetes occurs as a result of a natural hormone deficiency and when that hormone deficiency is addressed the patient will get better, without the need to take any drugs.

INTRODUCTION

Man took his first steps 5 million years ago. At that time, we had all the equipment to survive without all the medical care we have today. The inherent abilities of the human body have enabled our species to survive famine, plague, and our relentless poisoning of our own environment. So, rather than focusing upon the medical technology we have at our disposal, this paper will focus upon the body's ability to tackle diabetes itself with the help of bioidentical testosterone.

Diabetes has reached full-blown epidemic proportions. In 1950, an estimated five million individuals in the US had diabetes. Today, there are an estimated 30 million people suffering from this condition. Furthermore, for every person with diabetes, there are another two people with pre-diabetes. Diabetes is not just about amputations, ulcers, macular degeneration, and kidney dialysis. We now know that diabetes is a cause of heart disease and that it also significantly increases the risk of developing cancer.

A couple of years ago, a 50-year-old African-American man called Anthony from inner-city Detroit walked into my office. He had no regular source of work, food, or regular health care, and was living on junk food. He also had a history of homelessness. He was confused and disoriented, and testing revealed that his hemoglobin A1c (hbA1c) was 18 and his fasting blood sugar was 488. What would you want to do with this man? Send him to the hospital, refer him to an endocrinologist, or would you want to try and treat him – even if you are a board-certified gynecologist? Well, I decided to treat him, and within a month his hbA1c was down to 15.7. Two months later it was down to 11.7, and within five months of commencing treatment it had stabilized out at 7.4. What did I treat Anthony with? What was the key that kept our ancestors going? Our ancestors had to work hard to stay alive, thus they were extremely active. When you are active the body makes testosterone. Our ancestors had high levels of testosterone and it was testosterone that helped to keep them alive. The magic drug that I treated Anthony with was also testosterone, and the aim of this paper is to discuss how bioidentical testosterone can be used to conquer diabetes in men.

Ten years ago bioidentical hormones were seen as being the future of anti-aging medicine. The idea was to treat hormone deficiencies with hormones identical to those found in the body. When I started lecturing at meetings of the American Academy of Anti-Aging Medicine I introduced the concept of gender-specific hormones. This was vital because men and women are different. Just like there are gender differences in disease, there needs to be gender differences in treatment. You should not try to treat everybody exactly the same. Women need treating with natural estrogen, progesterone, and testosterone. Men need treating with natural testosterone. This paper will demonstrate that diabetes occurs as a result of a natural hormone deficiency and when that hormone deficiency is addressed the patient will get better, without the need to take any drugs.

The endocrine system is the key to our survival. If you imagine the endocrine system as a pyramid with a sun on top of it, the sun is the hypothalamus and the pineal gland tells us when to sleep. The top of the pyramid is the pituitary, which is there to instruct the four glands, the adrenal, the pancreas, the thyroid, and the ovaries. When the 12 hormones produced by these glands are in balance, we live longer and we have less disease. If you have diabetes, those hormones are unbalanced, and this imbalance can shorten your life by 10 to 15 years. All the diabetes drugs on the market today are simply treating the symptoms of diabetes, not the cause. The cause of diabetes is hormonal deficiencies.

CONQUERING THE DIABETES EPIDEMIC

As mentioned earlier, in 1950, an estimated five million individuals in the US had diabetes. Today, there are an estimated 30 million people suffering from this condition in the US, and at least 200 million worldwide. Diabetes is the leading cause of morbidity, mortality, heart disease, high blood pressure, cholesterol elevation, stroke, and obesity, and is responsible for a staggering 80% of non-cancer medical visits.

Diabetes is defined as a chronic disease characterized by excess sugar in the blood and urine – it is a wasting condition. There are only two causes of diabetes. The first is where the immune system destroys the pancreas, which gives rise to type I diabetes, and the second is insulin resistance, which gives rise to type II diabetes. So, type I diabetes is the inability to make insulin because of an immunological attack on the beta cells, whilst type-II diabetes is where the body is resistance to insulin, and this is typically caused by eating too many carbohydrates. The only defining test we have for diabetes is the hemoglobin A1c (HbA1c) test – if HbA1c level is 6 or more the patient is diabetic. However, an often forgotten test for diabetes is the glucose tolerance test.

The great thing about the glucose tolerance test is that it is dynamic. You get the patient to drink a glucose solution and then monitor their response. When the patient drinks the glucose solution their blood glucose levels should start at around 100, rise to approximately 150, and then begin to drop back down again. Thus, the dynamic of the blood glucose level going up and down defines the normal response of the body to the stress of glucose. However, what they did not teach us in medical school, and are still not teaching today, is that insulin levels are supposed to do exactly the same. They are supposed to start low at around 10, increase by fourfold in the first hour, and then drop by 50% back down to 20 within two hours. When glucose goes up, insulin should also go up, and when glucose goes down, insulin should also go down. Any deviation from that is metabolic syndrome, and an absence of insulin response signifies a burned out diabetic.

What kind of insulin response should we expect to glucose in type I insulin-requiring diabetes? The answer is none. No matter how much glucose you give them, their insulin response will be the same. 80% of people with type I diabetes that have been on oral agents for five years do not have an insulin response. Therefore, oral agents are worthless to 80% of your patients with type I diabetes. What is the benefit of giving people Micronase when they do not have an insulin response? Therefore you should give every diabetic patient a glucose tolerance test, and if they show no insulin response you can tell them to throw their oral agents away, because they are worthless. If you cannot produce insulin, there is no reason for an oral agent.

We teach our medical students that the aim of treatment in diabetes is to control hyperglycemia. So, for a person with type I diabetes the obvious answer is to give them insulin. But what about people with type II diabetes? Our medical students are taught to treat these patients by giving them oral agents, however all these oral agents actually do is squeeze more insulin out of the pancreas and force these patients into burned out type II diabetics, which, of course, means that they will have no insulin response, thus rendering the oral agents worthless.

So, we have a problem with standard medicine. It does not seem to work. The failure of evidence-based medicine is that we are treating the symptoms instead of the cause. This is what separates conventional medicine from anti-aging medicine – our aim is to treat the cause.

DIABETES AND TESTOSTERONE

Every diabetic male is testosterone-deficient. If men had higher levels of testosterone they would be significantly less lightly to develop diabetes. What's more, diabetes can be reversed with testosterone treatment. But, what does testosterone have to do with diabetes?

When glucose is presented to a cell for processing insulin needs to be present in order for the glucose to gain access to the cell. If there is no insulin present, the glucose will remain in the bloodstream. However, what is also needed is energy. It takes energy for glucose to move across the cell membrane. It is this energy requirement that links testosterone and diabetes, because testosterone plays a key role in the Krebs cycle, the biological reaction that is needed for the production of adenosine triphosphate (ATP), the source of cellular energy. If the glucose cannot be transported across the cell membrane, the membrane becomes stiff and resistant to glucose transport and the action of insulin. However, if there is enough energy, that glucose can be transported across the cell membrane and into the cell for processing. Thus, testosterone plays a key role in diabetes in the male because it is the source of energy.

However, testosterone also has a second role. We know that the cell membrane will change its physiology in the presence of insulin to facilitate the transport of glucose across the membrane. But, what very few people know is that testosterone bound to sex hormone binding globulin (SHBG) also facilitates the transport of glucose across the cell membrane. So, we have two keys that open the door for glucose to be transported across the cell membrane – insulin and testosterone bound to SHBG. Therefore, logic implies that if we want to improve glycemic control in men with type I diabetes, we need to be making sure that they have plenty of testosterone.

The Evidence

In 1997, a 72-year-old white male came to see me. He was taking 40 units of insulin per day, his blood glucose was 350, and he had a gangrenous foot. I gave him testosterone according to my T2 protocol. At the end of 11 weeks, his insulin requirement had dropped to seven units per day and his blood glucose had dropped to 70. Unfortunately, I could not fix his gangrenous foot and it had to be amputated. However, what this does show is that testosterone can help to improve glucose control even in the worst cases of diabetes.

In 2006, a 50-year-old man came to see me. His HbA1c was 18 and his fasting blood sugar was 488. I gave him testosterone, and six-months later his HbA1c was down to 7.2.

In 1997, I conducted a study of twelve male insulin-dependent diabetics with the Head of Endocrinology at Wayne State University. The participants each required more than 80 units of insulin per day. They were treated with either my T1 protocol or my once-a-month protocol, and after just three-months of treatment the insulin requirement of each and every one of them had dropped by 50%.

As well as helping to lower blood glucose and HbA1c levels, testosterone also prevents blood glucose levels from crashing. The main concern when trying to keep a patients blood glucose under tight control is that their blood glucose levels might drop too far and they might go into a diabetic coma. To prevent this from happening most doctors try to keep their patients blood glucose a little higher than it could be. However, testosterone keeps men from crashing. My patients do not crash and that means I can keep tighter control of their blood glucose levels, which means that I can save their lives – the difference between HbA1c level of 6 and 8 is a 16-fold increase in heart disease.

What is the Best Form of Testosterone for the Treatment of Diabetes?

Testosterone has to be injected. Why? Testosterone creams are aromatized to estrogen. If a patient uses testosterone cream for six months, their estrogen levels will rise dramatically. Therefore you do not want to use topical testosterone. Other options are injections of testosterone cypionate and testosterone pellets. The injections cost just $15 and are required once a month, however the testosterone used is not bio-identical, and once a man reaches 30 he will start aromatizing it. The pellets are bio-identical and FDA approved, however they are not popular with doctors or patients. The other option is a drug called Deca-Durabolin, or nandrolone, which is bioidentical and which cannot be aromatized. Unfortunately, the pharmaceutical company that made this recently stopped making it, however it is still possible to get hold of it.

Treating Diabetes with Testosterone

Every man with insulin-requiring diabetes has low levels of testosterone by definition; therefore the key to treating these men is testosterone replacement therapy. 100 mg of testosterone a week is the standard dose for replacement.

What about type II diabetes? Type II diabetes is really the same disease as type I diabetes. Patients develop the same complications – heart disease, retinopathy, and gangrene – and their life expectancy is approximately 10 years shorter than normal.

I had a 48-year-old patient called Joe who was 5'10" tall and weighed 295 pounds. He could not walk up a single flight of stair without being short of breath. He was diabetic with an abnormal glucose tolerance test. I put him on testosterone replacement therapy and a year and a half later his glucose tolerance test was normal, as were his insulin, fasting insulin, C-reactive protein, and SHBG levels and he was able to easily run for an hour-and-a-half on the treadmill. He is no longer diabetic. We physiologically reversed the disease.

Another man who came to me was taking 20 mg of Micronase. His blood glucose was 200. Nine weeks later, his blood glucose was 90 and we had him down to five units of Micronase.

Another example is Dan. Dan is a truck driver. When he first came to see me Dan had a HbA1c of 10.5. Being a truck driver, he did not get a lot of exercise and despite advice did not change his diet. I started to give him testosterone, and within five months he lost 15 pounds and his HbA1c dropped to 6.5 – by doing nothing more than embarking upon testosterone replacement therapy.

So, all men over the age of 40 are technically testosterone-deficient, however all diabetic men, men with heart disease, men with hypertension, and men with obesity are definitely testosterone-deficient. Men with insulin-dependent diabetes need testosterone and men with oral agent treated diabetes need testosterone.

How do you screen patients? The glucose tolerance test (looking at both glucose and insulin response) and HbA1c are the most effective tests you can give patients for diabetes. I am surprised by the sheer number of patients who come to see me who do not know they are diabetic. Approximately 15% of the men who walk in my office have an abnormal HbA1c with no history of diabetes at all. If the patient is diabetic you need to test for testosterone (free androgen index) – it should be greater than 450, estrogen – it should be less than 25, and SHBG – it should be less than 15.

It is important to remember that insulin resistance develops twenty years before diabetes. A normal glucose tolerance test has to be paired with a normal insulin response. If test results show an impaired glucose response, which means delays in the glucose tolerance test, the patient will have higher levels of insulin. Insulin resistance leads to a pre-diabetic phase, or metabolic syndrome, and then diabetes. Therefore when screening a patient for diabetes it is very important to run a glucose tolerance test as well as testing for HbA1c.

The media often say that testosterone causes prostate cancer. This is simply not true. A number of studies suggest that the reverse is actually true and that low testosterone levels correlate to higher levels of prostate specific antigen (PSA) and thus increased risk of prostate cancer. Furthermore, recent study results suggest that testosterone actually has little effect upon prostate tissue. Even so, it is always best to err on the side of caution, so do not treat men with a PSA of 2 and above.

CONCLUDING REMARKS

Testosterone is an effective treatment for diabetes in men. It costs just $15 a month. Oral agents are, on the whole, worthless. I only use oral sensitizing agents if I am trying to keep a patient off insulin, and then I use a compounded one that is far more effective than those offered by the pharmaceutical companies. We do not need insulin sensitizers. We do not need Byetta. We do not need all of the $300 a month drugs that are flooding the market. We need to look at the cause. We need to look at the physiology. We have to treat the cause of the disease and not the symptoms.

Every diabetic male should be tested for testosterone deficiency and every male who is low should be treated. I give everyone of my patients a battery of tests. I give them a full hormonal profile. I look at fasting insulin and I look at HbA1c. And over the years I have found that it is possible to treat most diseases, not just diabetes, simply by correcting core hormonal deficiencies with bio-identical gender-specific replacement to normal levels. Think simple. Do no harm. Fix the internal organism and let the body fix itself.

ABOUT THE AUTHOR

Dr. Edward Lichten completed his undergraduate degree at the University of Akron graduating summa cum laude and his medical training and residency in Obstetrics and Gynecology at Ohio State University College of Medicine. In private practice, he has been involved in resident and physician training for 30 years. His medical firsts include 1) a personal computer fetal monitor (1979), 2) surgical treatment for menstrual pain (1982), hormonal control of migraine (1991), hormonal replacement for men (1994) and testosterone for improved glycemic control in diabetic men (1996). He has established new protocols that will be made available to the public for the treatment of insomnia (2006) and intravenous vitamin/mineral therapy for asthma (2007). He has lectures on four continents giving more than 100 national and international lectures, published more than 35 peer review articles, and is a frequent speaker at the A4M Congresses.

Chapter 23
Successful Weight Management and Change in Body Composition With A Comprehensive Weight Management Program

Shari Lieberman, Ph.D., CNS, FACN
Founding Dean, New York Chiropractic College's MS Degree Program
in Applied Clinical Nutrition

ABSTRACT

Although more than 1000 diet books are available today and each year millions of Americans enroll in commercial self-help weight loss programs, the prevalence of obesity continues to rise. For weight loss to be meaningful and long lasting body fat loss must be maximized and muscle loss must be minimized. Unfortunately, the vast majority of self-help programs have focused merely on weight change instead of change in body composition. Lifestyle modification is also crucial, including low glycemic index (GI) food choices, specific exercise recommendations, and behavior modification. The foundation of anti-aging medicine is weight management and body composition and these must be addressed first in order for any further intervention to be successful – regardless of the health issue(s) needing to be addressed.

INTRODUCTION

Although more than 1000 diet books are available today and each year millions of Americans enroll in commercial self-help weight loss programs, the prevalence of obesity continues to rise. For weight loss to be meaningful and long lasting body fat loss must be maximized and muscle loss must be minimized. Unfortunately, the vast majority of self-help programs have focused merely on weight change instead of change in body composition. Lifestyle modification is also crucial, including low glycemic index (GI) food choices, specific exercise recommendations, and behavior modification. The foundation of anti-aging medicine is weight management and body composition and these must be addressed first in order for any further intervention to be successful – regardless of the health issue(s) needing to be addressed.

Bio-identical hormones, nutrition, and botanicals are all facets of anti-aging medicine, but the actual foundation is body composition and weight management. You will get very different results from an extremely overweight patient if you get that patient into tiptop shape. As we now know, body fat is the most hormonally active tissue that we have, and simply getting a patient to reduce their body fat can help them tremendously. Many diseases that are hormonally related, such as polycystic ovary disease, are much easier to treat if you get your patient into shape first.

THE FACTS

Unfortunately, anti-aging medicine now must extend to children. We are now seeing children with diseases of aging – everything from metabolic syndrome and type II diabetes to cardiovascular disease – and it is being predicted that this generation will be the first not to outlive their parents. So, anti-aging medicine is not just about Baby Boomers, it extends to children as well.

This is the first time in the history of this planet that the number of people who are obese outweighs the number of people who are starving. In Beijing, 50% of the population is now overweight, why? Not because they are eating their traditional Chinese diet, but because they have adopted a much more Western diet. The fact is that our Western lifestyle is spreading throughout the world and obesity is now a global epidemic.

58 million US citizens are overweight, 40 million are obese, and 3 million are morbidly obese. A staggering eight out of ten Americans over the age of 25 are obese, which is not too surprising considering the fact that 78% of Americans do not meet basic activity level recommendations. The biggest challenge, I have ever had in my practice is getting someone to exercise, and that is the most difficult challenge that we face. 25% of Americans never get off the couch – they are completely sedentary.

There has been a 76% increase in the incidence of type II diabetes in adults aged 30-40 since 1990. That is a staggering and very frightening increase. 80% of type II diabetes is related to obesity, 70% of cardiovascular disease is related to obesity, 42% of people diagnosed with breast and colon cancers are obese, 30% of gallbladder surgery is related to obesity, and 26% of obese people have high blood pressure, which is setting them up for all sorts of problems. Think of all the diseases and illnesses that are simply attributed to lifestyle, and that is why we cannot overlook this problem.

Obesity really is something that we have to take much more seriously when patients come into our offices. Physician office visits attributed to obesity alone cost $62.7 each year. Restricted activity days cost the economy $29.9 million each year, and bed-related days cost a phenomenal $89.5 million. On top of all that, employer insurances are skyrocketing. A lot of small businesses cannot even start up because insurance premiums are so expensive. Obesity puts people at a higher risk for disease than smoking, and I think that most people do not realize that.

4% of children were overweight in 1982, and by 1994, that figure had quadrupled to 16%. Now, approximately 30% of our children are either overweight or obese. If we look at different ethnic backgrounds we find that one in three white children and two in three Hispanic children are at risk of being obese or very overweight. Hospital costs associated with childhood obesity rose from $35 million in 1979 to $127 million in 1999, and by now that figure is probably closer to $200 million. 60% of children already have one risk factor for heart disease. The incidence of type II diabetes in children has risen from 4% in 1990 to 20% today, and 85% of children diagnosed with type II diabetes are obese. The statistics are clear, and it is time that we start to take notice of the obesity problem.

THE LOW GLYCEMIC INDEX

We regularly hear about the benefits of the Mediterranean Diet and the Japanese Diet. However, despite all the press that these diets may be good for us, the average American is not suddenly going to start adopting the same eating habits as traditional Italian or Japanese people. However, both the Mediterranean and the Japanese diets have something in common – they are both low glycemic index (GI) diets. In fact, the one fundamental thing that we all have in common – regardless of our ancestry – is that every single one of our ancestors ate a low GI diet.

A review of the scientific data clearly shows that a low GI diet appears to promote weight loss more effectively than other types of diets. The glycemic index is a measurement of the impact that a carbohydrate has on blood sugar levels. High GI foods (foods with a GI of 70 and above) such as sugar, white flour, and rice quickly raise blood sugar levels and insulin production. This throws the metabolic switch into fat storage mode – independent of calories. On the other hand, low GI foods (foods with a GI of 55 or less) give the body a steady stream of energy and promote weight loss whilst preserving lean muscle mass and increasing metabolic rate. A food with a GI index of between 56 and 69 is classed as moderate. Our ancestors ate a low GI diet, and we are genetically engineered to exist on a low GI diet.

It is very important not to confuse a low GI diet with a low carbohydrate diet. Simply restricting carbohydrates and treating them all the same still allows dieters to consume high GI carbohydrates, which will throw the metabolic switch to store more body fat. Low GI foods include beans, lentils, oats, yams, and sweet potatoes, as well as a host of other foods. Even most fruits such as apples, oranges, and grapefruit, which are all high in pectin, are low to moderate GI, which would make them permissible on a diet plan. The other beautiful thing about a low GI diet is you never have to restrict calories. When you teach someone how to eat a low GI ad lib diet, which means non-caloric restricted, they automatically adjust their calories and they eat a far better nutritionally profiled diet.

It is very important to begin educating our clients about the proper way to eat, because many people are confused. There are so many diets out there – the Atkins Diet, the Zone, the South Beach Diet – and the more people read the more confused they get. The best thing to do is forget all the other diets and concentrate on educating your clients on how to eat a low GI diet.

Low GI diets have been shown to be superior to the Step 1 American Heart Disease Association Diet for lowering of all blood lipids, and it is the best diet for weight management, cardiovascular disease prevention and treatment, prevention of stroke, treatment and prevention of metabolic syndrome and diabetes, and prevention and treatment of cancer.

Acceptance of the Low GI Diet

The American Diabetes Association, the American Heart Association, and the American Dietetic Association do not recognize the role of low GI food choices in health or disease prevention or treatment. In contrast, the joint Food and Agriculture Organization/World Health Organization Expert Consultation on Carbohydrates, the European Association for the Study of Diabetes, the Canadian Diabetes Association, and Diabetes UK, all encourage the application of the GI when choosing carbohydrate-containing foods.

Why is there such a conflict in acceptance? It is vital that we never lose sight of the fact that these associations are really businesses. I recently attended a seminar, which the American Heart Association happened to have sponsored, and one of the things that I was given was Ocean Spray Cranberry Cocktail, which contains high fructose corn syrup, and on the packaging was a stamp of approval from the American Heart Association. I don't really consider any of these associations, because they bow too much to industry pressure and money.

Diets Don't Work – But Low GI Does!

A landmark study was published in 2005. This study followed people on the Atkins diet, the Omish diet, the Weight-Watchers diet, and the Zone diet for a period of 12-months in order to compare their effectiveness. The results showed that none of the diets were particularly effective. Those who actually managed to stick to the diet for the whole 12-months lost, at best, 5% of their initial body weight. So, if you weighed 300 pounds at the start, by the end of the year, you would have lost 15 pounds. Whilst losing 15 pounds is better than nothing, it is not really significant if you are dealing with somebody who weighs 300 pounds, and that is why people find it hard to stick to these diets – they are not seeing results.

Crash dieting and fad dieting that induces "quick" weight loss generally promotes muscle and water loss and less fat loss. This keeps patients in the "yo-yo" syndrome since when they gain the weight back they gain it as fat – not muscle. Studies have shown that during low caloric intakes energy expenditure can be decreased by 10%. When normal food intake is resumed, it can further decrease by as much as 15%. Our bodies don't know we are cutting calories just to lose weight – they are programmed to reduce our metabolism to adjust for food shortages that occurred during our hunter-gatherer existence. Crash dieting leads to further slowing of metabolism since most of the weight is lost as muscle and water and later gained back as body fat. Therefore the end result is that instead of improving body composition, the yo-yo dieter ends up with greater and greater and greater amounts of body fat and lower and lower amounts of muscle mass.

Dieting can slow the metabolism by approximately 10-15%, but a calorie-restricted low GI diet will lower your metabolism much less, however by following a non calorie-restricted GI diet and taking regular exercise there will be absolutely no metabolic consequences. Furthermore, a low GI diet will help to improve insulin resistance and lower blood pressure, triglyceride levels, and C-reactive protein levels. Again, following a low GI diet does not mean eating a low carbohydrate diet – they are two completely different things. Eating a high GI carbohydrate diet containing high levels of sugar and starch and little fiber increases the risk of diabetes and obesity, whereas eating a low GI diet containing plenty of complex high fiber carbohydrates reduces the risk of disease. Therefore it is very important to remember that not all carbohydrates are created equal.

My colleagues and I devised the 12-week Lifestyle Intervention Study to determine the effects of a low GI diet and lifestyle changes. Participants ate a low GI diet, kept a food diary, followed exercise recommendations, and tried to reduce stress. They also took two specific dietary supplements supplied by Market America, which provided: chromium, Gymnema sylvestre, Gardinia cambogia, Bioperine, magnesium, wheat amylase inhibitor, Banaba leaf extract, vanadium, and bitter lemon. Participants attended weekly meetings where they watched DVD's on educational topics, such as food labeling and good and bad fats. Body weight, percentage body fat, and waist circumference were recorded at baseline, 4-weeks, 8-weeeks, and 12-weeks.

By the end of the 12-week study the mean weight loss was almost 14 pounds. Participants also lost an average of 4% body fat, and shaved an impressive 4 inches off their waist. Low GI diets do work!

Setting an Example

Results of a 15-year long study into the effects of eating fast food by Pereira *et al* found that eating fast food just twice a week was enough to cause a 10-pound weight gain and significantly increase the risk of diabetes. In the US, all people seem to eat is fast food. Never mind eating it twice a week, the average American eats fast food at least once a day.

In 2004 the NPD Group conducted a survey of 3,500 respondents to the question "What did I order at a restaurant today?" as part of a year-long diary of eating habits. Results showed that the top ten most popular foods consumed in restaurants by men were: 1) hamburger 2) French fries 3) pizza 4) breakfast sandwich 5) side salad 6) eggs 7) doughnuts 8) hash browns 9) Chinese food 10) main salad.

Whilst the top ten foods for women were: 1) French fries 2) hamburger 3) pizza 4) side salad 5) chicken sandwich 6) breakfast sandwich 7) main salad 8) Chinese food 9) chicken nuggets or strips 10) rice. Is it any wonder that eight out of ten Americans aged 25 and over are obese? What is even scarier is that our children are eating like this as well.

People have to learn healthier food choices and practitioners need to set the example. You have to practice what you preach. If you tell your patients to stop smoking and they smell cigarettes on your clothing they won't take any notice of your advice. If you tell them that they need to get in shape, but you are fat, they will be far less likely to listen to your advice than if you are healthy and fit. Be an example for you family, for your patients. It is very important that we practice what we preach.

The Glycemic Index and Children

Eating a low GI diet is not just for adults; children should be eating low GI foods as well. Unfortunately, that is not the case. Just like adults, children eat high GI foods, and just like us they crash and burn, their glucose levels skyrocket and then plummet. Would you want to teach a child a child with sky-high glucose levels? Would you want that child in your class? Would you want to sit next to that child on an airplane? It is easy to spot that child because he or she is the one that is hyperactive for no apparent reason. At the same time, would you want to teach or sit next to the child whose glucose levels have plummeted? It is easy to spot that child as well because he or she is the one that is screaming and crying for no apparent reason.

I sat next to a mom whose child was doing that. The mom apologized to me and I asked her what she had given the child to eat or drink before they got on the plane. She had given the child Coca Cola, which contains ten teaspoons of sugar. So, I asked her if she knew that Coca Cola contained ten teaspoons of sugar, and she confirmed that she did. And there lies the problem. Many parents know how bad the food they are feeding their children is, yet for some reason they want to ignore the facts and blame genetics for their child's weight problem and/or their behavior problem. Even with respect to attention deficit disorder and attention hyperactivity disorder, people still seem to think that a rogue gene has reared its ugly head all of a sudden. Could it be that our modern day love of high GI fast food is causing our children to pile on weight, be hyperactive, and not to pay attention in class?

Results of one study showed that teachers rated their classes' behavior more than 300 times worse after they had been given sugary beverages. Not 30% worse, 300% worse. Many parents answer to this is to give their children the diet version of their favorite fizzy drink instead; however giving children diet sodas is not healthy either. Aspartame is not a solution; it is part of the problem. Aspartame is metabolized in the body to its components: phenylalanine, aspartic acid, and methanol. Aspartic acid is an excitatory neurotransmitter and excitotoxin. In fact, aspartame has been linked to migraines, behavioral issues, and a whole host of diseases.

Furthermore, research at the University of Texas Health Science Center at San Antonio found that diet sodas themselves will not make you fat, however they also found that drinking diet soda in middle age dramatically increases the chance of gaining weight later on in life. Diet sodas have never been shown to induce weight loss, ever. There is a much larger body of evidence to show that diet sodas increase the risk of weight gain, because people get addicted to that intensely sweet taste and it interferes with their brain's ability to regulate food intake.

You Are What You Eat!

We need to teach people to buy fresh foods and avoid processed foods. They need to be taught to read labels and avoid foods containing sugars, high fructose corn syrup, hydrogenated oils, and trans fatty acids. Cereals should have no added sugar (or sugar should be one of the very last ingredients on the list) and should have at least eight grams of fiber per serving. Bread should contain at least three grams of fiber per slice. Get patients to clean the house of junk foods and to keep fresh fruit, fruit salad, and fresh vegetables on hand. Encourage them to make their own healthy snacks and fruit smoothies, and to eat dried fruit and raw or roasted (not salted) nuts.

As professionals, we know that children who are not nourished with healthy foods are less healthy, learn less, and are at increased risk of developing diseases of aging, and it is our job to do something about it. It is our job to educate our patients. Do not assume that they know what is healthy and what is not. We only have to look at the children in our country to know that many parents don't have a clue about nutrition. Numerous studies have shown that children who don't eat breakfast are fatter, learn less, and have behavioral issues. Yet there are many children out there who are still not eating a proper breakfast. Similarly there has been plenty of research, articles in newspapers, and items on television, showing that sugary beverages may cause severe behavioral changes in children. Yet there are many children out there whose parents are still giving them sugar-laden drinks.

Mahoney *et al* studied the effect of breakfast composition on cognitive processes in elementary school children. Results showed that eating a low GI oatmeal cereal had a significant impact on the children's learning and cognition. Spatial memory was enhanced in both boys and girls aged 6-11, and short-term memory improved in girls. In addition, auditory attention improved in both boys and girls aged 6-8. The researchers believe that the apparent cognitive benefits of eating oatmeal may be due to the fact that oatmeal provides a slower and more sustained source of energy due to its protein and fiber content, glycemic score (it is low GI), and rate of digestion. Such research shows that simply swapping a high GI food for a low GI food can have quite dramatic effects.

METABOLIC SYNDROME

The metabolic syndrome, a dangerous cluster of risk factors previously seen in adults and adolescents, is now appearing in elementary school aged children. The metabolic syndrome has become a prevalent condition in North America, affecting nearly one quarter of US men and women. An individual with the metabolic syndrome has three or more of the following factors: high blood pressure, high blood glucose, high plasma triglycerides, low HDL cholesterol, and high waist circumference. The metabolic syndrome is considered a precursor for type II diabetes, coronary artery disease, and premature mortality.

DuBose *et al* assessed nearly four hundred second and third grade children to determine the prevalence of the metabolic syndrome and its related components in this age group. The researchers developed metabolic syndrome screening protocol for the children, defined as the presence of three or more of the following components: 1) central obesity (high waist circumference) 2) elevated triglyceride concentration 3) low HDL cholesterol 4) elevated blood pressure 5) elevated fasting glucose levels. Results revealed that 5% of both boys and girls were identified as having the metabolic syndrome. Half of the children had no components, and 45% had at one or two components, with elevated blood pressure being the most common component. The prevalence of metabolic syndrome dramatically increased among children who were overweight, with one in five overweight children having the condition. The researchers say that their results show the need for early prevention since components of the metabolic syndrome track into adulthood.

CONCLUDING REMARKS

We have to get serious with our patients about changing their diet and lifestyle. We have to get back to basics. Bioidentical hormone replacement and nutritional intervention are both extremely valuable anti-aging tools, however we need to deal with the fundamental issue first, which is getting people who have large amounts of body fat to lose that excess body fat.

A review of the scientific literature reveals that the best diet to follow for life is a low GI diet. It can be followed indefinitely and helps correct many of the metabolic alterations that overweight and obese people must overcome. It is time to change the paradigm and move away from quick-fix fashionable diets that are focused on weight loss alone and towards a program that incorporates a low GI diet and exercise, which will help people to lose weight and improve their body composition.

REFERENCES

Dansinger ML, Gleason JA, Griffith JL, Selker HP, Schaefer EJ. Comparison of the Atkins, Ornish, Weight Watchers, and Zone diets for weight loss and heart disease risk reduction: a randomized trial. *JAMA*. 2005;293:43-53.

DuBose KD, Stewart EE, Charbonneau SR, Mayo MS, Donnelly JE. Prevalence of the metabolic syndrome in elementary school children. *Acta Paediatr*. 2006;95:1005-1011.

Dulloo AG, Girardier L. Adaptive changes in energy expenditure during refeeding following low-calorie intake: evidence for a specific metabolic component favoring fat storage. *Am J Clin Nutr*. 1990;52:415-420.

Mahoney CR, Taylor HA, Kanarek RB, Samuel P. Effect of breakfast composition on cognitive processes in elementary school children. *Physiol Behav*. 2005;85:635-645.

Pereira MA, Kartashov AI, Ebbeling CB, Van Horn L, Slattery ML, Jacobs DR Jr, Ludwig DS. Fast-food habits, weight gain, and insulin resistance (the CARDIA study): 15-year prospective analysis. *Lancet* 2005;365:36-42. Erratum in: *Lancet* 2005;365:1030.

ABOUT THE AUTHOR

Dr. Shari Lieberman earned her Ph.D. in Clinical Nutrition and Exercise Physiology from The Union Institute, Cincinnati, OH and her M.S. degree in Nutrition, Food Science and Dietetics from New York University. She is a Certified Nutrition Specialist (C.N.S.); a Fellow of the American College of Nutrition (FACN); President of the American Association for Health Freedom. She is the recipient of the National Nutritional Foods Association 2003 Clinician of the Year Award and a member of the Nutrition Team for the New York City Marathon. Her newest book, *Transitions Glycemic Index Food Guide* (Square 1 Publishers 2006) was just recently released. Dr. Lieberman's best-selling book *The Real Vitamin & Mineral Book* is now in its 3rd Edition (Avery/Penguin Putnam 2003). Dr. Lieberman is the Founding Dean of New York Chiropractic College's MS Degree in Clinical Nutrition; an industry consultant; a contributing editor to the American Medical Associations' *5th Edition of Drug Evaluations*; a peer reviewer for scientific publications; a published scientific researcher and a presenter at numerous scientific conferences. Dr. Lieberman is a frequent guest on television and radio and her name is often seen in magazines as an authority on nutrition. She has been in private practice as a clinical nutritionist for more than 20 years.

Chapter 24
An Integrative Approach to the Treatment of Cancer

Shari Lieberman, Ph.D., CNS, FACN
Founding Dean, New York Chiropractic College's MS Degree Program
in Applied Clinical Nutrition

ABSTRACT

The aim of this paper is to dispel the myth that antioxidants interfere with chemotherapy and radiotherapy by reviewing the medical literature. The role of vitamin C as an adjunct to chemotherapy, and as a chemotherapy agent itself, will be discussed. Several cases supporting the use of Poly-MVA (lipoic acid-palladium complex) in the treatment of a number of different types of cancer will be presented.

INTRODUCTION

The aim of this paper is to dispel the myth that antioxidants interfere with chemotherapy and radiotherapy. Since the 1970's, 280 peer-reviewed in vitro and in vivo studies, including 50 human clinical randomized or observational trials involving 8,521 patients – 5,081 of whom were given beta-carotene, vitamins A, C, and E, selenium, cysteine, B vitamins, vitamin D, vitamin K, and glutathione as single agents or in combinations – have consistently shown that non-prescription antioxidants and other nutrients do not interfere with therapeutic modalities for cancer. Furthermore, these nutrients enhance the efficacy of therapeutic modalities for cancer, decrease their side effects, and protect normal cells from damage. In fact, 15 human studies involving 3,738 patients who took non-prescription antioxidants and other nutrients, have shown that these patients are more likely to survive.[1]

Block *et al* reviewed 845 articles and of those 19 trials met the inclusion criteria for their study. The antioxidants evaluated were glutathione (7), melatonin (4), vitamin A (2), an antioxidant mixture (2), vitamin C (1), N-acetylcysteine (1), vitamin E (1), and ellagic acid (1). The subjects of the majority of these studies had advanced or relapsed disease. None of the trials reported evidence of significant decreases in efficacy from antioxidant supplementation during chemotherapy, and many of the studies suggested that antioxidant supplementation resulted in increased survival and/or increased efficacy of treatment, as well as reduced toxic side effects of treatment.[2] The authors of this study concluded that their results suggested that large, well-designed studies of the use of antioxidant supplementation as an adjunct to chemotherapy are warranted.

A phase II study involving 44 patients with advanced cancer and adherence to a regimen including high amounts of dietary and supplementary antioxidants was found to increase body weight, lean body mass, and appetite, decrease pro-inflammatory cytokines (IL-6 and TNF-alpha), and improve quality of life over a period of four months. The participants in this study received 400 mg a day of polyphenol through their diet and they took alpha lipoic acid (300 mg), carbocysteine lysine salt (2.7 g), vitamin E (400 mg), vitamin A (30,000 IU), vitamin C (500 mg), as well as an omega-3 supplement. The participants kept taking their prescription medications as normal. By the end of the study 22 of the 39 patients were responders or high responders.[3] These results suggest that an integrated program including high amounts (not RDA) of antioxidants in the diet and through supplementation may provide a safe and effective means of improving symptoms of decreased appetite, weight loss, and diminished quality of life in patients with advanced cancer.

So, there seems to be plenty of research out there to suggest that antioxidant supplementation may well be of benefit to cancer patients. If this is the case, why are oncologists still telling their patients that they must not take antioxidants in conjunction with chemotherapy or radiotherapy? There is no excuse for these oncologists not to know about every single thing that they can do to improve their patients' survival time.

VITAMIN C AND CHEMOTHERAPY

There is an increasing body of evidence to suggest that vitamin C itself could be used as a chemotherapy agent. Results of a human study by Chen *et al* suggest that intravenous ascorbic acid (vitamin C) in pharmacologic concentrations could well have an unanticipated role in cancer treatment.[4] The goal of this study was to test whether ascorbate killed cancer cells selectively, and if so to determine how it did so. Results showed that ascorbic acid does selectively kill cancer cells, but not normal cells, and that cell death was mediated via apoptosis, pyknosis, and necrosis. It is important to note that the results of this study suggest that the concentration of ascorbic acid needed to have this effect upon cancer cells can only be achieved by intravenous administration.

Intravenous vitamin C is safe in most patients except, of course, for those with the glucose 6 phosphate dehydrogenase (G6PD) deficiency (which every patient should be tested for), and the best thing about this is that vitamin C is associated with virtually no toxic side effects. Complementary and alternative medicine practitioners worldwide currently use ascorbic acid intravenously in doses as high as 70 g over several hours. Because ascorbic acid is easily available to people who seek it, a phase I safety trial on patients with advanced cancer is justified and is currently underway.

LIPOIC ACID/PALLADIUM COMPLEX – A DIETARY SUPPLEMENT

Of great interest is a dietary supplement called Poly-MVA, which contains a lipoic acid/palladium complex (LAPd). Poly-MVA was developed by Dr Merrill Garnett. Its main active ingredient LAPd has several patents as "synthetic reductase". The initials MVA stand for minerals, vitamins, and amino acids. Poly-MVA is a proprietary formulation that contains palladium, alpha-lipoic acid, thiamine, riboflavin, cyanocobalamin, formyl-methionine, and acetylcysteine. LAPd is the main active ingredient in Poly-MVA.

There have been no large-scale clinical trial of Poly-MVA; however there are many cases where this dietary supplement has been used with great sucess in people with different types of cancer, some of these cases are discussed below.

Multiple Myeloma

DW was diagnosed with stage IV multiple myeloma in May 2006 at 65 years of age. He had multiple lesions in his ribs and compression fractures in several vertebrae (T11-L2). He was hospitalized and offered either very aggressive or lighter chemotherapy. He opted for the lighter chemotherapy: bortezomib (Velcade), doxil, and decadron. He refused radiation. He was told that he had rapidly progressive multiple myeloma and he was being prepared for an autologous bone marrow transplant. He was released from the hospital and continued to be treated as an outpatient every three days for four months. On May 15th he started taking Poly-MVA, and he quickly went up to 12 teaspoons a day. He had severe neuropathy from the chemotherapy and as a result his dose of decadron was reduced from 40 to 20 mg, and his dose of Velcade was cut from 1 mg/mm to 0.7 mg/mm. His dose of Doxil remained the same. In June, he increased his dose of Poly-MVA to 16 teaspoons a day. His last dose of chemotherapy was on the 31st July 2006.

At the time of diagnosis, DX's IgG was elevated at 7369 mg/dl, and his beta-2-microglobulin was elevated at 3.7 mg/l. By July, his IgG was normal at 1232 mg/dl, and his beta-2-microglobulin was normal at 1.6 mg/l. Basically, he was in remission. His oncologist said that he had never seen this happen with multiple myeloma, and still wanted to prepare him for an autologous bone marrow transplant. DX refused.

By September 2006, DX reduced his dose of Poly-MVA to 4 teaspoons a day. His follow-up readings remained normal. He took pamidronate IV 90 mg/month. His bones healed. He did not need a kyphoplasty. He was physically and mentally active and his quality of life was 100%.

On the 1st January 2007 all of his lab results were normal. For some reason he decided to cut his dose of Poly-MVA down to 2 teaspoons a day, and he often missed the dose altogether. By May, his lab results were elevated. His beta-2-microglobulin was 2.5 mg/l and his IgG was very elevated – it went up to over 3600 mg/dl. I spoke to him in August and he told me that he had been under severe emotional and physical stress between May and July, and he was not feeling at all well. I told him to increase his dose of Poly-MVA to 16 teaspoons. He also was not feeling well. After a very short time, he felt great, and he had no back pain.

I received an e-mail off DX recently. He is traveling. He feels absolutely fantastic, but his tumor markers have gone up again. However, he feels great, he is traveling, he is living a full life, he does not have any symptoms, and his oncologist does not understand why he does not feel sick and he is still pushing for him to have treatment, but DX is once again refusing treatment and wants to stick with the poly-MVA.

Non-Small Cell Lung Cancer

Non-small cell lung cancer (NSCLS) is associated with a very poor prognosis. FA was diagnosed with stage IV NSCLC in July 2004, when she was 61 years of age. She was given Taxol and carboplatin from July to September 2004. Her follow-up CT scan showed that the tumors had shrunk to about half their original size. She had two heart attacks in 2004. The chemotherapy had destroyed part of her heart muscle and the heart attacks themselves also did some damage. As a result, she had to be managed with medication, as she could not have bypass surgery because of the destruction of the heart muscle.

Her oncologist prescribed her Iressa. However, she could not afford it and her insurance did not cover it, so she never took it. Instead, she opted for Poly-MVA, which she started in October 2004, at a dose of 8 teaspoons a day. Five months later, her CT scan showed no tumors. The lung cancer had completely cleared. She has regular checkups and scans. She is now taking just one teaspoon of Poly-MVA a day, and she has been in complete clinical remission. If she has any recurrence, she will simply increase the dose of Poly-MVA up to 8 teaspoons a day or more. FA's oncologist told her that only 10% of patients with NSCLC go into remission, and that figure is even lower in people with stage IV NSCLC. On her last check up in May she was give the all-clear with both the CT scan and lab results.

BB was diagnosed with stage IV NSCLC in June 2005 when she was 74 years old. She had a compression fracture (which was from the malignancy) and was scheduled to have kyphoplasty. The surgery was canceled because an x-ray showed a nodule in her lung. Her oncologist recommended 10 radiation treatments to her vertebrae and Tarceva, which she started immediately after the diagnosis. This was for palliative care. Her daughter was told that she had approximately eight months to live.

BB started taking poly-MVA at approximately the same time as her radiotherapy and chemotherapy treatment started. She started on a dose of eight teaspoons a day. On August 29, 2005, her follow-up CT and PET scan showed that the tumor was stable and no growth had occurred. The oncologist was pleased and actually rather shocked. She was monitored every two months. She started Zometa in September 2005. In October, her CT scan revealed complete resolution of the tumor. Her oncologist was amazed. The conventional therapy he had prescribed was only an attempt to slow progression of her cancer – Tarceva and radiation does not cure stage IV NSCLC. Her subsequent CT and bone scans both in 2006 and 2007 still demonstrate complete remission of the cancer, including the metastases to the lumbar and thoracic lesions, and many lymph nodes. Her quality of life is superb. She still takes two teaspoons of Poly-MVA a day, and visits her oncologist every four to six months.

Prostate Cancer

This is an interesting case because the laboratory that actually makes Poly-MVA told me that it does not work with prostate cancer patients. However, I have tracked several cases that show excellent results. AH is 45-year-old man who was diagnosed with early-stage prostate cancer in December 2006. His biopsy was positive, his PSA was 5.8, and his Gleason's score was 6. Due to the early detection, he was told that he could have nine months of watchful waiting to think about his treatment decision. His urologist was encouraging him to have a radical prostatectomy. After reading the potential side effects of the procedure, including impotence and incontinence, he decided that he wanted to try something else.

He decided to use his nine months to try some integrative noninvasive treatment. He found an integrative physician that evaluated his nutritional status, and he was given omega-3, fatty acids, methionine, and glutamic acid. He was also given calcium EDTA after a challenge for toxic metal showed that he had elevated heavy metals. In January 2007 he started taking Poly-MVA at a dose of 16 teaspoons a day. He kept taking Poly-MVA at this dose until June 2007 when he reduced the dose to 8 teaspoons a day. He was also given vitamins and minerals which were supportive, including antioxidants and omega-3s, coenzyme Q10, Angiostop (a Chinese herbal formula), and immune 26 as a part of his comprehensive plan. In addition, he had a weekly Myers cocktail (intravenous vitamins and minerals) and intravenous glutathione from January through to April 07. He also received hyperbaric oxygen therapy three times a week from January to March 2007, and in June 2007 he purchased his own hyperbaric oxygen chamber and increased the treatment to two to three hours per day.

At the time of diagnosis in December 2006, AH's PSA was 5.8. In March 2007, his PSA was reduced to 2.3, and by June 2007 it had dropped to 1.5. In July 2007, he flew to San Francisco to have a high-resolution ultrasound. The ultrasound did not show any trace of prostate cancer. He has not yet had a repeat biopsy. In July 2007, he reduced his intake of Poly-MVA to four teaspoons a day. He feels great and has no prostate or urological symptoms.

Breast Cancer

JB was diagnosed with infiltrating ductal carcinoma moderately differentiated with micro-lymphatic invasion of the right breast at age 55 in November 2000. She underwent a modified radical mastectomy in December 2000, and also underwent reconstructive surgery. The mastectomy also revealed a 0.9 cm moderately differentiated infiltrating ductal carcinoma with 14 lymph nodes being free of disease. She was staged at 0 -1, and her breast cancer was estrogen and progesterone positive. She was given tamoxifen, but stopped taking it after just 10 days because of a severe adverse reaction. In January 2001, she had her ovaries removed because they were cystic.

All appeared to be well until February 2005 when she found a lump along the right breast near the nipple. She was in Europe and she had to wait until she got home in May 2005. Her doctor thought that it was scar tissue and performed a biopsy. Unfortunately, it turned out to be a local recurrence and it was the exact same breast cancer; the same that she was diagnosed with at the beginning. Both the tumor and some surrounding tissue was removed. Even though it was a small tumor of 0.5 cm, the margins were still not clear and she underwent surgery again to remove more tissue. A biopsy sample was also taken in several different locations in the right breast. Her PET scan in June 2005 did not show any enhanced uptake and was clear. However, results of the biopsy revealed that cancer had been found in two of the five areas sampled, thus making the cancer diagnosis multifocal. She refused chemotherapy and radiation.

JB heard about Ply-MVA in October 2005, and immediately started taking it at a dose of 8 teaspoons a day. She stayed on this protocol until June 2006 when she had a follow-up CT scan and brain MRI, both of which were clear. After getting a clean bill of health she cut down to a maintenance dose up to two teaspoons twice a day. Her physician sees her every three months and follow-up testing is performed. Her last CT and mammography in January 2007 were normal. Her exam and labs on in August 07 were normal.

She then began to feel very tired. Fatigue can oftentimes be the first presenting symptom of a recurring cancer – long before anything will show up on test results. Therefore, JB immediately upped her dose of Poly-MVA to eight teaspoons a day again, and within two weeks she felt much better. Her latest tests and scans show that she is still in remission.

Glioblastoma

JS was diagnosed with stage IV glioblastoma in December 2003 at the age of 48. He was told that his cancer was very aggressive, and that the tumor doubles in size every 7 to 14 days. He had surgery where the visible tumor was removed. In the same month he had surgery, where all of the visible brain tumor was removed. He also underwent 33 rounds of intensity modulated radiation therapy and rotating gamma. He had completed his treatment by February 2004. He refused chemotherapy and Temador, and his oncologist informed him that the Christmas he had just celebrated would be his last. The oncologist also told him that even if he changed his mind and went ahead with the follow-up chemotherapy and Temador it was unlikely that he would survive for more than a year.

He started taking Poly-MVA in January 2004, and quickly increased his dose to eight teaspoons a day. In September 2004, his PET scan was completely clear with no positive uptake findings. In October 2004, he had a grand mal seizure. His surgeon told him that the glioblastoma was back; however, his oncologist suggested that the seizure may have been caused by radiation damage. His surgeon disagreed. However, whatever the problem was, it was causing more intense and frequent grand mal seizures, slurring of speech, and impairment of motor skills. Exploratory surgery was performed in October 2004. The pathology report revealed that 98% of the tissue was necrotic (due to radiation damage), and the remaining 2% of the tissue was "unknown." There was no evidence of cancer. The surgeon could not believe the results and ordered three more pathology reports – all came back negative for cancer. JS was in remission, and is still in remission today. He remains on a maintenance dose of 2 teaspoons a day.

CONCLUDING REMARKS

In conclusion, there is an abundance of evidence to show that non-prescription antioxidants and other nutrients do not interfere with therapeutic modalities for cancer. In fact, as has been shown in this paper, there is evidence to suggest that such nutrients may actually increase the efficacy of chemotherapy, reduce its toxic side effects, and increase patients' chances of survival. We have also learnt that vitamin C may well prove to be a chemotherapy agent in its own right. Furthermore, there is compelling evidence to suggest that the dietary supplement Poly-MVA may be of benefit to patients with a number of different types of cancer, including multiple myeloma, NSCLC, prostate cancer, breast cancer, and glioblastoma, when used alongside conventional treatment, alongside other integrative treatment, and in some cases by itself.

REFERENCES

1. Simone CB 2nd, Simone NL, Simone V, Simone CB. Antioxidants and other nutrients do not interfere with chemotherapy or radiation therapy and can increase kill and increase survival, part 1. *Altern Ther Health Med*. 2007;13:22-8. Review.
2. Block KI, Koch AC, Mead MN, Tothy PK, Newman RA, Gyllenhaal C. Impact of antioxidant supplementation on chemotherapeutic efficacy: A systematic review of the evidence from randomized controlled trials. *Cancer Treatment Reviews*. 2007;33:407-418.
3. Mantovani G, Macciò A, Madeddu C, *et al*. A phase II study with antioxidants, both in the diet and supplemented, pharmaconutritional support, progestagen, and anti-cyclooxygenase-2 showing efficacy and safety in patients with cancer-related anorexia/cachexia and oxidative stress. *Cancer Epidemiol Biomarkers Prev*. 2006;15:1030-1034.
4. Chen Q, Espey MG, Krishna MC, Mitchell JB, Corpe CP, Buettner GR, Shacter E, Levine M. Pharmacologic ascorbic acid concentrations selectively kill cancer cells: action as a pro-drug to deliver hydrogen peroxide to tissues. *Proc Natl Acad Sci U S A*. 2005;102:13604-13609. Epub 2005 Sep 12.

ABOUT THE AUTHOR

Dr. Shari Lieberman earned her Ph.D. in Clinical Nutrition and Exercise Physiology from The Union Institute, Cincinnati, OH and her M.S. degree in Nutrition, Food Science and Dietetics from New York University. She is a Certified Nutrition Specialist (C.N.S.); a Fellow of the American College of Nutrition (FACN); President of the American Association for Health Freedom. She is the recipient of the National Nutritional Foods Association 2003 Clinician of the Year Award and a member of the Nutrition Team for the New York City Marathon. Her newest book, *Transitions Glycemic Index Food Guide* (Square 1 Publishers 2006) was just recently released. Dr. Lieberman's best-selling book *The Real Vitamin & Mineral Book* is now in its 3rd Edition (Avery/Penguin Putnam 2003). Dr. Lieberman is the Founding Dean of New York Chiropractic College's MS Degree in Clinical Nutrition; an industry consultant; a contributing editor to the American Medical Associations' *5th Edition of Drug Evaluations*; a peer reviewer for scientific publications; a published scientific researcher and a presenter at numerous scientific conferences. Dr. Lieberman is a frequent guest on television and radio and her name is often seen in magazines as an authority on nutrition. She has been in private practice as a clinical nutritionist for more than 20 years.

Chapter 25
The Effects of Hormones on Breast Cancer: How to Use Them to Reduce the Risk

Khalid Mahmud, M.D., FACP, ABAAM
Medical Director, Innovative Directions in Health;
Former Medical Director of Oncology, North Memorial Medical Center
(Minneapolis, Minnesota USA)

ABSTRACT
Conventional practice of medicine has done very little to prevent breast cancer – the one disease women dread the most. The usual emphasis is on self-exam and mammogram, which is early detection, not prevention. By the time cancer is found on a mammogram it, as a rule, has been slowly growing for up to 15 years. Many factors influence the appearance and growth of cancer cells positively or negatively, and these factors could be manipulated to inhibit the initiation and growth of tiny cancers during this period of time. Hormones are one such factor. The aim of this paper is to consider how different hormones affect breast cancer and how to use them to reduce its risk.

INTRODUCTION
Conventional practice of medicine has done very little to prevent breast cancer – the one disease women dread the most. The usual emphasis is on self-exam and mammogram, which is early detection, not prevention. By the time cancer is found on a mammogram it, as a rule, has been slowly growing for up to 15 years. Many factors influence the appearance and growth of cancer cells positively or negatively, and these factors could be manipulated to inhibit the initiation and growth of tiny cancers during this period of time. Hormones are one such factor (Table 1). The following is a discussion of how different hormones affect breast cancer and how to use them to reduce its risk.

Estrogens	Melatonin
Progesterone, Progestins	Oxytocin
Testosterone	Insulin
DHEA	Thyroid (Tri-iodothyronine)
	Human growth hormone

Table 1. Hormones that affect breast cancer

ESTROGENS THAT CAN PROMOTE BREAST CANCER
Estradiol (E2) and Estrone (E1)
It is well known that these two strong estrogens stimulate the growth of breast cancer cells. They do so by acting on the estrogen receptor alpha (ER-alpha) on these cancer cells (Figure 1). ER-negative breast cancer cells are not affected by these hormones.

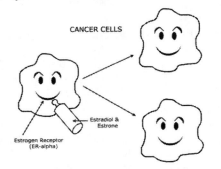

Figure 1. Cancer Promotion by Estradiol (E2) and Estrone (E1)

The Importance of E1 and E2 Manufactured by the Breast Fat Cells

Although it is commonly recognized that postmenopausal women with breast cancer tend to have higher blood levels of estrogens,[1] what is generally not appreciated is the fact that post-menopausal women have much higher levels of these estrogens in the breast – 10 to 50 times higher than in the blood.[2, 3] Fat cells, around a post-menopausal breast cancer, have been found to have high aromatase activity, generating estrogen locally to fuel the growth of cancer. (Figure 2).[4] The blood level is merely a reflection of the estrogen being generated by the aromatase in the fatty tissues, such as the breast, and not directly involved in stimulating the cancer.

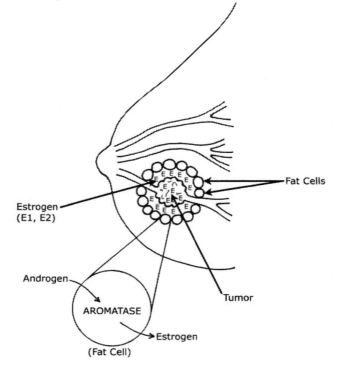

Figure 2. Breast fat cells producing estrogen to fuel cancer growth.

Does Estrogen Treatment for Menopause Increase Risk of Breast Cancer?

Scientific evidence does not support the notion that estrogen treatment for menopause increases the risk of breast cancer. The Women's Health Initiative (WHI) and Women's Health Initiative Lund Area, Sweden (WHILA) studies revealed that post-menopausal women receiving estrogen only (without Provera) did not have any increase in the occurrence of breast cancer.[5, 6] Only women who had received Provera (PremPro) had an increased risk of breast cancer. In fact, a Swiss HRT study of 23,000 women who were using more natural forms of estrogen (estradiol and estriol) showed an actual 25% decrease in breast cancer risk.[7] Furthermore, results of two studies of estrogen use in women with prior history of breast cancer showed a decrease in recurrence rate compared with control subjects.[8, 9] The obvious explanation for these findings is that a modest increase in E2 in the blood with estrogen administration does not make any difference to the estrogen level in the breast, which is locally produced and many times higher than what is in the blood. In addition, a study of baboons has revealed that in ovariectomized females (similar to post-menopausal women) estrogen administration causes a sharp and significant drop in the breast tissue aromatase level,[10] which should decrease the risk of cancer. This finding suggests that, like in other endocrine systems, the breast fat cells are affected by a negative feedback loop, so that externally administered estrogen actually acts as an 'aromatase inhibitor' in the breast, thus explaining the decrease in breast cancer in the larger studies mentioned above.

It should be mentioned that the greatest reduction in breast cancer occurred in the Swiss study where most women received E2 and E3 in more natural forms. The protection has been less obvious in the Premarin studies. This may have to do with the fact that Premarin blocks glutathione S-transferase, an important phase 2 enzyme in the detoxification of carcinogens.[11]

16 Alpha-Hydroxyestrone (16 alpha-OHE)
16 alpha-hydroxyestrone is an estrogen metabolite that stimulates the growth of breast cancer cells, and has been shown to increase the risk of breast cancer in several studies.[12, 13] 16 alpha-OHE levels can be lowered by eating less foods containing animal fat and eating more vegetables, particularly the cruciferous varieties, such as broccoli, brussels sprouts, cabbage, and cauliflower.

ESTROGENS THAT INHIBIT BREAST CANCER
Estriol (E3)
There is considerable evidence suggesting that estriol (E3) is protective against breast cancer. Estriol is a weak estrogen that binds to ER-alpha, thus keeping the stronger cancer promoting estrogens, E1 and E2, away from the cancer cells.[14] Estriol levels decrease in menopause. Asian women have higher estriol levels than Western women and a lower rate of breast cancer. Women with breast cancer tend to have lower levels of this estrogen.[15]

Henry Lemmon, a gynecologic oncologist at the University of Nebraska spent years studying estriol. He was able to prevent the induction of carcinogen and radiation induced breast cancer in animals by using estriol.[16]

Pregnancy is associated with very high levels of estriol and provides protection against breast cancer. A 40-year follow up of 15,000 pregnant women showed that those with the highest pregnancy levels of estriol had a 58% lower rate of breast cancer compared with those that had the lowest levels.[17] In the Swiss study cited above, many women received estriol.

Based on such evidence, it makes a great deal of sense to include estriol in hormone replacement therapy preparations. Unfortunately, pharmaceutical estrogen preparations have always excluded estriol.

I believe Biest [E2, 20% + E3 80%] to be the most logical estrogen preparation for women in menopause. Biest should act as an aromatase inhibitor in the breast tissue as well as block ER-alpha to the action of E2. I use Biest cream rather than oral preparations because, unlike oral estrogens, transdermal preparations do not increase clotting factors and CRP,[18] thus reducing the risk of thromboembolism and cardiovascular events. I teach patients to adjust the amount they use and to use just enough to control hot flashes without developing any breast tenderness.

2-Hydroxyestrone (*2-OHE)
2-hydroxyestrone is a good estrogen metabolite. Acting as a week estrogen, it blocks ER-alpha.[19] Several studies have shown its protective action, especially the ORDET study (Hormones and Diet in the Etiology of Breast Cancer), an Italian study of 10,760 women.[20] 2-OHE levels can be increased by eating more vegetables and fruits and less animal fat. Indole 3-Carbinol, an extract of broccoli, has been shown to increase its levels and is a popular supplement for the prevention of breast cancer. I use it in heavy-set women who do not consume enough vegetables.

Progesterone
I believe that progesterone is an anti-cancer hormone. As well as having anti-breast cancer properties it also has an overall anti-cancer effect. Let us look at the evidence:

1. In 1981, researchers at Johns Hopkins University reported a 13-33 year follow up on approximately 1000 infertile women. These women were divided into two groups: progesterone deficient women and an all-other-cause of infertility group. The progesterone deficient women had five times more breast cancer than the all-other-causes group. Furthermore, the death rate from all types of cancers was ten times higher in the progesterone deficient group than the other group.[21]

2. Fromby and Wiley from the Sansum Medical Research Institute, California, have performed and reported studies demonstrating that progesterone upregulates *p53* (tumor suppressor gene) and downregulates *bcl-2* and *survivin* (tumor promoter genes) in progesterone receptor-positive breast cancer cells, thus resulting in apoptosis of cancer cells.[22, 23] These findings have been corroborated by other researchers and reported in the *International Journal of Cancer.*[24]

3. Application of progesterone gel to breast has been shown to reduce mitotic activity in the breast glands.[25]

4. A National Cancer Institute study revealed that premenopausal women with the highest third week-of-cycle progesterone levels had a 60% decrease in subsequent breast cancer compared with those who had the lowest levels.[26] A French study from International Agency for Cancer Research showed the same results.[27]

5. Breast cancer surgery studies reveal that surgical treatment during the follicular part of menstrual cycle (low progesterone levels) results in higher metastases and death rate compared to surgery during the luteal part (higher progesterone levels) of the menstrual cycle.[28]

6. A large 2005 French study of 54,548 menopausal women revealed that women who took estrogen and Provera had a 40% increase in breast cancer. However, those who took estrogen and natural progesterone had a 10% decrease.[29]

It must be emphasized that only natural bioidentical progesterone has these anti-cancer effects, not the artificial progestins such as Provera (Medroxyprogesterone). Unfortunately, the majority of medical literature does not distinguish between bioidentical and artificial progesterone. Many practitioners of medicine tend to brush these differences aside with statements like: "*a hormone is a hormone is a hormone – they are all the same.*" To understand such beliefs, one has to go back into the history of steroid hormone discovery and synthesis (Figure 3).

In the 1930s, Russel Marker, a brilliant scientist at Penn State University, set out on a quest to manufacture exact replicas of human steroid hormones by a process of degeneration of similar molecules in plants. Eventually he found one such molecule in the Mexican Yam that could be chemically degraded to produce an exact copy of human progesterone. His discovery was ridiculed in the United States, so he moved in with a small Mexican lab and started producing bioidentical progesterone on a large scale. Subsequently, other bioidentical hormones, such as testosterone and estrogen could be produced.

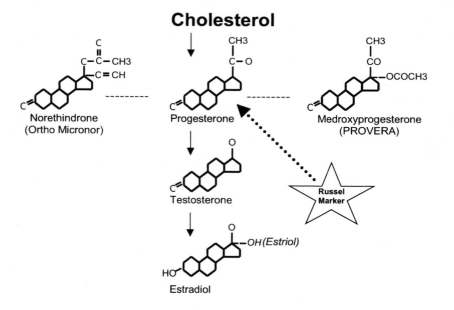

Figure 3. Natural and artificial hormones.

When the large US drug companies got into the action, there was no profit motive in marketing the bioidentical, or real hormones, as these hormones could not be patented. The drug houses therefore modified the molecules to create artificial hormones, which are patentable drugs, and marketed those to US physicians as hormones. They called drugs like Provera "Progestins" and made the physicians believe that it was the same thing as progesterone. Similarly, Premarin, a horse estrogen was marketed as a replacement for human estrogen despite the fact that the molecules are very different.

The pharmaceutical companies should have known that a minimal change in the natural molecule – like the minimal change that turns progesterone into testosterone, and testosterone into estrogen – changes the entire action and function of the molecule, and that these molecules act in the human body only by attaching to their specific and exact receptors (Figure 4). Yet, they proceeded to blur the difference between the real and the artificial and proceeded to market these substances to US doctors and US women.

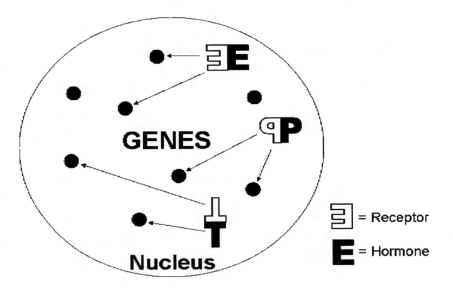

Figure 4. Steroid hormones working in the nucleus of the cell.

Many billions of dollars worth of these "hormones" were sold to women for many years until the WHI studies showed that these drugs resulted in increased cardiovascular complications, strokes, dementia, and breast cancer. Most of these complications appear to be related to Provera (medroxy-progesterone), which has been demonstrated to cause endothelial damage, inflammation, and insulin resistance,[30-32] all of which increase the risk of cardiovascular problems, strokes, dementia, and cancer. Real progesterone is protective against these problems.

It must be mentioned that the same companies also manufacture real, "bioidentical", hormones under government regulations, and sell them to compounding pharmacists who can mix and dispense these according to physician's orders for individual patients, and much less expensively. It is up to the physicians to learn how to prescribe the real hormones. Unfortunately, most physicians do not have the time or the desire to do so.

Testosterone

Testosterone exerts a direct anti-breast cancer effect. An NIH study clearly demonstrated that testosterone reduced the ER-alpha activity on breast cells in monkeys and reduced the proliferation rate of the cells.[33] Researchers at the University of Calabria in Italy have shown that testosterone inhibits breast cancer cells through its own androgen receptor, *AR*.[34] A recent report on 624 breast cancer patients at the National Cancer Institute has indicated that testosterone or DHEA levels did not increase the risk of breast cancer.[35]

However, it is important to point out that testosterone can get converted into estrogen by aromatase in the breast tissue, and some reports suggest that women with higher estrogen plus testosterone have more breast cancer. So, what is the bottom line? I believe that menopausal women should receive testosterone, if their levels are low and symptomatic, but only in small doses, and in the form of testosterone creams. I monitor their testosterone levels and make every effort not to exceed their levels beyond the 60th percentile. I do not believe in giving women testosterone injections as they lead to high peak levels of testosterone and potentially high conversion to estrogen in the fatty tissues such as the breast.

DHEA

DHEA inhibits the growth of breast cancer cells in mice.[36, 37] It also inhibits the growth of human breast cancers transplanted on to mice.[38] Patients with low DHEA levels and breast cancer have more metastases.[39]

Low DHEA levels have been associated with higher breast cancer risk in pre-menopausal women, conversely, high DHEA levels have been associated with more post-menopausal breast cancer.[40] It has been shown that if one infuses a large amount of DHEA into Petri dishes containing breast cancer cells, after about 4 days some of it eventually gets converted into estrogen, which can stimulate breast cancer cells.[41]

I recommend that women with low DHEA levels receive DHEA, but with caution, and only with blood level monitoring to ensure that you do not to exceed the 60th percentile of the reference range.

Melatonin

Melatonin is not just a sleep hormone. It plays a major role in the integrity of the neuroendocrine and immune systems. Melatonin levels begin to drop after the age of 15. By the time we reach our 60th birthday we have only one-tenth of our youth levels of melatonin.

Melatonin has multiple anti-cancer effects (Figure 5). It upregulates *p53* and *p21* tumor suppressor genes and reduces the concentration of ER-alpha on the tumor cells.[42] Linoleic acid (LA) can promote cancer cell growth. Melatonin has been shown to block the entry of LA into cancer cells.[43, 44] Melatonin protects cells against the effect of radiation.[45] It also increases superoxide dismutase (SOD), glutathione, and catalase levels in cells, thus protecting them from cancer promoting free radicals.[46] Melatonin also has anti-inflammatory properties,[47] and thus may also help to prevent cancer by combating inflammation.

Blind women have higher levels of melatonin and a significantly lower rate of breast cancer than non-blind women.[48] Conversely, night shift workers such as nurses, radio-telephone operators, and flight attendants tend to have lower melatonin levels and higher rates of breast cancer.[49] Some studies have now appeared showing that the addition of melatonin to conventional treatments of cancer result in superior results.[50]

I believe melatonin should be given to all women having sleep difficulties, especially those at higher risk for breast cancer.

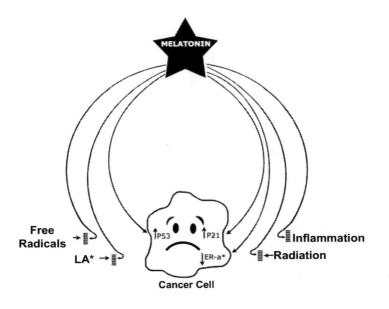

Mechanisms of Melatonin Anti-Cancer Action
*LA: Linoleic Acid   *ER-a: Estrogen Reception-alpha

Figure 5. Inhibitory effects of melatonin on breast cancer.

Oxytocin

Oxytocin is the pituitary hormone that lets the milk down in lactating mothers. It also has anti-cancer effects. It contracts the milk ducts thus propelling the free radical laden fluid out of the ducts. Free radicals in this fluid have been implicated in the initiation and stimulation of cancer.[51] Oxytocin inhibits many types of cancer cells through its own oxytocin receptor (*OR*) on these cells.[52] It also inhibits ER-alpha.[53] Studies from many countries have shown that breastfeeding reduces the risk for breast cancer.[54] Most likely this benefit is due to higher oxytocin levels during lactation. It makes a great deal of sense to breastfeed babies as long as possible, not just for breast cancer prevention but also for many other benefits to mother and child.

Oxytocin is not only increased with breastfeeding but also with breast and nipple stimulation. A 10-minute stimulation increases oxytocin levels by 100%.[55] Alcohol tends to block this release of oxytocin. Frequent breast and nipple stimulation, performed hygienically, seems to make sense and may reduce the risk of breast cancer.[56]

Insulin

By acting as a growth factor insulin promotes cancer cells by increasing levels of tyrosine kinase.[57] A Vanderbilt study has shown that women with higher insulin levels are more likely to develop breast cancer.[58] Whilst other studies have demonstrated that breast cancer patients with high insulin levels have more metastases.[59] Finally, the large Nurses Health Study has revealed a higher incidence of breast cancer in the presence of diabetes.[60]

I believe insulin resistance (metabolic syndrome) should be managed and controlled before the onset of frank diabetes. It will not only reduce breast cancer and other cancers, but also reduce hyperlipidemias, hypertension, and cardiovascular events. I use agents like chromium or metformin in addition to appropriate nutrition and exercise to achieve these ends.

Tri-iodothyronine (T3)

T3 has many unappreciated anti-cancer effects. As we age our natural killer (NK) cells (the first defense against cancer cells) decline. T3 increases NK cell activity.[61] It increases interleukin-2 (IL-2), an important cytokine in the defense against cancer, which has been used effectively in many cancer treatment protocols.[62] Tenacin C, a proliferative protein in cancer cells, is inhibited by T3.[63] *Cyclin D1* and *Cyclin T1* genes are turned on in breast cancer cells. T3 suppresses these genes.[64] It has been shown to directly inhibit MCF-7 (common type of breast cancer cells) in tissue cultures,[65] to decrease aromatase in breast cancer cells,[66] and to increase oxytocin production which inhibits cancer cells.[67] T3 also increases sex hormone binding globulin (SHBG), which has an anti-breast cancer effect.[68] T3 is also involved in DNA repair, which is important for our defense against cancer.[69]

Hypothyroidism is associated with increased breast cancer risk.[70] It is T3 and not T4 or TSH that has anti-cancer activity. Unfortunately, most physicians check TSH and maybe T4, but not T3. Synthroid contains T4 only, and does not increase T3 adequately in many patients. Armour thyroid has both T3 and T4 in more natural proportions. I prefer to give my patients Armour thyroid, and I monitor their T3 levels regularly.

Human Growth Hormone (HGH)

HGH increases the production of insulin-like growth factor (IGF), which, like insulin, can stimulate the growth of cancer cells.[71, 72] However, HGH has many anti-cancer actions (Figure 6). HGH administration increases IGFBP-3, a protein which binds IGF. IGFBP-3 inhibits estrogen-induced proliferation of breast cancer cells as well as promoting apoptosis of cancer cells.[73] HGH repairs DNA damage inflicted to cells by carcinogens and radiation.[74] It increases the activity of NK cells.[75] It stimulates the thymus gland and modulates the secretion of thymic hormones, improving the overall immune response.[76, 77] Its effect on the function of monocytes is inhibitory to cancer cells.[78] Nuclear Factor Kappa B (NFKB) is a proliferator of cancer cells. HGH inhibits NFKB in cancer cells by increasing glutathione.[79] It also increases levels of vitamin D, which has been shown to be inhibitory to cancer cells.[80] Low-dose HGH therapy, unlike high-dose HGH therapy, has been shown to reduce visceral fat and actually improve insulin resistance,[81] which should have an anti-cancer effect.

Unfortunately, the academia accentuates the one cancer stimulatory effect of HGH, but fails to mention any thing about its multiple anti-cancer effects. Studies of HGH administration to adults have not shown cancer as a risk.[82] Recently, a western clinic that had treated some 2000 adults with HGH over several years communicated the results at the annual A4M meeting. There had been only one case of cancer. Acromegalics with sky-high HGH levels do not have increased rates of cancer; except for a somewhat higher risk for colon cancer.[83] They do not have any increase in the rate of breast cancer.

I do not believe that HGH therapy should be withheld for fear of cancer if clear cut indications for such therapy exist.

196

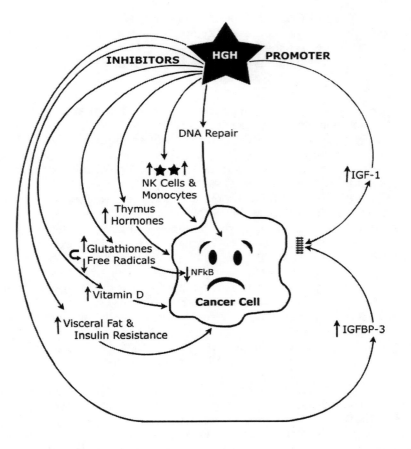

Figure 6. Effects of HGH on Breast Cancer.

CONCLUDING REMARKS

Many factors influence the appearance and growth of cancer cells positively or negatively, and these factors can be manipulated to inhibit the initiation and growth of tiny cancers during this period of time. There are a number of things that you can do to help reduce your patient's risk of developing breast cancer:

- For HRT use only bioidentical hormones
- For estrogen use Biest [4:1 ratio of E3 to E2]. Monitor patient and blood levels. Control hot flashes, but avoid breast tenderness. If breast tenderness develops back off on the dose. It may mean that the breast is not manufacturing much estrogen and the treatment E2 is entering the breast more than desired amounts. Use cream rather than oral preparations, thus avoiding an increase in clotting factors and c-reactive protein. Also, cream dose is easier to adjust.
- Increase 2/16 E ratio by encouraging patients to eat more vegetables and fruits, and less animal fat. Give Indole 3 Carbinol to patients with a high risk of breast cancer.
- Avoid Provera. Use only natural bioidentical progesterone.
- In pre-menopausal women with PMS, check E2 and progesterone levels on day 21 of cycle. If there is E2 dominance or Progesterone deficiency, give progesterone from day 14-28 of cycle. You will relieve PMS and very likely reduce the risk of breast cancer.
- In women with DHEA or T deficiency use DHEA or T cream and monitor levels not to exceed 60th percentile of the reference range.
- Treat insulin resistance rather than waiting for frank diabetes to develop (nutrition, exercise, chromium, DHEA, metformin, etc.)

- Increase oxytocin levels (breastfeeding, breast and nipple stimulation, alcohol reduction).
- Pay attention to free T3 in patients with symptoms of hypothyroidism. Use Armour thyroid rather than Synthroid when needed.
- Don't be afraid to use HGH for fear of cancer, when clear indications for HGH exist.

REFERENCES

1. Mady EA, Ramadan EE, Ossman AA. Sex steroid hormones in serum and breast tissue of benign and malignant breast tumor patients. *Dis Markers*. 2000;16:151-157.
2. Pasqualini JR, Gelly C, Nquyen BL, Vella C. Importance of estrogen sulfates in breast cancer. *J Steroid Biochem*. 1989;34:155-163.
3. Jefcoate CR, Liehr JG, Santen RJ, *et al*. Tissue-specific synthesis and oxidative metabolism of estrogens. *J Natl Cancer Inst Monogr*. 2000;(27):95-112.
4. Brueggemeier RW, Richards JA, Petrel TA. Aromatase and cyclooxygenases: Enzymes in breast cancer. *J Steroid Biochem Mol Bio*. 2003;86:501-507.
5. Chelbowski RT, Hendrix SL, Langer RD, *et al*. Influence of estrogen plus progestin on breast cancer and mammography in healthy post-menopausal women. The women's health initiative randomized trial. *JAMA*. 2003;289:3243-3253.
6. Jernstrom H, Bendahl PO, Lidfeldt J, *et al*. A prospective study of different types of hormone replacement therapy use and the risk of breast cancer: the women's health in the Lund area (WHILA) study (Sweden). *Cancer Causes Control*. 2003;14:673-680.
7. Schairer C, Adami HO, Hoover R, Persson I. Cause-specific mortality in women receiving hormone replacement therapy. *Epidemiology*. 1997;8:59-65.
8. Vassilopoulou-Sellin R, Asmar L, Hortobagyi GN, *et al*. Estrogen replacement therapy after localized breast cancer. Clinical outcome of 319 women followed prospectively. *J Clin Oncol*. 1999;17:1482-1487.
9. Vassilopoulou-Selin R, Cohen DS, Hortobagyi GN, *et al*. Estrogen replacement therapy for menopausal women with a history of breast carcinoma: results of a 5 year prospective study. *Cancer*. 2002;95:1817-1826.
10. Nakamura J, Lu Q, Aberdeen G, Albrecht E, Brodie A. The Effect of Estrogen on Aromatase and Vascular Endothelial Growth Factor Messenger Ribonucleic Acid in the Normal Nonhuman Primate Mammary Gland. *J Clin Endocrinol Metab*. 1999;84:1432-1437.
11. Chang M, Zhang F, Shen L, *et al*. Inhibition of glutathione S-transferase activity by the quinoid metabolites of equine estrogens. *Chem Res Toxicol*. 1998;11:758-765.
12. Kabat GC, Chang CJ, Sparano JA, *et al*. Urinary estrogen metabolites and breast cancer: a case control study. *Cancer Epidemiol Biomarkers Prev*. 1998; 6:505-509.
13. Ursin G, London S, Stanczyk FZ, *et al*. Urinary 2-hydroxyestrone/16 alpha-hydroxyestrone ratio and the risk of breast cancer in post-menopausal women. *J Natl Cancer Inst*. 1999;91:1067-1072.
14. Lemon HM, Wotiz HH, Parsons L, Mozden PJ. Reduced estriol excretion in patients with breast cancer prior to endocrine therapy. *JAMA*.1966;196:1128-1136.
15. Lemon HM. Oestriol and prevention of breast cancer. *Lancet*. 1973;1:546-547.
16. Lemon HM. Pathophysilogic considerations in the treatment of menopausal patients with oestrogens; the role of oestriol in the prevention of mammary carcinoma. *Acta Endocrino Suppl (copenh)*. 1980;233:17-27.
17. Siiteri PK. Pregnancy hormone estriol may reduce risk for breast cancer. Doctor's Guide 2002 Sept 30: www.pslgroup.com/
18. Vehkavaara S, Silveira A, Hakala-Ala-Pietala T, *et al*. Effects of oral and transdermal estrogen on markers of coagulation, fibrinolysis, inflammation and serum lipids and lipoproteins in postmenopausal women. *Thromb Haemost*. 2001;85;619-625.
19. Bradlow HL, Telang NT, Sepkovic DW, Osborne MP. 2-hydroxyestone: the 'good' estrogen. *J Endocrinol*. 1996;150 suppl:S259-265.
20. Muti P, Bradlow HL, Micheli A, *et al*. Estrogen metabolism and the risk of breast cancer: a prospective study of the 2:16alpha-hydroxyestrone ratio in premenopausal and post menopausal women. *Epidemiology*. 2000;11:635-640.
21. Cowan LD, Gordis L, Tonascia JA, Jones GS. Breast cancer incidence in women with a history of progesterone deficiency. *Am J Epidemol*. 1981;114:209-217.

22. Formby B, Wiley TS. Progesterone inhibits growth and induces apoptosis in breast cancer cells: inverse effects on Bcl-2 and p53. *Ann Clin Lab Sci.* 1998;28:360-369.

23. Formby B, Wiley TS. Bcl-2, surviving and variant CD44 v7-v10 are downregulated and p53 is upregulated in breast cancer cells by progesterone: inhibition of cell growth and apoptosis. *Mol Cell Biochem.* 1999;202:53-61.

24. Leo JC. Gene regulation profile reveals consistent anticancer properties of progesterone in hormone-independent breast cancer cells transfected with progesterone receptor. *Int J Cancer.* 2005;117:561-568.

25. Barrat J, de Lignieres B, Marpeau L, *et al.* The in vivo effect of the local administration of progesterone on the mitotic activity of human ductal breast tissue. Results of a pilot study. *J Gynecol Obstet Biol Reprod (Paris).* 1990;19:269-274.

26. Micheli A, Muti P, Secreto G, *et al.* Endogenous hormones and subsequent breast cancer in premenopausal women. *Int J Cancer.* 2004;112:312-318.

27. Kaaks R, Berrino F, Key T, *et al.* Serum sex steroids in premenopausal women and breast cancer risk within the European Prospective Investigation into Cancer and Nutrition (EPIC). *J Natl Cancer Institute.* 2005;97;755-765.

28. Jatoi I. Timing of surgery for primary breast cancer with regard to the menstrual phase and prognosis. *Breast Cancer Res Treat.* 1998;52:217-225.

29. Fournier A, Berrino F, Riboli E, Avenel V, Clavel-Chapelon F. Breast cancer risk in relation to different types of hormone replacement therapy in the E3N-EPIC cohort. *Int J Cancer.* 2005;114:448-454.

30. Sorensen MB, Collins P, Ong PJ, *et al.* Long-term use of contraceptive depot medroxyprogesterone acetate in young women impairs arterial endothelial function assessed by cardiovascular magnetic resonance. *Circulation.* 2002;106:1646-1651.

31. Clarkson TB. Progestogens and cardiovascular disease. A critical review. *J Reprod Med.* 1999;44(2Suppl):180-184.

32. Kahn HS, Curtis KM, Marchbanks PA. Effects of injectable or implantable progestin-only contraceptioves on insulin-glucose metabolism and diabetes risk. *Diabetes Care.* 2003;26:216-225.

33. Dimitrakakis C, Zhou J, Wang J, *et al.* A physiologic role for testosterone in limiting estogenic stimulation of the breast. *Menopause.* 2003;10(4):292-298.

34. Ando S, De Amicis F, Rago V, *et al.* Breast cancer: from estrogen to androgen receptor. *Mol Cell Endocrinol.* 2002;193:121-128.

35. Key TJ, Appleby Pn, Reeves GK, *et al.* Body mass index, serum sex hormones, and breast cancer risk in postmenopausal women. *J Natl Cancer Inst.* 2003;95:1218-1226.

36. Luo S, Labrie C, Belanger A, Labrie F. Effect of dehydroepiandrosterone on bone mass, serum lipids and dimethylbenz(a)anthracene-induced mammary carcinoma in the rat. *Endocrinology.* 1997;138:3387-3394.

37. Green JE, Shibata, MA, Shibata E, Moon RC, Anver MR, Kelloff F, Lubet R. 2-difluoromethylornithine and dehydroepiandrosterone inhibit mammary tumor progression but not mammary or prostate tumor initiation in C3(1)SV40 T/t-antigen transgenic mice. *Cancer Res.* 2001;61:7449-7455.

38. Couillard S, Labrie C, Belanger A, Candas B, Pouliot F, Labrie F. Effect of dehydroepiandrosterone and the anti-estrogen EM-800 on growth of human ZR-75-1 breast cancer xenografts. *J Natl Cancer Inst.* 1998;90:772-780.

39. Lissoni P, Rovelli F, Giani L, *et al.* Dehydroepiandrosterone sulfate secretion in early and advanced solid neoplasms: selective deficiency in metastatic disease. *Int J Biol Markers.* 1998;13:154-157.

40. Johnson MD, Bebb RA, Sirrs SM. Uses of DHEA in aging and other disease states. *Ageing Res Rev.* 2002;1:29-41.

41. Schmitt M, Klinga K, Schnarr B, Morfin R, Mayer D. Dehydroepiandrosterone stimulates proliferation and gene expression in MCF-7 cells after conversion to estradiol. *Mol Cell Endocrinol.* 2001;173:1-13.

42. Sanchez-Barcelo EJ, Cos S, Fernandez R, Mediavilla MD. Melatonin and mammary cancer: a short review. *Endocr Relat Cancer.* 2003;10:153-159.

43. Blask DE, Sauer LA, Dauchy R, Holowachuk EW, Ruhoff MS. New actions of melatonin on tumor metabolism and growth. *Biol Signals Recept.* 1999;8:49-55.

44. Blask DE, Dauchy RT, Sauer LA, Krause JA, Brainard GC. Light during darkness, melatonin suppression and cancer progression. *Neruo Endocrino Lett.* 2002;23 Suppl 2:52-56.

45. Vijayalaxmi, Reiter RJ, Tan DX, Herman TS, Thomas CR Jr. Melatonin as a radioprotective agent: a review. *Int J Radiat Oncol Biol Phys.* 2004;59:639-653.

46. Rodriguez C, Mayo JC, Sainz RM, Antolin I, Herrera F, Martin V, Reiter RJ. Regulation of antioxidant enzymes: a significant role for melatonin. *J Pineal Res.* 2004;36:1-9.

47. Cuzzocrea S, Reiter RJ. Pharmacological actions of melatonin in acute and chronic inflammation. *Curr Top Med Chem.* 2002;2:153-165.

48. Coleman MP, Reiter RJ. Breast cancer, blindness and melatonin. *Eur J Cancer.* 1992;28:501-503.

49. Anisimov VN. The light-dark regimen and cancer development. *Neuro Endocrino Lett.* 2002;23Suppl 2:28-36.

50. Panzer A, Viljoen M. The validity of melatonin as an oncostatic agent. *J Pineal Res.* 1997;22:184-202.

51. Chen G, Djuric Z. Detection of 2,6 cyclolycopene-I,5-diol in breast nipple aspirate fluids and plasma: a potential marker of oxidative stress. *Cancer Epidemiol Biomarkers Prev.* 2002;11:1592-1596.

52. Cassoni P, Catalano MG, Sapino A, *et al.* Oxytocin modulates estrogen receptor alpha expression and function in MCF7 human breast cancer cells. *Int J Oncol.* 2002;21:375-378.

53. Cassoni P, Marrocco T, Deaglio S, Sapino A, Bussolati G. Biological relevance of oxytocin and oxytocin receptors in cancer cells and primary tumors. *Ann Oncol.* 2001;12 Suppl 2:S37-39.

54. Collaborative group on hormonal factors in breast cancer. Breast cancer and breast feeding: collaborative reanalysis of individual data from 47 epidemiological studies in 30 countries. *Lancet.* 2002;360:187-195.

55. Coiro V, Alboni A, Gramellini D, *et al.* Inhibition by ethanol of the oxytocin response to breast stimulation in normal women and the role of endogenous opioids. *Acta Endocrinol (Copenh).* 1992;126:213-216.

56. Murrell TG. Epidemiological and biochemical support for a theory on the cause and prevention of breast cancer. *Med Hypotheses.* 1991;36:389-396.

57. Boyd DB. Insulin and Cancer. *Integr Cancer Ther.* 2003;2:315-329.

58. Malin A, Dai Q, Yu H, Shu XO, GAO YT, Zheng W. Evaluation of the synergistic effect of insulin resistance and the insulin-like growth factors on the risk of breast carcinoma. *Cancer.* 2004;100:694-700.

59. Goodwin PJ, Ennis M, Pritchard KI, *et al.* Fasting Insulin and outcome in early-stage breast cancer: results of a prospective cohort study. *Journal of Clinical Oncology.* 2002;20:42-51.

60. Michels KB, Solomon CG, Hu FB, *et al.* Type 2 diabetes and subsequent incidence of breast cancer in the nurses' health study. *Diabetes Care.* 2003;26:1752-1758.

61. Kmiec Z, Mysliwska J, Rachon D, Kotlarz G, Sworczak K, Mysliwski A. Natural Killer cell activity and thyroid hormones in young and elderly persons. *Gerontology.* 2001;47:282-288.

62. Nakanishi K, Taniguchi Y, Onji M. Triiodothyronine enhancesw expression of the interleukin-2 receptor alpha chain. *Endocr J.* 1999;46:437-442.

63. Gonzalez-Sancho JM, Alvarez-Dolado M, Caelles C, Munoz A. Inhibition of tenascin-C epression in mammary epithelial cells by thyroid hormone. *Mol Carcinog.* 1999;24:99-107.

64. Gonzalez-Sancho JM, Figueroa A, Lopez-Barahona M, Lopez E, Beug H, Munoz A. Inhibition of proliferation and expression of T1 and Cyclin D1 genes by thyroid hormones in mammary epithelial cells. *Mol Carcinog.* 2002;34:164.

65. Martinez MB, Ruan M, Fitzpatrik LA. Altered response to thyroid hormones by prostate and breast cancer cells. *Cancer Chemother Pharmacol.* 2000;45:93-102.

66. Gregoraszczuk EL, Slomczynska M, Wilk R. Thyroid hormone inhibits aromatase activity in porcine thecal cells cultured alone and in combination with granulose cells. *Thyroid.* 1998;8:1157-1163.

67. Adan RA, Vox JJ, van Kats JP, Burbach Jp. Thyroid hormone regulates the oxytocin gene. *J Biol Chem.* 1992;267:3771-3777.

68. Krotkiewski M, Holm G, Shono N. Small doses of triiodothyronine can change some risk factors associated with abdominal obesity. *Int J obes Relat Metab Disord.* 1997;21:922-929.

69. Antipenko Aye, Antipenko YN. Thyroid hormones and regulation of cell reliability systems. *Adv Enzyme Regul.* 1994;34:173-198.

70. Smyth PP. The thyroid and breast cancer: a significant association. *Ann Med.* 1997;29:189-191.

71. Furstenberger G, Senn HJ. Insulin-like growth factors and cancer. *Lancet Oncol.* 2002;3:298-302.
72. Schernhammer ES, Holly JM, Pollak MN, Hankinson SE. Circulating levels of insulin-like growth factor 1 and risk of breast cancer. *Lancet.* 1998;351:1393-1396.
73. Pratt SE, Pollak MN. Insulin like binding protein 3 (IGFBP-3) inhibits estrogen-stimulated breast cancer cell proliferation. *Biochem Biophys Res Commun.* 1994;198:292-297.
74. Madrid O, Varea S, Sanchez-Perez I, et al. Growth hormone protects against radiotherapy-induced cell death. *Eur J Endocrinol.* 2002;147:535-541.
75. Crist DM, Kraner JC. Supplemental growth hormone increases the tumor cytotoxicity activity of natural killer cells in healthy adults with normal growth hormone secretion. *Metabolism.* 1990;39:1320-1324.
76. Savino W, Smaniotto S, Binart N, Postel-Vinay MC, Dardenne M. In vivo effects of growth hormone on thymic cells. *Ann NY Acad Sci.* 2003;992:179-185.
77. Khorram O, Yeung M, Vu L, Yen SS. Effects of growth hormone releasing hormone (GHRH) administration on the immune system of aging men and women. *J Clin endocrine Metab.* 1997;82:3590-3596.
78. Serri O, St-Jacques P, Sartippour M, Renier G. Alteration of monocyte function in patients with growth hormone deficiency: effect of substitutive GH therapy. *J Clin Endocrine Metab.* 1999;84:58-63.
79. Cherbonnier C, Deas O, Carvalho G, *et al.* Potentiation of tumor apoptosis by human growth hormone via glutathione production and decreased NF-Kappa B activity. *Brit J Cancer.* 2003;89:1108-1115.
80. Wright NM, Papadea N, Wentz B, Hollis B, Willi S, Bell NH. Increased serum 1,25-dihydroxyvitamin D after growth hormone administration is not parathyroid hormone mediated. *Calcif Tissue Int.* 1997;61:101-103.
81. Nam SY, Kim KR, Cha BS, Song YD, Lim SK, Lee HC, Huh KB. Low dose growth hormone treatment combined with diet restriction decreases insulin resistance by reducing visceral fat and increasing muscle mass in obese type 2 diabetic patients. *Int J Obes Relat Metab Disord.* 2001;25:1101-1107.
82. Abs R, Bengtsson BA, Hernberg-Stâhl E, Monson JP, Tauber JP, Wilton P, Wüster C. GH replacement in 1034 growth homone deficient hypopituitary adults: demographic and clinical characteristics, dosing and safety. *Clin Endocrino (Oxf).* 1999;50:703-713.
83. Webb SM, Casanueva F, Wass JA. Oncologic complications of excess GH in acromegaly. Pituitary. 2002;5:21-25.

ABOUT THE AUTHOR

Dr. Khalid Mahmud is board certified in Internal Medicine, Hematology and Oncology, as well as in anti-aging medicine by the American Board of Anti-Aging & Regenerative Medicine (ABAARM). He is a Fellow of the American College of Physicians. Formerly, Dr. Mahmud has served as the Chief of Medicine, North Memorial Medical Center, Minneapolis, MN; and also as the Medical Director of Oncology North Memorial Medical Center, Minneapolis, MN (serving in this capacity for more than 10 years). He is the author of Keeping a Breast: Ways to Stop Breast Cancer [AuthorHouse, 2005], which details lifestyle, hormonal balance, and appropriate supplementation in the prevention of breast cancer. A frequent national speaker on numerous health related topics, including management of menopause with the use of bio-identical hormones, Dr. Mahmud is currently in full-time practice of anti-aging and preventive medicine.

Chapter 26
Energy Medicine and Matrix Regeneration
James L. Oschman, Ph.D.[1]; Judy Kosovich[2]
[1]President, Nature's Own Research Association
[2]Associate, Law firm of Swankin and Turner

ABSTRACT

Energy medicine includes a variety of diagnostic and therapeutic tools that are becoming increasingly popular worldwide and that are steadily entering mainstream medicine. Matrix Regeneration is an approach that is emerging from our increasing understandings of how various forms of energy are used by the human body to regulate living processes such as healing. For example, an injury results in an electrical wave called the injury potential that triggers healing and regeneration; a number of modern therapeutic devices introduce comparable electric waves that stimulate natural tissue repair processes. It has also been discovered that injured cells emit light that is sensed by other cells and that light triggers both cell division and cell migration to an injury site. These biophysical phenomena also help explain how various hands-on and device-based therapies stimulate healing.

The "living matrix" is the largest organ system in the human body. It consists of the extracellular matrix, i.e. the connective tissues and myofascial systems, and their extensions into the cytoskeleton and nuclear matrix of every cell. The matrix forms a continuous semiconducting network reaching into every nook and cranny of the body. Neurons, skin, the intestinal lining, capillary walls, arteries, immune cells, and even DNA are all components of this matrix. As a whole-body substrate for chemical, electronic, and mechanical signaling, as well as access to genetic information, the quality and integrity of the living matrix is a major factor in maintaining optimal health, vitality and longevity. This article summarizes the scientific basis for a variety of technologies that enable the physician to interrogate the entire matrix and to detect and correct imbalances and thereby resolve health issues. Of particular interest is the application of the Vascular Autonomic Signal (VAS) to detect areas of the body that are physiologically stressed or that are in early stages of disease onset, when they are easier to correct.

Keywords: connective tissue, longevity, energy medicine, frequency, spontaneous healing, inflammation, living matrix, physiological balance, matrix

INTRODUCTION

Anti-aging medicine is becoming a major discipline in health care worldwide, as evidenced by the growing popularity and global spread of the A4M conferences. Energy medicine is also growing in popularity because it includes techniques that are often capable of resolving medical issues that are difficult to diagnose or treat by other means. The public is attracted to energy medicine because the techniques provide excellent healing in all stages of disease, from pre-symptomatic to chronic and intractable. Moreover, the treatments are very cost-effective, are generally non-invasive and have few if any lingering side effects. After a long period of skepticism, the science behind energetic approaches is emerging as a rich and fascinating topic with major implications for prevention and longevity.

As with anti-aging medicine, there are several major categories of practices in energy medicine. To be specific, energy medicine encompasses both hands-on or manipulative therapies (Table I) as well as an increasing number of therapeutic devices. Some approaches involve a combination of hands-on and therapeutic instruments. Basic biophysics and the living matrix concept are providing scientific understandings of the effectiveness of these approaches.

Table 1. Applications of Energy Medicine

Acupuncture	Alexander	Biodynamics	Body Talk
Bowen	Chiropractic	Consegrity	Cranial-sacral
Feldenkrais	Healing touch	Holographic Repatterning	Homeopathy
Massage	Osteopathy	Palates	Pranic Healing
Polarity therapy	Reiki	Rolfing/Structural Integration	Therapeutic touch
Yoga	Zero Balancing		

This essay focuses on therapeutic approaches that utilize biofeedback that informs both patient and practitioner. Such systems are instructive for the practitioner because they involve the integration of both branches of energy medicine: touch and technology. There is a basis for these devices in the Vascular Autonomic Signal (VAS), which is increasingly being utilized for diagnostic purposes. The VAS is a sensitive indicator of the condition of a variety of systems within the body. The article begins with a description of the VAS and continues with consideration of its application as part of diagnostic and treatment protocols.

THE VASCULAR AUTONOMIC SIGNAL

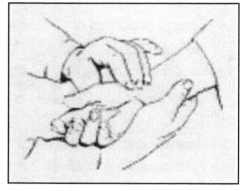

Figure 1. The radial artery pulse.

A discussion of the VAS begins with the work of French physician, Dr. Paul Nogier, who taught neurology at the medical school in Lyon, France. Nogier also studied Traditional Oriental Medicine, which includes sophisticated methods of analyzing the radial artery pulse (Figure 1). In 1966, Nogier discovered that the Vascular Autonomic Signal was evoked in the radial pulse (termed the RAC in French, for Réflexe Auriculo-Cardiaque or Autonomic Circulatory Reaction) when he touched certain points on the ear of a patient. Subsequently, he discovered that the arterial system responds in a reproducible manner to a variety of changes to key physiological systems in the body. To be specific, the VAS is a rapid change in the tone of the smooth muscles in the walls of the arterial system throughout the body, mediated by sympathetic and parasympathetic neurons.[1,2]

Distinct changes in the amplitude and other characteristics of the pulse take place when certain points on the ear are stimulated. This occurs consistently and is both repeatable and measurable by modern equipment. The response that is felt by the practitioner is a qualitative variation in the perception of the pulse that begins from 1 to 3 cycles after the stimulus begins and continues for about 8 to 15 cardiac cycles.[3] Nogier found that there are four pulse responses to stimuli: no response, the weakening of the pulse signal (negative V.A.S.), increase of the pulse signal (positive V.A.S.), and a sharp pulse spike. These responses occur from colors, magnetically induced currents, sound frequencies, light waves, emotions, touch, substances, and electromagnetic frequencies. There is considerable medical interest in the VAS, as evidenced by five International Symposia, the most recent one held in Lyon, France in 2006. Several United States Patents[4] and several diagnostic and therapeutic tools are based on the phenomenon. The method is sometimes referred to as Peripheral Arterial Tonometry.

Although the term "signal" as in the "Vascular Autonomic Signal" is widely used, many who use the system consider the term "response" as more accurate. A response is an answer to a question, and the VAS is the body's reaction or answer to a question posed by the introduction of stimulation into the body or into its energy field. For a discussion of the term, "energy field," see Oschman.[5]

The VAS is extremely sensitive, and can be used to discover both the best treatment for a symptom as well as more subtle levels of disturbances in the organism. These can include blockages to the healing response, layers of pathology, the appropriate priority for treatment and even subclinical issues. The VAS can be used both before and after a treatment to determine the accuracy of the diagnosis and the success of the treatment. In essence, the VAS is a very sensitive way of "listening" to the body. A wide variety of therapeutic schools around the world train practitioners to read the VAS and use it to define areas of the body under stress, the causes of the stress, chemical intolerances and the degree of success of interventions. The VAS can also provide early warnings of subclinical issues and therefore provide the practitioner with the opportunity to reverse developing conditions at an early stage.[6]

DIAGNOSTIC APPLICATIONS OF THE VASCULAR AUTONOMIC SIGNAL

A number of devices based on the VAS are being incorporated into mainstream medical practice. They are generally non-invasive and are extremely sensitive for detecting the location of elusive pathologies or serious medical conditions that are in early stages of development. The implications of these techniques for anti-aging and longevity are obvious.

One system is based on Peripheral Arterial Tonometry, an autonomic response of the cardiovascular system that can provide an early warning of cardiovascular disease.[7] This application of VAS is a device that is worn at home while sleeping. It diagnoses factors contributing to obstructive sleep apnea syndrome.

A second device, by Itmar, is used as an early warning for coronary artery endothelial dysfunction, before symptoms begin to manifest.[8] This system uses continuous monitoring of the pulse in the fingertip with a preprogrammed calibration as determined by medical practitioners. It measures temporary changes in the cardiovascular pulse that occur naturally throughout the body when the autonomic nervous system is stressed.

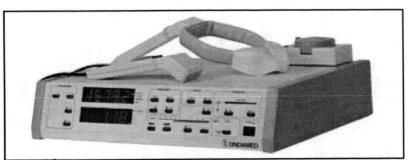

Figure 2. The Ondamed® system, with components on the top, including the hand held applicator (front), the neck applicator and the frequency regulator.

A third technology (Figure 2) has very broad applications.[9] It consists of a non-invasive system that detects cardiovascular responses to electromagnetic stimulation at various frequencies ranging from 0.1Hz to 32,000Hz. The device supplements a physician's decision-making process, and is used in conjunction with knowledge of a patient's history and other clinical findings. The device is a computerized programmable system that is used by a medical practitioner to deliver weak magnetic pulses of various frequencies to the body, during which time the practitioner detects temporary changes in the radial artery pulse or VAS. This pulse response indicates which frequencies stimulate the autonomic nervous system, leading to a VAS.

Many frequencies and ranges of frequencies have been correlated with particular conditions, tissues, organs, or areas of the body. The practitioner scans through the entire range of frequencies delivered by a neck applicator (see Figure 2) to determine the frequencies most important to a patient. The location of the tissue or area that is most responsive to a particular frequency can be determined by moving the Hand-held Applicator (Figure 3) over areas of the body. One advantage of the system is that sometimes the VAS can be detected before a condition has begun to manifest symptoms. This is particularly important for conditions that may prove life threatening if not caught early.

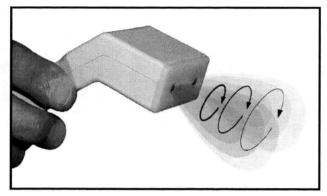

Figure 3. Hand-held Area Applicator.

The frequencies can, in principle, be applied at any point on the body. In practice, however, it is convenient to use two magnetic coils, wound in opposite spirals, in an applicator that rests loosely around the neck of a reclining patient. The system is designed in such a way that no current flows directly from the device to the patient. Instead, microcurrents are induced in the tissues of the body by a pulsing magnetic field delivered through the magnetic applicators that are encased in non-conducting plastic. There is therefore no transcutaneous flow of current and no risk of electrical shock. The magnetic fields used are comparable in strength to those naturally present in the body and in the environment due to the magnetic field of the earth. Hence there is no known risk of movement of metallic objects or implants in the body. The system has been used internationally for more than a decade without reports of adverse effects. There is considerable anecdotal evidence showing positive results, and the system has been used in small-scale trials and is in the early stages of clinical testing.

There are two primary mechanisms by which magnetic fields can introduce energy (microcurrents) within the body, whether for diagnostic or treatment purposes. The usual textbook explanation involves the laws of induction: a time-varying magnetic field will cause charges in surrounding regions to move. In living systems the primary charge carriers for low frequency electric currents are thought to be electrolytes: the charged ions such as sodium, potassium and chloride, which are abundant in blood and other body fluids. Another mechanism that becomes more important at higher frequencies involves much smaller charged particles such as electrons and protons (hydrogen ions) that can be semiconducted through the living matrix, to be described below. Semiconduction and magnetic effects arise in part because of the Hall Effect, an important physical phenomenon discovered in 1879 by Harvard Physicist Edwin H Hall.

Biophysical studies have shown that cells and tissues can respond to electrical signals that are far weaker than those needed to depolarize neurons, produce heating or cause ionization.[10] Moreover, magnetic fields can cause dipolar molecules (molecules that do not have a net electrical charge but that have an uneven distribution of charges) to bend or rotate or change their configuration. In other words, enzymatic processes and cell behavior are both field-sensitive.[11]

THE LIVING MATRIX

The living matrix is a continuous physical network reaching into every part of the body. While this "organ of form" has not attracted the same attention in biomedical research circles as other major systems, such as the nervous, circulatory, reproductive, digestive, immune, and other systems, the living matrix is actually the fundamental material that forms all of the systems, organs, tissues, and cells in the body. The living matrix concept evolved from the discovery that molecules called integrins traverse cell surfaces, joining the cytoskeleton of every cell with the extracellular or connective tissue matrix.[12,13] Deep inside every cell, the cytoskeleton also connects to the nuclear matrix and to the genome.[14]

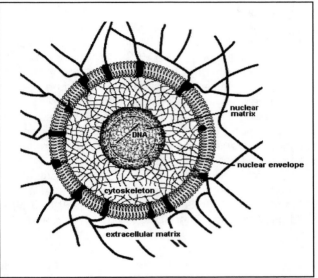

Figure 4. A cell and its surrounding matrix.

Figure 4 shows a cell and its surroundings. Note the nuclear matrix within the cytoplasmic matrix within the extracellular matrix. Molecular biologists have described the thousands of different molecules comprising this matrix system. A prominent scientist from Johns Hopkins University School of Medicine in Baltimore, Donald Coffee, and his colleague, KJ Pienta, wrote about this system:

> *Cells and intracellular elements are capable of vibrating in a dynamic manner with complex harmonics, the frequency of which can now be measured and analyzed in a quantative manner ...These vibrations can be altered by growth factors and the process of carcinogenesis ...a tissue matrix system consisting of the nuclear matrix, the cytoskeleton, and the extracellular matrix...is poised to couple the biological oscillations of the cell from the peripheral membrane to the DNA...*[15]

Fascinating research from Donald Ingber and his colleagues at Harvard Medical School shows that tensions in the matrix are as significant as chemical factors in regulating cellular activities.[16] And the research summarized above indicates the significance of electrical and magnetic factors. Taken together, the matrix and its energetic properties provide a mechanism for the semiconduction of electrons and protons at various frequencies throughout the body.

One of the most prominent scientists to research electronic biology was Albert Szent-Györgyi, who received the Nobel Prize in 1937 for the synthesis of Vitamin C. He observed that living processes are too rapid and subtle to be explained only by slow moving chemical reactions and nerve impulses.[17] To account for the speed and subtlety of living processes, he described in detail how the double bonds in the backbone of protein molecules contribute free or mobile or delocalized electrons that can move extremely rapidly throughout the body. He viewed the protein fabric as the "circuitry" that conducts mobile electrons and protons. His key contribution was the identification of proteins as semiconductors.[18] Migration of electrons can take place within the matrix far faster than the random diffusion of chemicals and nerve conduction that is measured in meters per second. Signaling with electronic and electromagnetic signals can be virtually instantaneous.

Until recently, these ideas have had little experimental support and even less impact in the fields of physiology and biomedicine. This has changed, however, because the reality of the semiconducting nature of proteins and other components of the matrix is providing the basis for a nanoelectronics industry, which is producing molecular and atomic circuitry.[19, 20] In other words, an entire global industry is turning to biology for inspiration in miniaturization of electronic devices.

ENERGY MEDICINE IN THERAPEUTICS

The above descriptions of the VAS and the living matrix lead to a consideration of how oscillating fields can be introduced into the body for diagnostic and therapeutic purposes. Once the critical frequencies have been identified with the VAS, various signals can be introduced for therapeutic purposes. For example, shortly after his discovery of the VAS, Nogier described a set of frequencies and their harmonics that could be used constantly in routine medical practice, as they are preferentially recognized by the body. They enter into resonance with specific tissues and exert specific effects. Thus, frequencies can be varied for diagnosis or selected for treatment.[21]

The Ondamed® system described above (Figures 2 and 3) has applicators of various shapes and sizes that allow the magnetic pulses to be delivered to particular areas, e.g., the neck, the abdomen, a joint, the spine, an organ, a gland, or a muscle.

The use of a range of frequencies of electromagnetic pulses to provide therapeutic stimulation is well known. The first devices to be approved by the Food and Drug Administration for this purpose were developed in the early 1980's by Brighton, Bassett and others, who demonstrated that fracture 'non-unions' could be stimulated to heal using tiny electric and magnetic fields. A review of this widely used technology was published by Bassett in 1995.[22] The methods were so successful that they were tested on other tissues. It was found that each tissue responds to a different frequency.[23] Currently a variety of pulsed electromagnetic field and implantable electrical stimulators are available to stimulate the repair of delayed union of fracture (improper healing within 6 months) or fracture nonunion (failure of union after 6 months). There are now hundreds of devices for electromagnetic stimulation at various frequencies for nerve and muscle, pain relief, incontinence, evoked responses, bone and wound healing, and reduction of stress. Some of these are biofeedback systems.

CONCLUDING REMARKS

Optimum health, vitality and longevity depend on maintaining the structural and functional integrity of our internal energetic systems. Technologies employing the Vascular Autonomic Signal (VAS) can be used to diagnose subtle levels of disturbances in the organism and determine the best treatment. This diagnosis can include blockages to the healing response, layers of pathology, the appropriate priority for treatment, and even subclinical issues. In essence, the VAS is a very sensitive way of "listening" to the body. A wide variety of therapeutic schools around the world train practitioners to read the VAS and use it to define areas of the body under stress, the causes of the stress, chemical intolerances and the most beneficial interventions. The VAS can also provide early warnings of subclinical issues and therefore provide the practitioner with the ability to reverse developing pathologies.

REFERENCES

[1] James L. Oschman, PhD, Nature's Own Research Association, PO Box 1935, Dover, New Hampshire 03821, USA.

[2] Judy Kosovich, c/o Swankin - Turner, 1400 16th Street NW, Suite 101, Washington, D.C. 20036, judy@swankinturner.com

[3] http://www.sedatelec.com/english/acupauri.htm

[4] United States Patent 6,942,622, issued September 13, 2005, for Method for monitoring autonomic tone.

[5] Oschman JL. Energy Medicine: the scientific basis. Edinburgh; Churchill Livingstone/Harcourt Brace: 2000.

[6] Agnes M. Toward an Integral Energy Medicine Model for Understanding the Vascular Autonomic Signal. Ph.D. Thesis, Greenwich University - Holos University: 2002.

[7] Bonetti PO, Pumper GM, Higano ST, Holmes DR, JR, Kuvin JT, Lerman A. Noninvasive Identification of Patients With Early Coronary Atherosclerosis by Assessment of Digital Reactive Hyperemia. Journal of the American College of Cardiology 44(11): 2137–21 41: 2004

[8] Bonetti PO Pumper GM Higano ST Holmes DR Kuvin JT Lerman A. Noninvasive identification of patients with early coronary atherosclerosis by assessment of digital reactive hyperemia. J Am Coll Cardiol. 44(11):2137-41: 2004.

[9] http://www.ondamed.net/

[10] Adey WR. A growing scientific consensus on the cell and molecular biology mediating interactions with environmental electromagnetic fields. In: Ueno S (ed) Biological effects of magnetic and electromagnetic fields. Plenum Press, New York Ch. 4, pp. 45-62: 1996.

[11] Westerhoff HV Kamp F Tsong TY Astumian RD. In Blank M Findl E (eds) Mechanistic approaches to interactions of electric and electromagnetic fields with living systems. Plenum Press, New York, pp. 203-215: 1987.

[12] Bretscher M. C-Terminal region of the major erythrocyte sialoglycoprotein is on the cytoplasmic side of the membrane. *J Mol Biol.* 1975;98:831-833.

[13] Horwitz AF. Integrins and health. Discovered only recently, these adhesive cell surface molecules have quickly revealed themselves to be critical to proper functioning of the body and to life itself. *Scientific American.* 1997;276:68-75.

[8] Maniotis AJ, Chen CS, Ingber DE. Demonstration of mechanical connections between integrins, cytoskeletal filaments, and nucleoplasm that stabilize nuclear structure. *Proc Natl Acad Sci USA.* 1997;94:849-854.

[15] Pienta KJ, Coffey DS. Cellular harmonic information transfer through a tissue tensegrity-matrix system. *Medical Hypotheses.* 1991;34:88-95.

[16] Ingber DE. The riddle of morphogenesis: a question of solution chemistry or molecular cell engineering. *Cell* 1993;75:1249-1252.

[17] Szent-Györgyi A. See: Oschman JL. *Energy Medicine: the scientific basis.* Edinburgh: Churchill Livingstone/Harcourt Brace; 2000.

[18] Szent-Györgyi A. Towards a New Biochemistry? Science 93:609-11:1941.
[19] Stroscio MA, Dutta M. Integrated biological-semiconductor devices. Proceedings of the IEEE. 2005;93:1772-1783.

[20] Hush NS. An overview of the first half-century of molecular electronics. *Annals of the New York Academy of Sciences.* 2003;1006;1-20.

[21] Nogier P Nogier R. The man in the ear. Maisonneuve, 255 p.: 1979.

[22] Bassett CAL. Bioelectromagnetics in the service of medicine. In: Blank M (ed) Electromagnetic fields: biological interactions and mechanisms. Advances in Chemistry Series 250, American Chemical Society, Washington DC: pp. 261-275: 1995.

[23] Sisken BF Walker J. Therapeutic aspects of electromagnetic fields for soft-tissue healing. In: Blank M (ed) Electromagnetic fields: biological interactions and mechanisms. Advances in Chemistry Series 250, American Chemical Society, Washington DC, pp. 277-285: 1995.

ABOUT THE AUTHORS

Dr. James L. Oschman is the President of Nature's Own Research Association, and is a leading authority on the science behind a wide variety of energy medicine therapies. He has a BS degree in biophysics and a Doctoral degree in biology from the University of Pittsburgh. He has worked in major research labs around the world, and his scientific papers have been published in the world's leading journals. Jim is also the author of *Energy Medicine: The Scientific Basis*, published by Churchill Livingstone. This book gives the most ardent skeptic a logical and scientifically sound basis for a variety of therapies. Elsevier Health Sciences published Jim's second book, *Energy Medicine in Therapeutics and Human Performance*. This research provides new insights into the ways the body can function in peak athletic or artistic performances and in profound therapeutic encounters. Jim's research has led to useful insights that can help all health care professionals better understand and advance their work and explain it to others. He has also become involved in the development of cutting-edge medical devices and other applications of the emerging concepts of energy medicine. Jim is a member of the Scientific Advisory Board for the National Foundation for Alternative Medicine, and is the recipient of their Founders Award. He has also received a Distinguished Service Award from the Rolf Institute. You can learn more about his work on his website: http://www.energyresearch.us/

Judy Kosovich is an Associate with the law firm of Swankin and Turner in Washington, D.C. Her work includes the areas of patents, health policy, and FDA's regulation of medical devices, especially in the area of energy medicine.

Chapter 27
Energy Medicine and Longevity
James L Oschman, Ph.D.[1]
President, Nature's Own Research Association

ABSTRACT

After much skepticism, energy medicine and the science behind it are emerging as rich and fascinating topics with major implications for anti-aging medicine. The public is attracted to energetic techniques because they are cost-effective, are relatively non-invasive, and have few if any side effects. Those who follow the emerging field of energy medicine are exposed to entirely new vistas about how the human body works in health and disease. Some of the major new perspectives will be considered here: the cell is not a "bag of solution"; biochemistry in living cells is very different from biochemistry in a test tube; because of resonance, molecules do not have to touch to interact; and bioenergetic fields are real and important in the healing process. The "bag of solution" model has been replaced with a matrix model that incorporates the latest findings of cell biology: the trans-membrane proteins or integrins are key elements in a continuous molecular fabric or living matrix that extends throughout the living body in the form of connective tissue and throughout the cell as the cytoskeleton and nuclear matrix. Many biochemical reactions take place in highly ordered systems called metabolons, sequences of enzymes ordered along the matrix. Regulation by signal molecules randomly diffusing to receptors must be very slow, and is undoubtedly supported in life by non-contact resonant electromagnetic interactions between regulatory molecules and their receptors. Energy fields are measurable in the spaces around the body using technologies such as magnetocardiography and magnetoencephalography. Taken together, these concepts help us understand new diagnostic/therapeutic technologies. Well-documented and widely used examples include: scanning the body with microcurrents to evaluate the condition of organs and systems and even to image tiny tumors; the use of pulsing electromagnetic fields (PEMF) to stimulate bone growth and the healing of soft tissue injuries; and a technology called ONDAMED® that combines PEMF with pulse biofeedback to establish treatment frequencies on a patient-by-patient basis. The system is extremely sensitive for detecting elusive pathologies and serious medical conditions in the earliest stages of development. The implications for prevention and longevity are profound.

Keywords: connective tissue, longevity, energy medicine, regulation, living matrix, resonance

INTRODUCTION

After much skepticism, energy medicine and the science behind it are emerging as rich and fascinating topics with major implications for anti-aging medicine. The public is attracted to energetic techniques because they are cost-effective, are usually non-invasive, and have few if any side effects. This article begins by updating some long held and widely taught concepts of communication and control in living systems and what modern science is revealing about them. We then move on to consider some of the remarkable technologies that are emerging from this established scientific base.

The reason energy medicine has been so controversial is a lack of appreciation of the research that has gone into the subject over the past century. With a little background in physics and biophysics, energy medicine ceases to be a mystery. In fact, it is an exciting area of research and clinical practice that has opened up new vistas in patient care and longevity.

The author was introduced to this subject through the work of Albert Szent-Györgyi, MD, PhD, who received the Nobel Prize in 1937 for the synthesis of vitamin C and for his fundamental research on biological oxidation. His work was instrumental in establishing the dominant paradigms of western biomedicine, biochemistry, and molecular biology, and their practical applications provided by pharmacology. In spite of this success, Szent-Györgyi continued to recognize that chemistry is but one piece of a much larger puzzle, and that energy provides the key to unraveling the mysteries of life and health.

> *The cell is a machine driven by energy. It can thus be approached by studying matter, or by studying energy.*
> ~Albert Szent-Györgyi, MD, PhD

Others who stepped back to look at the organism and its environment in their entirety arrived at similar perspectives. From a leading German scientist:

...the materialistic views of the world only deals with...one billionth of reality.
~Dr. Wolfgang Ludwig

And from a leading science educator:

Some say there is no such thing as energy medicine. They have not been listening to the physicists, who tell us that there is nothing but energy in the universe.
~Deane Juhan

Those who follow the emerging field of energy medicine are quickly exposed to entirely new vistas about how the human body works in health and disease. Some of the major new perspectives we will consider here:

- The cell is not a "bag of solution".
- Biochemistry in living cells is very different from biochemistry in a test tube.
- Because of resonance, molecules do not have to touch to interact.
- Bioenergetic fields are real and important in the healing process

REGULATION BY RANDOM DIFFUSION OF SIGNAL MOLECULES

A theme for looking at living processes emerged from Szent-Györgyi's realization that life is much too rapid and subtle to be explained by slow moving chemical reactions and nerve impulses. For example, our conventional chemical models of biological communications and regulations are based on the activities of a variety of types of messenger molecules. These include hormones, neurohormones, neurotransmitters, antigens, cytokines, growth factors, and intracellular messengers such as cyclic AMP. The extracellular messengers are viewed as being transported throughout the body via the circulatory system, and then through extracellular fluids by diffusion. The latter is a slow and random process because there is no motivation for the molecules to move in any particular direction, i.e. toward or away from their respective receptors, so they tend to bump and stagger about in all directions. Eventually, after a long and irregular journey, signal molecules may encounter receptors on the surfaces of cells (Figure 1). Given the randomness of the process, it has to be a matter of luck for a signal molecule to actually encounter its respective receptor. Once this fortunate and rare coincidence occurs, it triggers changes in cell behavior mediated by randomly diffusing intracellular "second messengers" which, in turn, regulate enzymatic processes. Processes are regulated up and down, depending on the concentration of the messenger molecules. Similar processes are thought to take place within cells, which are often inaccurately viewed as bags filled with a solution of dissolved enzymes and substrate molecules which are envisioned to diffuse about until they have a random chance collision which brings them together so that a reaction can take place.

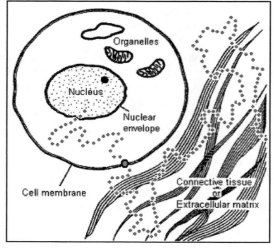

Figure 1. The theory that cellular regulation is controlled by the random diffusion of signal molecules.

THE "LOCK AND KEY" MODEL

The interaction of messengers with receptors, enzymes with substrates and antibodies with antigens has been analogized with a simple lock and key model (Figure 2). The messenger is the key and the receptor is the lock. Within the cell, the metabolic substrate is the key and the enzyme is the lock. Since everyone has used keys and locks, the image is easy to grasp. But is it a complete and accurate image?

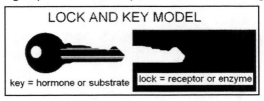

Figure 2. The lock and key model.

With the molecular lock and key model we are dealing with entities that we cannot see because they are too small, so we have to infer the reality from various kinds of evidence obtained with molecular and biochemical techniques. We can isolate hormones and receptors, and we can isolate enzymes and substrates, for example, and we can determine that their molecular structures physically match in ways that allow them to bind together. But we must always remember that when we isolate the components of a living system we are no longer dealing with an intact living system. And when we study the behavior of the components in a certain way, other modes of behavior become invisible. We always need to ask if the intact living system really behaves the way we think it does from study of the parts in isolation; we must always ask if our method of observation limits our perspectives on the process. The mature scientist knows the answers to these questions.

What the lock and key model leaves out is another level of interaction that arises because all molecules at a temperature above absolute zero, −273.15 °C, are vibrating intensely. The components of molecules are charged particles, and when such particles vibrate they inevitably give off electromagnetic fields. We know this because it is the basis for spectroscopy, a well established and highly refined technology that enables us to determine the detailed structure of atoms and molecules. Spectroscopy is so refined that we know the wavelengths of the emission spectra of the various elements to a hundredth of an Ångström, a unit of measure that represents one ten-millionth of a millimetre, or 1×10^{-10} metres. If you ask a chemist to identify an unknown material, their first step will be to obtain an absorption or emission spectrum of the substance and determine the molecular/atomic structure from the frequencies emitted. Each peak in the spectrum is indicative of the presence of a particular element or a particular type of chemical bond.[1]

What this means in terms of communication and control in living systems is that the well-characterized regulatory molecules, second messengers, metabolic substrates, and antibodies, and their respective receptors, enzymes, or antigens, can interact at a distance through electromagnetic resonance.

Molecules do not have to touch each other to interact.
Energy can flow through the electromagnetic field…
~Albert Szent-Györgyi, 1988[1]

In other words, there can be no doubt that organisms possess another matrix or web of molecular intercommunication employing electromagnetic interactions rather than direct physical contact between molecules. Here we are talking about the mechanisms involved in the major regulatory and biochemical pathways in the organism.

Hence we see that the "lock and key" model is accurate but incomplete because it leaves out electromagnetic biocommunication and its subtle aspects. It is obvious that if regulatory processes and chemical reactions depended completely on such a slow and random process as diffusion, we could simply not respond to the world around us rapidly enough to survive.

The problem has been eloquently stated by Professor Guenther Albrecht-Buehler from Northwestern Medical School in Chicago in a classic paper entitled, "In defense of 'nonmolecular' cell biology." Albrecht-Buehler asks us to take a close look at the space around a cell. If one makes the reasonable assumption that the extracellular volume around the cell is about 26 times the volume of the cell itself, a signal molecule with a concentration of 1 pM (6×10^{-11} molecules/liter) will have a concentration of about 8 molecules in the region adjacent to the cell. In the region around the receptor, the hormone concentration will be essentially zero. Albrecht-Buehler concludes that our usual concept of concentration is virtually meaningless.[2] For regulatory molecules to interact with receptors in a timely fashion, and regulate cell behavior in a concentration-dependent manner, electromagnetic communication must be present, and is probably the dominant mechanism. Hence we suggest the electronic car key (Figure 3) as the appropriate analogy for regulatory interactions. Yes, you can insert the key into the lock on your car door; and a hormone can activate a cell by touching the receptor. But you can also unlock the door from a distance of 30 or so feet by pressing the button on the key. And cell behavior can be changed with a tiny field of the appropriate frequency, delivered by a vibrating molecule a distance from a receptor or even a distance from the organism. And metabolic pathways within cells must be explored in terms of highly specific and extremely rapid (possibly instantaneous) resonant interactions between enzymes and substrates.

Figure 3. For regulatory molecules to interact with receptors in a timely fashion, and regulate cell behavior in a concentration-dependent manner, electromagnetic communication must be present, and is probably the dominant mechanism. Hence we suggest the electronic car key (Figure 3) as the appropriate analogy for regulatory interactions.

To complete the analogy, your electronic car key opens your car only, and not other cars that are nearby. What is the basis for this specificity of interaction? It is the specific frequency signature encoded in the electromagnetic field. The equivalence of molecules and their fields has been well worked out by Cyril W. Smith. There is no difference between the biological effects of a molecule and the biological effects of the energy field emitted by that molecule. Smith calls upon us to identify the specific frequencies that regulate biological processes:

> *What is urgently needed is to be able to read the language of electromagnetic biocommunication to complement our understanding of the genetic code.*
> ~C.W. Smith, 1994[2]

Research in energy medicine is exploring this fascinating concept, and is leading to highly effective diagnostic and therapeutic tools.

LIVING CELLS VERSUS REACTIONS IN TEST TUBES

Cells are not bags of solution. Instead, they contain a pervasive framework, the cytoskeleton. The cytoplasm is not a solution of reactants. It is a special form of gel where reactions are highly ordered and extremely rapid, rather than rate-limited by slow and random and non-directed diffusion. Key research by Ahmed Zewail, who received the Nobel Prize in Chemistry in 1999, showed that metabolic sequences operate as fast as a rifle bullet. For this kind of metabolic velocity, the enzymes have to be organized close together in sequence so substrates and reaction products are passed from enzyme to enzyme in rapid succession. These enzymatic units have been characterized; they are called metabolons.[3] In other words, the rates of biochemical reactions in cells vastly exceed those *in vitro*. Extreme caution should be taken when extrapolating experimental results acquired in dilute solutions *in vitro* to function in the intact cell!

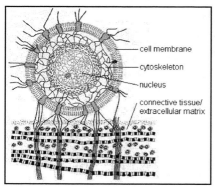

Figure 4. A cell and its surrounding matrix.

A key study by Mark Bretscher showed that some of the membrane proteins actually span the membrane from the inside to the outside.[3] It has been discovered that such trans-membrane proteins are widespread, and that they have vital roles in communicating energy and information between the cell and its environment and *vice versa*. Hence we have a new image of the cell and its environment (Figure 4) that includes the well characterized extracellular matrix elements, primarily collagen and hyaluronin, and equally thoroughly studied intracellular scaffolds called microtubules, microfilaments and microtrabeculae. Termed the living matrix, this all pervasive system is composed of semiconducting molecules with remarkable properties. With its extensions into every cell and nucleus, the living matrix is the largest organ-system in the body, as it is the material that forms all biological structures. The connective tissue is composed primarily of collagen, the most abundant protein in nature. It is a triple helical molecule, and has a helical layer of water associated with it. And the collagen molecules are highly organized into molecular arrays that can best be described as crystals. Likewise, muscles are composed of extended arrays of the helical proteins, actin and myosin. Finally, cell membranes are molecular arrays best described as being crystalline. The connective tissue, muscle and cell membranes are all, in fact, liquid crystals, making them among the most remarkable and mysterious and fascinating materials found in nature. The materials making up these structural components are piezoelectric semiconductors, enormously amplifying to their biophysical agility.

BIOENERGETIC FIELDS ARE REAL AND ARE IMPORTANT IN THE HEALING PROCESS

Physicians are familiar with the electrocardiogram, electroencephalogram, and electromyograms. These are technologies that measure the bioelectrical fields of the heart, brain, and muscles, respectively. When the heart muscle contracts, for example, electrical currents flow through the tissues and can be picked up with electrodes on the skin surface.

It has been known since the work of Hans Christian Ørsted in 1820 that electric currents create measurable magnetic fields in the surrounding space. The principle has led to a fundamental law of electromagnetism known as *Ampère's Law*. On the basis of this law, the electrical currents within organisms must create magnetic fields around the body.

A few years after Ørsted discovered that electric currents in conductors produce magnetic fields, Faraday in England discovered the opposite effect: magnetic fields can cause currents to flow in nearby conductors. This is known as *Faraday's Law of Induction*, and is another fundamental law of electromagnetism. The phenomena discovered by Ampère and Faraday provide the basis for a variety of electromagnetic therapy devices. These two laws of physics account for many of the phenomena taking place in complementary and alternative medicine and are the basis for a number of devices.

For a long time, sensitive therapists had been talking about a palpable energy field that surrounds human beings, but the idea was generally met with disbelief. However, in the early 1960's, scientists at the Massachusetts Institute of Technology began measuring these fields with sensitive magnetometers.[3] We now know that biomagnetic fields can be measured and that they contain information on the condition of the organs that generate them. For each bioelectrical measurement there is now a corresponding biomagnetic measurement:

- Electroencephalogram / Magnetoencephalogram
- Electrocardiogram / Magnetocardiogram
- Electromyogram / Magnetomyogram

Harold Saxton Burr (1889-1973), Professor of Anatomy at Yale University School of Medicine, researched the energy fields of organisms, and published 93 papers on biological electricity between 1932 and 1956. He discovered that measurable imbalances in the electrical field of an organ precede the onset of pathology and that if the electrical imbalance is corrected, the disease does not manifest. While little attention was given to this remarkable discovery, subsequent research has confirmed it. Modern therapeutic technologies are able to detect and correct energetic imbalances. The implications for disease prevention and longevity are obvious and profound.

ENERGY MEDICINE IN ACTION

Now we look at examples of technologies incorporating the concepts described above. Electrical interstitial scanning, shown in Figure 5, involves passing tiny currents at different frequencies between sets of points on the body surface to determine the conductance of various tissues and organs. The physiological condition of a wide range of systems can be determined in this manner.

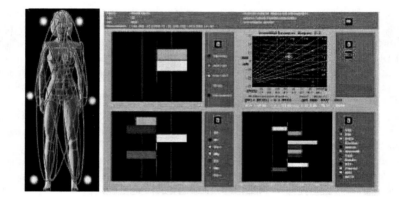

Figure 5. Electrical interstitial scanner

Figure 6 shows an application of this concept, the Trans-Scan 2000. This scanner can develop an image of a tiny breast tumor on the basis of the discovery that the conductance of tumors is seven times (7x) higher than normal tissues at 106-108 Hz. The technology shows the potential of frequency-based medicine in diagnosis.

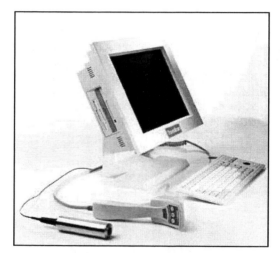

'Figure 6. Trans-Scan 2000

Figure 7 illustrates pulsing electromagnetic field therapy, an established procedure used by orthopedic surgeons for stimulating the repair of bony non-unions. The method has been in use since the 1980's and has been proven to be safe and effective. A frequency of 7 Hz pulsed from a coil into a fracture site induces a tiny current flow through the bone and "jump starts" the healing process.[3] The method was so successful, and its scientific basis so well established, that researchers began applying it to soft tissue injuries as well. It was soon discovered that each tissue responds to a specific frequency, i.e. nerves to 2 Hz, ligaments to 10 Hz, and capillaries and skin to 15 Hz.[4] Subsequent research revealed therapeutic frequencies between 0.5 and 27,000,000 Hz. Remember from above the significance of molecular resonance. Many difficult disorders arise because of problems with regulatory systems, which involve a variety of signal molecules and their receptors. A problem is that the optimal therapeutic frequencies must be determined individually.[4]

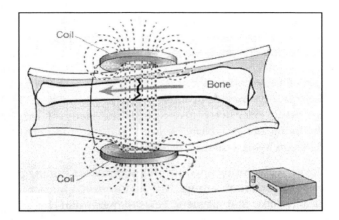

Figure 7. Pulsing Electromagnetic Field Therapy for treating bone non-union.

This issue is resolved with the technology shown in Figure 8. This is the ONDAMED®. The device scans the body with different frequencies and determines which ones are appropriate for the individual. This is accomplished through the use of pulse biofeedback, a very sensitive indicator of changes inside or outside of the body. The arterial pulse gives rise to the vascular autonomic signal, or VAS, which can be used for a variety of purposes:

- Optimize treatments for each patient
- Detect very early stages of serious medical conditions
- Detect elusive pathologies
- Locate blockages to the healing response
- Detect layers of pathology
- Determine the appropriate priority for treatments
- Determine the success of interventions

Pulse biofeedback determines which systems are imbalanced. The device remembers the relevant frequencies and delivers the corresponding resonant therapeutic frequencies, selected on a patient-by-patient basis. The frequencies are delivered using pulsing electromagnetic fields that induce minute currents flows in the tissues. A hand applicator locates which area of the body is responding to the stimulus. This is another form of biofeedback, since it reveals to the patient the real location of their energetic imbalance. ONDAMED® is being used by many physicians in the USA and elsewhere. The outcome: healthier patients with even more respect for their doctors.

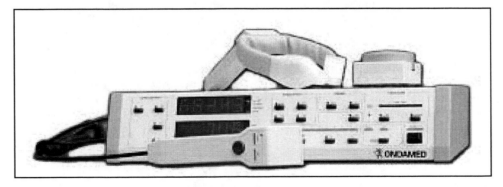

Figure 8. The Ondamed® system, with the hand-held applicator (front), the neck applicator, and the frequency regulator.

CONCLUDING REMARKS

Energy medicine adds another dimension to biochemistry and molecular biology: the body can also be viewed as an electronic circuit composed of molecular semiconductors. Sophisticated technologies have been developed on the basis of the energetic concepts presented here. The condition of the systems and organs can be evaluated and energetic imbalances can be detected and corrected without reference to specific diseases. This is a new and more gentle kind of medicine, in which "You have a disease that we can treat," is replaced with "You had an imbalance that we have corrected." While there is no medical approach that can treat every problem, these technologies are achieving success for the patient who has tried every other method and simply run out of options. Because they can correct imbalances long before disease has developed, these methods are profoundly effective in promoting longevity.

REFERENCES

1. James L. Oschman, PhD, Nature's Own Research Association, PO Box 1935, Dover, New Hampshire 03821, USA.
2. These values can be found in tables in the Handbook of Chemistry and Physics, CRC Press, Boca Raton, FL.
3. Szent-Györgyi A. To see what everyone has seen, to think what no one has thought. *Biological Bulletin.* 1988;175:191-240.
4. Albrecht-Buehler G. In defense of 'nonmolecular' cell biology. *International Review of Cytology.* 1999;120:191-241.
5. Smith CW. Biological effects of weak electromagnetic fields. In: Ho MW, Popp FA, Warnke U, (eds). *Bioelectrodynamics and biocommunication.* Singapore: World Scientific; 1994 81-107.
6. Sere PA. The metabolon. *Trends in Biochemical Sciences.* 1985;10:109-110.
7. Bretscher M. Major human erythrocyte glycoprotein spans the cell membrane. *Nature New Biology.* 1971;231:229-232.
8. Cohen D. Magnetic fields around the torso: production by electrical activity of the human heart. *Science.* 1967;156:652-654.
9. Bassett CAL. Bioelectromagnetics in the service of medicine. In: Blank M (ed). *Electromagnetic fields: biological interactions and mechanisms. Advances in Chemistry Series 250.* Washington DC: American Chemical Society; 1995;261-275.
10. Sisken BF, Walker J. Therapeutic aspects of electromagnetic fields for soft-tissue healing. In: Blank M (ed). *Electromagnetic fields: biological interactions and mechanisms. Advances in Chemistry Series 250.* Washington DC: American Chemical Society; 1995:277-285.
11. Peters TK, Koralewski HE, Zerbst EW. The evolution strategy--a search strategy used in individual optimization of electrical parameters for therapeutic carotid sinus nerve stimulation. *IEEE Transactions in Biomedical Engineering.* 1989;36:668-675; Peters TK, Koralewski HE, Zerbst EW. Search for optimal frequencies and amplitudes of therapeutic electrical carotid sinus nerve stimulation by application of the evolution strategy. *Artificial Organs.* 1989;13:133-143.

ABOUT THE AUTHOR

Jim Oschman has published about 30 papers in leading scientific journals, and about an equal number in complementary medicine journals. He has also written two books on energy medicine, and lectures internationally on this subject. Jim's investigations of the living connective tissue matrix provide the basis for powerful anti-aging techniques.

Chapter 28
Anti-Aging Nutraceuticals

Harry G. Preuss M.D., MACN, CNS[1]; Bobby Echard MT[1];
Debasis Bagchi Ph.D., FACN, CNS[2]; Shari Lieberman Ph.D., FACN, CNS[3];
Nicholas V. Perricone M.D., FACN[4]

[1] *Department of Physiology, Georgetown University Medical Center (Washington, D.C. USA)*
[2] *Department of Pharmacy Sciences, Creighton University Medical Center (Omaha, NE USA)*
[3] *New York Chiropractic College, School of Applied Clinical Nutrition (Seneca Falls, NY USA)*
[4] *Michigan State University College of Human Medicine (East Lansing, MI USA)*

ABSTRACT

Avoiding perturbations in many metabolic-endocrine systems that occur in aging may play a prominent role in extending healthful lifespan. For example, we previously hypothesized that preventing insulin resistance by means other than caloric restriction might prolong longevity in a more acceptable manner. Accordingly, we examined various effects of niacin-bound chromium (NBC) compared to control over the lifespan of Zucker rats that have a proclivity toward developing metabolic syndrome. At six months, neither abnormalities nor differences were noted in hematology; but in the treatment group, circulating glucose levels were significantly lower. Systolic blood pressure (SBP) was consistently lower in the NBC group after 10 weeks. The first control rat died at 8 months followed by two more deaths at 9 and 10 months. The first deaths in the NBC group occurred in the tenth month. After all control rats had died, four in the NBC group continued to live at least a month beyond. The NBC group compared to control showed increased average lifespan by 19.1%, median lifespan by 12.2%, 30th percentile survival by 19.6% and maximum lifespan by 22%. Further work revealed that NBC also affects the renin-angiotensin system (RAS). Decreases in SBP, circulating angiotensin 2 levels (A2), and in the circulating converting enzyme activity and lesser response to losartan challenge indicate a lower activity of the RAS. With recent reports concerning the adverse role of circulating A2 on cardiovascular health, this may be another factor in the increased longevity emanating from NBC intake. We conclude that NBC can increase lifespan without caloric restriction. There was no evidence of blood dyscracias or renal and liver perturbations from NBC over the lifespan of the Zucker rats. NBC and other safe natural supplements may influence healthful lifespan via their ability to prevent age-related changes in various metabolic endocrine systems such as glucose-insulin and RAS. Additional recent work has also shown the ability of astaxanthin to affect RAS favorably. Fortunately, there are many safe, natural supplements that favorably influence the glucose-insulin and RAS systems.

Keywords: longevity, rats, insulin resistance, chromium, niacin-bound, lifespan, niacin-bound chromium, aging

ANTI-AGING NUTRACEUTICALS

Caloric restriction significantly increases the lifespan of rodents. Many years ago, McCay *et al* pioneered the concept that partial restriction of food intake overcomes, ameliorates, and/or slows the progression of age-related perturbations and increases lifespan.[1] Aging, caloric-restricted rodents compared to aging, *ad libitum*-fed rodents remain healthier – maintaining better cardiovascular fitness, more efficient glucose utilization, and stronger immune responses.[2] Although most of the original work on caloric restriction and longevity was performed in rodents (Fig. 1),[3-8] more recent studies strongly suggest that primates are affected similarly. In Rhesus Monkeys, every measurable index indicates that dietary restriction increases fitness and slows the aging process.[9] Also, changes in biomarkers of health suggest that low caloric intake in humans favorably influences the aging process.[10] Thus, it is not surprising that caloric-restriction has been used extensively to examine the pathogenesis behind aging.[11, 12]

**INFLUENCE OF FOOD RESTRICTION ON LONGEVITY
OF MALE FISCHER 344 RATS**

	Ad Libitum Fed Rats n = 115	Food Restricted rats n = 115
Median Length of Life (days)	711	1046 (47%)
Age 10th percentile survivors (days)	797	1236 (55%)
Maximum length of life (days)	963	1435 (49%)

Food restricted rats received approximately 60% of mean food intake of
Ad libitum rats.

Yu et al J Gerontol 40:657, 1985

Figure 1. Influence of calorie restriction on longevity of male Fischer 344 rats.

One popular theory is that caloric-restriction slows aging by preventing or, at least, ameliorating the development of deleterious insulin resistance (IR) associated with aging.[13-19] Masoro et al examined the circulating levels of glucose and insulin over the lifespan of the shorter-lived, ad libitum fed and the longer-lived, caloric restricted rats.[13] Caloric restricted rats consistently maintained 24-hour glucose concentrations 15% below those of ad libitum fed rats (Fig 2). Further, plasma insulin levels remained about half of control. Dilman and Anisimov[20] and Anisimov et al [21] reported that biguanide drugs such as phenformin and metformin, insulin sensitizing agents, are potential anti-aging agents as well.

MEAN 24-HOUR PLASMA GLUCOSE CONCENTRATION (mg/dl)

Age (months)	n	Ad Libitum	n	Food Restricted
3-7	21	136+2	21	119+2
9-13	21	147+2	21	126+2
15-19	21	149+2	21	131+2
21-25	15	148+3	19	135+3
27-31			13	127+3

Mean + SEM

Massoro et al J of Gerontology 47:B202, 1992

Figure 2. Influence of calorie restriction on 24-hour plasma glucose levels.

Concerning underlying pathogenic mechanisms, how could the IR that develops with aging influence lifespan? IR at certain stages is associated with hyperglycemia and hyperinsulinemia.[16] In the case of hyperglycemia, Cerami has proposed that chronically elevated circulating glucose levels hasten the aging process via glycosylation of proteins and DNA.[22, 23] While IR with or without accompanying hyperinsulinemia can cause damage through glycosylation of proteins and DNA and increased production of damaging free radicals, higher circulating levels of insulin are frequently associated with hormonal imbalances in renin-angiotensin, cortisol, catecholamines, and DHEA (Figure 3).[24] As a final point, high sucrose diets, associated with IR, have shortened lifespan in certain strains of rats.[25-27]

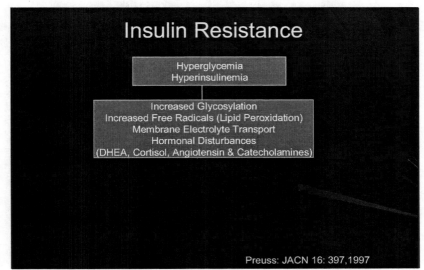

Figure 3. Does insulin resistance play a role in aging?

In an earlier paper, we postulated, "manipulation of diet by influencing the glucose/insulin system may favorably affect lifespan and reduce the incidence of chronic disorders associated with aging".[28] This hypothesis was based upon earlier reports suggesting that the ability of caloric restriction to augment longevity was associated with favorable effects on the glucose-insulin system[13] and that phenformin, a recognized insulin-sensitizer, prolonged lifespan of rodents.[20] Natural insulin-sensitizing supplements are ubiquitous and include certain forms of trivalent chromium, soluble fibers, mushroom extracts, cinnamon, and certain antioxidants, etc.[29] When we followed rats consuming niacin-bound chromium (NBC) and two antioxidants for more than a year, many biomarkers of good health in the test rats were better than in control.[30] In more recent work, we postulated that NBC and fraction SX, another insulin-sensitizer extracted from the maitake mushroom, alone and combined, produced results suggesting that they could increase longevity of rats.[31]

Accordingly, we examined various effects of NBC (n=12) compared to control (n=10) over the lifespan of Zucker Fatty Rats (ZFR), which have a proclivity toward developing metabolic syndrome. At six months, hematology and blood chemistries were analyzed. No abnormalities were noted in hematology. In the treatment group, circulating glucose levels were significantly lower. Systolic blood pressure (SBP) was consistently lower in the NBC group after 10 weeks. The first control rat died at 8 months followed by two more deaths at 9 and 10 months. The first deaths in the NBC group occurred in the tenth month. After all control rats had died, four in the NBC group continued to live at least a month beyond. The NBC group compared to control showed increased average lifespan by 19.1%, median lifespan by 12.2%, 30th percentile survival by 19.6% and maximum lifespan by 22% (Fig. 4).

EFFECTS OF NBC ON LIFESPAN OF ZUCKER RATS

Parameters	Control	NBC
Average Length of Life (Days)	436+23.8	531+21.4* (21.8%)
Median Length of Life (Days)	447	510 (14.1%)
Age 30th Percentile Survival	519+11.8	621+15.5* (19.6%)
Maximum Length of Life (Days)	542	661 (22%)

•Statistically significantly different from control. Average or
average + SEM shown.

Figure 4. Effects of niacin-bound chromium on the lifespan of Zucker rats.

Many recent studies have indicated that the renin-angiotensin system (RAS) may have a significant effect on longevity.[32-34] Could the RAS also play a role in the ability of NBC to extend longevity? Three means to assess the activity of the RAS suggest that there was a decrease when NBC was ingested. The greater decrease in SBP after losartan challenge, an angiotensin receptor blocker, in the control group suggests that the RAS was more active in the control group compared to the NBC group.[35, 36] When estimating the ACE activity in the serum of rats,[37] the latter was found to be lower in the NBC group compared to control. In fact, the lowering was of the same magnitude as seen in the additional group of rats receiving the drug captopril as the positive control (Fig. 5). Captopril reduced the levels of circulating angiotensin-2 significantly, and there was a trend to see a lowering in the NBC group (p=0.06). Although the latter did not achieve statistical significance, the trend along with the positive lowering seen in the losartan challenge and the ACE activity test suggest a relative decrease in the activity of the RAS compared to control. In addition to NBC, we have recently found that astaxanthin, a powerful antioxidant, can also decrease the activity of the RAS.

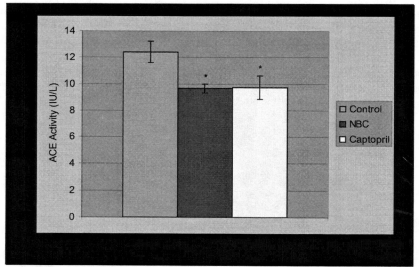

Figure 5. Effect of niacin-bound chromium on ACE activity in the serum of rats.

CONCLUDING REMARKS

Over the last century, man has made great strides to increase his longevity. Much of this has come about through better hygiene, availability of better nutrients, and medical advancements. We present information here that suggests that amelioration of IR, which would lower glycosylation, free radical formation, and membrane transport alterations, would also be beneficial. It is generally recognized that type 2 diabetes is increasing, and this is mainly attributed to the increase in the overweight state and obesity. In turn, the latter is attributed to the increased consumption of calories and less exercise that is typical of society today. Lessening of the activity of the RAS could also be important for a healthful longevity. How the glucose-insulin and RAS interact is uncertain. In any case, we hope the current paper will encourage a better life style.

REFERENCES

1. McCay C, Crowell M, Maynard L. The effect of retarded growth upon the length of life and upon ultimate body size. *J Nutr*. 1935;10:63-79.
2. Hopkin K. Aging in focus. Caloric restriction may put the brakes on aging. *J NIH Res*. 1995;7:47-50.
3. Coleman GL, Barthold SW, Osbaldiston GW, Foster SJ, Jonas AM. Pathological changes during aging in barrier-reared Fischer 344 male rats. *J Gerontol*. 1977;32:258-278.
4. Bertrand HA, Lynd FT, Masoro EJ, Yu BP. Changes in adipose mass and cellularity through the adult life of rats fed *ad libitum* a life-prolonging restricted diet. *J Gerontol*. 1980;35:827-835.
5. Yu BP, Masoro EJ, Murata I, Bertrand HA, Lynd FT. Lifespan study of SPF Fischer 344 male rats fed *ad libitum* or restricted diets: longevity, growth, lean body mass, and disease. *J Gerontol*. 1982;37:130-141.
6. Yu BP, Masoro EJ. McMahan CA. Nutritional influences on aging of Fischer 344 rats: 1. physical, metabolic, and longevity characteristics. *J Gerontol*. 1985;40:657-670.
7. Maeda H, Gleiser CA, Masoro EJ, Murata I, McMahan CA, Yu BP. Nutritional influences on aging of Fischer 344 rats: II. pathology. *J Gerontol*. 1985;40:671-688.
8. Iwasaki K, Gleiser CA, Masoro EJ, McMahan CA, Seo EJ, Yu BP. The influence of dietary protein source on longevity of age-related disease processes of Fischer rats. J Gerontol. 1988;43:B5-B12.
9. Roth GS: Ingram DK, Lane MA. Caloric restriction in primates and relevance to humans. *Ann NY Acad Sci*. 2001;928:305-315.
10. Walford RL, Harris SB, Gunion MW. The calorically restricted low-fat nutrient-dense diet in Biosphere 2 significantly lowers blood glucose, total leucocytes count, cholesterol and blood pressure in humans. *Proc Natl Acad Sci USA*. 1992;89:11533.
11. Harman D. Aging; prospects for further increases in the functional lifespan. *Age* 1994;17:119-146.
12. Knight JA. The process and theories of aging. *Annals Clin Lab Sci*. 1995;25:1-12.
13. Masoro EJ, McCarter RJM, Katz MS, McMahan CA: Dietary restriction alters characteristics of glucose fuel use. *J Gerontol*. 1992;47:B202-B208.
14. Masoro EJ. Assessment of nutritional components in prolongation of life and health by diet. Proc Soc Exper Biol Med. 1990;193:31-34.
15. DeFronzo R. Glucose intolerance and aging. *Diabetes Care*. 1981;4:493-501.
16. Reaven GM, Chen N, Hollenbeck C, Chen YDI. Effect of age on glucose tolerance and glucose uptake in healthy individuals. *J Am Ger Soc*. 1989;37:735-740.
17. Broughton DL, Taylor RL. Review: deterioration of glucose tolerance with age: the role of insulin resistance. *Age and Aging*. 1991;20:221-225.
18. Shimokata H, Muller DC, Fleg JL, Sorkin J, Ziemba AW, Andres R. Age as independent determinant of glucose tolerance. *Diabetes* 1991;40:44-51.
19. DeFronzo RA, Ferinimmi E. Insulin resistance: a multifaceted syndrome responsible for NIDDM, obesity, hypertension, dyslipidemia, and atherosclerotic cardiovascular disease. *Diabetes Care*. 1991;14:173-194.
20. Dilman VM, Anisimov VN. Effect of treatment with phenformin, dyphenylhydantoin, or LDOPA on lifespan and tumor incidence in C3H/Sn mice. *Gerontology 1980;*26:241-245.
21. Anisimov VN, Semenchenko AV, Yashin AI. Insulin and longevity: antidiabetic biguanides as geroprotectors. *Biogerontology* 2003;4:297-307.
22. Cerami A, Vlassare H, Brownlee M. Glucose and aging. *Scientific American* 1987;256:90-96.
23. Cerami A. Hypothesis. Glucose as a mediator of aging. *J Am Ger Soc*. 1985;33:626-634.

24. Krieger DR, Landsberg L. Mechanisms in obesity-related hypertension: role of insulin and catecholamines. *Am J Hypertension.* 1988;1:84-90, 1988.
25. Preuss HG, Zein M, Areas JL, Podlasek SJ, Knapka J, Antonovych TT, Sabnis SG, Zepeda H: Effects of excess sucrose ingestion on the lifespan of hypertensive rats. *Ger Nephrol.and Urol.* 1991;1:13-20.
26. Preuss HG, Knapka JJ. Sugar-induced hypertension in Fischer 344 and F1-hybrid at different ages. *Ger Nephrol and Urol.* 1994;4:15-21.
27. Preuss HG. Effects of diets containing different proportions of macronutrients on longevity of normotensive Wistar rats. *Ger Nephrol Urol.* 1997;7:81-86.
28. Preuss HG. Effects of glucose/insulin perturbations on aging and chronic disorders of aging: the evidence. *J Amer Coll Nutr.* 1997;16:397-403.
29. Preuss HG, Bagchi D. Nutritional therapy of impaired glucose tolerance and diabetes mellitus. In: Bronner F (ed). *Nutritional Aspects and Clinical Management of Chronic Disorders and Diseases.* Boca Raton FL: CRC Press; 2002:69-91.
30. Preuss HG, Montamarry S, Echard B, Scheckenbach R, Bagchi D. Long-term effects of chromium, grape seed extract, and zinc on various metabolic parameters of rats. *Molecular and Cellular Biochemistry.* 2001;223:95-102.
31. Talpur N, Echard B, Yasmin D, Bagchi D, Preuss HG. Effects of niacin-bound chromium, maitake mushroom fraction SX and a novel (-)-hydroxycitric acid extract on the metabolic syndrome in aged diabetic Zucker Fatty Rats. *Molec Cell Biochem.* 2003;252:369-377.
32. Ruiz-Ortega M, Lorenzo O, Ruperez M, Estaban V, Suzuki Y, Mezzano S, Plaza JJ, Egido J. Role of the renin-angiotensin system in vascular diseases. Expanding the field. *Hypertension* 2001;38:1382-1387.
33. Basso N, Paglia N, Ines S, de Cavanagh EM, Ferder L, Arnaiz MRL, Inserra F. Protective effect of the inhibition of the renin-angiotensin system on aging. *Regulatory Peptides.* 2005;128:247-252.
34. deCavanagh EM, Piotrkowski B, Fraga CG: The interaction between the reninangiotensin system and peroxisome proliferators activated receptors: a hypothesis including the participation of mitochondria in aging. *Front Biosci.* 2007;12:1049-1062.
35. Wong PC, Price WA Jr, Chiu AT, Ducia JV, Carini DJ, Wexler RR, Johnson AL, Timmermans PB. In vivo pharmacology of DuP 753. *Am J Hypertens.* 1991;4:288S-298s.
36. Mohamadi A, Jarrell ST, Dadgar-Dehkordi A, Bushehri N, Shi S-J, Andrawis NS, Myers A, Clouatre D, Preuss HG. Effects of wild garlic on blood pressure and other parameters of hypertensive rats: Comparison with cultivated garlics. *Heart Disease* 2000;2:3-9.
37. Aviram M, Dornfeld L. Pomegranate juice consumption inhibits serum angiotensin converting enzyme activity and reduces systolic blood pressure. *Atherosclerosis* 2001;158:195-198.

ABOUT THE AUTHOR

Primary author Dr. Harry Preuss is a Professor of Physiology, Medicine, and Pathology at Georgetown University Medical Center. He is a past President of the Certification Board for Nutrition Specialists (CNS), past President and ninth Master of the American College of Nutrition (ACN), former Established Investigator of the American Heart Association, past member three NIH councils, a member of the National Cholesterol Education Program, and the author of more than 600 medical publications.

Chapter 29
The Nuts and Bolts of Anti-Aging Medicine: How to Prescribe Bioidentical Hormones

Ron Rothenberg, M.D.
Clinical Professor, Family and Preventive Medicine, University of California San Diego School of Medicine; Founder, California Healthspan Institute

ABSTRACT

This paper will focus on the practical aspects of hormone replacement therapy for adult hormone deficiencies. For each hormone the symptoms of deficiency, best method of delivery, dose, possible side effects, protocol for follow-up, and any controversy surrounding the hormone will be discussed.

INTRODUCTION

This paper is concerned with the nuts and bolts of prescribing bioidentical hormones. The first thing we should remember is that we should not rush to throw hormones at people. Hormone optimization is the finishing touch. A good anti-aging physician should first consider the patient's lifestyle, including: nutrition, detoxification, exercise, stress reduction, antioxidants, and nutraceuticals. Of course, hormones should be used to treat a deficiency disease, and if hormone replacement is necessary it should be with bioidentical hormones titrated to youthful levels.

The aim of this paper is to review how to prescribe testosterone, DHEA, thyroid hormone, estrogen, progesterone, growth hormone (GH), cortisol. For each hormone the symptoms of deficiency, best method of delivery, dose, possible side effects, protocol for follow-up, and any controversy surrounding the hormone will be discussed.

PRESCRIBING BIOIDENTICAL HORMONES

Before even thinking about prescribing hormone replacement to a patient it is necessary to gather some data and determine the patient's baseline panel. You need to determine their complete blood count (CBC), their metabolic panel, their lipid panel or VAP, their hormone panel, their C-reactive protein (CRP) level, their homocysteine level, their AA (arachidonic acid) / EPA (eicosapentaenoic acid) ratio, their fasting insulin level and cancer screens such as PSA and CA-125. Evaluation of their baseline hormone levels is important, including the free or bioavailable if possible. Advanced testing could include levels of the cytokines interleukin-6 (IL-6), tumor necrosis factor-alpha (TNF-α), and interleukin-1 beta (IL-1β). Once you have all that data to hand, you can sit down and begin to develop their personal anti-aging preventive medicine program.

TESTOSTERONE

Testosterone replacement therapy (TRT) is safe and it provides dramatic benefits. Testosterone decreases inflammation, which is linked to many diseases, including heart disease, cancer, and neurodegenerative diseases. Testosterone also improves quality of life.

The male menopause is called the andropause, and androgen deficiency in the aging male is a very real phenomenon. It may be less sudden than the female menopause, but it is severe. The cause of andropause is decreased levels of bioavailable testosterone. In studies by Araujo et al, decreasing testosterone levels leads to increased aging of the heart and circulation, increased myocardial infarction and stroke, decreased hemodynamic function, increased brain aging, decreased memory, increased dementia and Alzheimer's disease, decreased cognitive function and cognitive impairment – even without dementia, and loss of drive and competitive edge. The general inflammatory state of low testosterone levels produces a general feeling of stiffness and pains in the muscles and joints. Fitness levels fall, and workouts are not as effective as they used to be – if you don't have the anabolic hormone to take that protein and put it in the muscle, it's not going to work. Fatigue, depression, irritability, decreased libido, decreased erectile tension, and increased refractory period between orgasms are all symptoms of the male menopause. All of these lead to an impaired quality of life.

Is andropause a deficiency disease? The simple answer is yes. According to Korenman et al, half of healthy men between the ages of 50 and 70 years have a bioavailable testosterone level below the lowest level seen in healthy men aged 20 to 40 years old. Thus, a normal 50 year old has a deficiency disease compared to a 20 year old. That is the rationale for replacing testosterone, not to normal-for-age levels but to optimal levels.

The first test that needs to be done when considering TRT is total testosterone. Total testosterone is a measure of the testosterone floating around in the blood, a lot of it is stuck onto the sex hormone binding globulin (SHBG) and you cannot use it. The range goes from about 350 to 1030 nanograms per decilitre (ng/dl) in men (optimal 700-1000 ng/dl) and 10 to 75 ng/dl (optimal 50-75 ng/dl) in women. It is important to check with the lab you use as some use different units. Sometimes it is reported in nanomoles per liter (nMol/l). The conversion factor is 10.4 nMol/l=33 ng/dl. Remember, these are reference ranges. Normal ranges are not optimal ranges, and you have to explain this to the patients when they see the results. It is a reference range. That is just statistics. It does not talk about optimal health. There is a circadian pattern to testosterone secretion, so draw blood for total testosterone in the morning.

Total testosterone may not correlate with bioavailable or free testosterone, depending on SHBG and albumin. SHBG holds on to sex steroids. It holds onto testosterone, tighter than estrogen. Normal SHBG levels are 20 to 60 nMol/l in males and 40 to 120nMol/l in females. If this number is high or low is does not necessarily mean that something is wrong and that you have got to fix it, but it does explain things. Thyroid increases SHBG. We are treating a lot of patients with thyroid. Estrogens and progesterone increase SHBG. Aging itself increases it. Testosterone, glucocorticoids, growth hormone, and insulin decrease SHBG.

The optimal range for free testosterone is in the region of 18-24 ng/dl for men and 5-8 picograms per milliliter (pg/ml) for women. Free testosterone is the fraction that is not stuck to SHBG or albumin. There are two main problems with free testosterone. First, the portion stuck to albumin comes off and it is usable. Second, it is a difficult test to do and most doctors don't ask the lab what method they used. The analogue ligand radioimmunoassay (RIA) technique is notoriously inaccurate. While the research methods like equilibrium dialysis or ultracentrifugation are good, they are not usually done.

The most useful test is the one for bioavailable testosterone. The reference ranges for bioavailable testosterone are 120 to 500 ng/dl for men, and 10-30 ng/dl for women. Bioavailable testosterone is a measurement of the amount of free testosterone plus the testosterone loosely bound to albumin. Bioavailable testosterone is a calculated number. The higher it is the better, and the optimal range is 300-500 ng/dl for men and 10-30 ng/dl for women.

Dihydrotestosterone (DHT), some people measure it, some do not. In the US, DHT is considered to be bad and is blamed for hair loss, BPH, and even prostate cancer. However, in Europe DHT is used often as androgen replacement. So is it good or is it bad? We just do not know. Either way, the reference range is 30 to 85 ng/dl in men and 4 to 22 (ng/dl) in women. There is no need to routinely measure DHT.

It is a different story with estradiol. It is important to measure and control estradiol levels in men. Men need estradiol. You cannot let it drop to zero, but you cannot let it get high either. This is what separates the men from the boys and the women from the girls in TRT. The reference range for estradiol in men is 15 to 45 pg/ml; the optimal range is 15 to 25 pg/ml. Controlling estradiol is the key. If you do not do that, you will be chasing your own tail.

When you think about TRT it is important to remember you are not just thinking about testosterone, you also have to consider DHT and estradiol. You have got to remember that. There are three or four options when it comes to TRT. One method of TRT is by giving injections of testosterone enanthate or testosterone cypionate. These are bio-identical because the ester hydrolysis that takes place in the blood leaves you with bio-identical testosterone. In the past, patients were typically given 200 mg every two to three weeks. It was a bad roller coaster ride as the patient got sky-high supraphysiological levels at the initial injection, a lot of which was aromatized to estradiol, and by the end of the two to three weeks testosterone levels had plummeted to lower than baseline levels. However, if you shorten the interval to a weekly dose of 100 to 150 mg you have got a pretty smooth result and when given all the different options, most of my patients actually prefer giving themselves an IM shot once a week. It has got to be given IM gluteal. Sometimes it hurts in the anterior thigh. The advantage of this method is that it gives you more physiologically stable levels and there is less aromatization to estradiol.

Oral TRT is not good. The FDA allows women to use methyltestosterone in Estratest but does not allow it to be given to men. In fact, no one should be using it, as it is hepatotoxic. There is an oral form of testosterone undecanoate called Andriol that is not associated with hepatotoxicity; however this is not available in the United States. That is no great loss, as it does not work too well anyway.

Another method of giving TRT is by using subcutaneous pellets. To implant the pellets you simply need to give the patient a local anesthetic and make a nick with a scalpel. Most of the pellets last for two or three months, but some last for up to six months. Pellets are good for people who are going traveling and do not want to take needles or gels with them, and for those who do not like injecting themselves. But the majority of patients are not that keen on pellets and think it is easier just to go ahead and give themselves the IM once a week.

The other main method of TRT is by using transdermal testosterone. Transdermal testosterone is available in the form of AndroGel or custom made from a compounding pharmacy. Transdermal testosterone is well absorbed in most men, but not everybody. Some patients just do not absorb transdermal testosterone in my experience. I do not know why. I think AndroGel is the wrong strength because it is 1%, which is the female dose. You need to apply 5-10 Gms at a time with dosing. It is better to get your transdermal testosterone from a compounding pharmacy, first because it is cheaper, and second, because you have complete control over the strength.

If you decide to go with transdermal testosterone there are a few precautions you need to tell your patients about. It is important to keep it off the scrotum if you do not like DHT. Warn patients about not getting the gel on women and children. It can increase hair growth in the area where you rub it in both men and women. Unfortunately, this is not the case on the head. It is also important to warn patients that free testosterone can actually decrease with transdermal testosterone.

Through the miracle of biology, the alpha sub unit of human chorionic gonadotropin (hCG) is the same as the alpha subunit of luteinizing hormone (LH). This means that you can give men the female pregnancy hormone hCG, and if their Leydig cells still work (this technique works better in 40 to 50 year olds than 70 to 80 year olds) they will be instructed to make more testosterone. So this is an option. One of the side effects of testosterone is a 10 to 15% decrease in testicle size. Men do not want that. So hCG is an option if it will still work. It is also a good option if they want to keep their sperm count up, as hCG has no effect on sperm count. Zitzman et al supports a typical dose of hCG is between 1000 to 5000 units per week given subcutaneously. It is possible to use just hCG as TRT (you obviously need to monitor free testosterone to check that it is working) or you can cycle it with more traditional TRT every 6-months. Another alternative is combining testosterone and hCG. This involves giving IM testosterone ester cypionate once a week on day 1. On day 5 and 6 you will have a little bit of drop off and you can give a small dose (i.e. 250 units) of hCG subcutaneous on those two days. If you go with this method you maintain testicle size and you maintain sperm count.

If a patient has high levels of follicle stimulating hormone (FSH) and LH, then hCG is probably not going to work because their body is already trying to tell the Leydig cells to make more testosterone and it is not happening. So, that gives you a clue as whether to use it or not.

Does testosterone replacement increase prostate cancer risk or risk of benign prostatic hyperplasia? No it does not. Morgantaler discusses this issue in detail in his 2006 article in the European Journal of Urology. Are there any other side effects of testosterone replacement that need treatment? The only significant side effect that needs to be treated is increased red cell mass, or polycythemia. Estrogen control may be needed if estradiol gets too high. However, these potential risks can be kept minimal with comprehensive anti-aging medical care.

The major adverse effect of testosterone replacement is polycythemia. Polycythemia is more likely with injections than with gel. However, it is something that can easily be managed. Some people suggest that you should just stop testosterone replacement; however you can just do a phlebotomy, or better yet, tell your patient to donate blood if their hematocrit starts hitting around 55. Either way it is important to stay on top of this, and certainly in the first few years of managing balanced hormone optimization, it is advisable to test patient's blood levels every three months. People with COPD, smokers, and men with sleep apnea are at increased risk of developing polycythemia. There has never been a case report of increased red cell mass causing a thromboembolic event. However, it still needs to be controlled.

Gynecomastia is a potential side effect of testosterone replacement, thus it is important to monitor estradiol levels and control them with aromatase inhibitors when needed. Fluid retention is rare. Does testosterone replacement accelerate male pattern hair loss? To be truthful, there is no data one way or another. Testosterone replacement can lead to a decrease in testicle size. With prolonged treatment a decrease of 10% to 15% can be expected. Testosterone is a form of male birth control because you're suppressing FSH and LH, thus testosterone replacement does lead to a lower sperm count.

A comprehensive evaluation of the patient is vital before prescribing a patient testosterone replacement. This should include a physical exam, a digital rectal exam, cardiac risk factors, fitness evaluation, bone density, body composition, cognitive function tests, and laboratory tests – including all hormone levels, testosterone levels, free testosterone levels, PSA, sex hormone binding globulin (SHBG), follicle stimulating hormone (FSH), and luteinizing hormone (LH).

If a patient's PSA is greater than four, or just seems higher than it should for the patient's age, or there is abnormal digital rectal exam, or any other suspicion of prostate cancer, refer the patient to urology for evaluation and possible biopsy. If there is PSA velocity, meaning that the patient's PSA levels has increased by more than 1.0 in a year, you should repeat the lab test, then if velocity is still evident refer the patient to urology. If PSA is greater than 4.0 and a biopsy is negative, testosterone replacement is ok. There is no need to withhold testosterone treatment once a negative biopsy result has been obtained. If the patient has had prostate cancer and has had a radical prostatectomy, and two or three years their PSA is still at zero, or at close to zero, then it is fine to go ahead with testosterone replacement. What about a patient with active prostate cancer? Well, this goes so much against conventional wisdom that it is advisable not to prescribe patients with active prostate cancer TRT.

The first follow-up appointment should be at three months. In fact, for the first couple of years, it is a good idea to conduct quarterly lab tests of all the parameters – testosterone, estradiol, hemoglobin, and PSA.

What about their testosterone levels? Have they increased? Are they too high? What is too high? Ideally, you want to see a total testosterone level of between 700 and 1000 ng/dl. Are they too low? What is too low? If it is still less than 600 ng/dl or so they will not really be getting any benefits. So, if it is too high or too low you need to think about adjusting the dose. Are they polycythemic? If their hematocrit is approaching 55 get them to donate blood. Is their estradiol level too high? The ideal estradiol level in men is approximately 20, but anywhere between 15 and 30 is good. You do not want to let it get over 50 because levels that high will start to cause estrogenic side effects, such as tingling nipples and gynecomastia. On the other hand you cannot let it drop to zero either – if it drops to zero your patient will start losing bone. If their estradiol is too high encourage them to try and lose any excess abdominal fat and try giving them chrysin. If that does not work, then try giving them anastrozole (Arimidex®). The dose needed is usually small, 0.5 mg two or three times a week is often enough and that way you can optimize. Do they have an increase in male pattern baldness or hair loss? Is there any PSA velocity? You need to answer all of these questions.

Testosterone Replacement in Women

Women obviously need some testosterone. It is needed for sense of well-being, strength (especially upper body strength), nipple and clitoral sensitivity, body composition, and bone density. Sometimes you get better results on bone density with TRT than with Fosamax, etc. DHEA can increase testosterone somewhat in women but not in men. This is because DHEA in men is mostly testicular and in women it is half ovarian and half adrenal. If the ovaries are not making it, it is all coming from the adrenal gland. Thus, you can have relative androgen deficiency with normal levels in women. Women's testosterone levels decrease by as much as 50% by the time they reach their 60's. HRT, either bio-identical or old-fashioned Prempro, increases SHBG and decreases free testosterone.

Symptoms of female androgen deficiency syndrome (FADS) include: impaired sexual function, loss of libido, energy loss, loss of well-being, and depression. Thus, the symptoms of FADS are just like those of low testosterone in men.

Testosterone deficiency is not just about sex in men and it is not just about sex in women either, Kaczmarek et al showed that decreased testosterone and free testosterone is associated with coronary artery disease in women independent of other risk factors. So just as in men, low testosterone, because of its anti-inflammatory effect, is associated with more coronary artery disease. Meanwhile, Dimitrakasis et al found that women given traditional HRT plus TRT had a lower incidence of breast cancer than those given HRT alone. It seems that testosterone balances some of the estrogenic effects, just like progesterone does.

What do you do if a woman has symptoms of FADS or if their bioavailable testosterone is too low? First, measure it. The reference range for bioavailable testosterone in young women is 10-30 ng/dl. In saliva, the reference range is 4.5 to 40 pg/ml, the optimal range is 30 to 50 pg/ml, and the therapeutic range is 30 to 60 pg/ml. If it is low you treat them.

A compounded cream or a gel is the best method of delivery for women. Doses range from 1.25 to 10 mg a day; however you need to teach the patient to titrate the dose in order to prevent androgenic side effects. You have got to dance very delicately around androgenic side effects with women. Too much testosterone has androgenic side effects. Fortunately, there is a sequence of events and the first thing is acne. It could be caused by testosterone or could be caused by DHEA. So you can play with both. After the patient gets acne, hirsutism, clitoromegaly, and a deepening voice will follow. So, you need to make your patient aware of these side effects, and tell them to decrease their dose if they get acne, and that will prevent any of the other side effects from appearing. It is also important to tell your patients that the gel could cause increased hair growth on the place you rub it in. Advise her to rotate spots and put it on an area where she might shave anyway. A few women do not absorb creams or gels and may be better off with 10 mg of cypionate a week, again titrating the dose if side effects start to make an appearance.

There are no serious safety considerations concerning the use of testosterone in women, if the women is very hirsute to begin with, you might not want to use it, the same is true if she has male pattern baldness. What about giving testosterone to women with breast cancer? Of course, if you do treat a women with testosterone, some of that testosterone will be converted to estrogen by aromatization. So, whether you choose to go ahead and use testosterone depends upon both your philosophy and hers.

DHEA

There are no unique symptoms of DHEA deficiency, but low levels are associated with obesity. Type 2 diabetes, immune dysfunction, autoimmune disease, cancer, hypertension, cardiovascular disease, depression and loss of well-being, low libido, erectile dysfunction, and osteoporosis.

Von Muhlin et al found that DHEA is an anti-aging steroid because it is stimulatory to the immune system, and has anti-diabetes, anti-atherosclerosis, anti-dementia, anti-obesity, anti-osteoporosis, and anti-cancer properties. DHEA is a neurosteroid. Numerous animal studies suggest that DHEA appears to make them smarter. Oelkers et al, found that DHEA balances cortisol, and even the conventional literature is now saying that patients treated with corticosteroids should also be treated with DHEA. DHEA is also anti-inflammatory. It lowers IL-6 and TNF-α.

DHEA is always measured as DHEA-sulfate (DHEAS). The optimal ranges in serum are 400-600 micrograms/dl for men and 150-300 micrograms/dl for women. In saliva, the optimal level is approximately 250 pg/dl for men and 200 pg/ml for women.

If you do not want downstream metabolites of DHEA (in women DHEA increases testosterone) the best thing to do is use 7-keto DHEA. 7-keto DHEA is great because it is a bioidentical hormone that will give you all the benefits of DHEA without the problem of unpredictable biotransformation into androgens or estrogens.

A typical dose of DHEA ranges between 25-100 mg for men and 12.5-25 mg for women. For 7-keto DHEA, typical doses range between 25 and 200 mg. I would recommend 25 mg for women and 100 mg for men. It is important to remember that you may well need to titrate the dose of DHEA in women in order to avoid androgenic side effects; alternatively you can avoid them altogether by prescribing 7-keto DHEA instead.

Patients with autoimmune disease are likely to benefit from DHEA, and even the conventional literature is now saying that patients treated with corticosteroids should also be treated with DHEA. DHEA is contraindicated in people with prostate cancer, breast cancer, and reproductive cancers, although DHEA is really an anti-cancer hormone, so those are hypothetical contraindications.

THYROID HORMONE

Symptoms of hypothyroidism include: weight gain, difficulty losing weight, lowered body temperature, cold intolerance, a lack of energy, fatigue, cognitive dysfunction, dry skin, constipation, and fluid retention.

What laboratory tests are needed to determine whether or not your patient is suffering from hypothyroidism? When it comes to thyroid hormones, T3 is where the action is. Thus the most important thing to check is the patient's free level of T3. Free T4 does not really tell you anything because T4 is a pro-hormone. What about thyroid stimulating hormone (TSH)? That is a standard test for hypothyroidism, right? No. This is the analogy. Would you test levels of luteinizing hormone (LH) to check the testosterone status of a patient, and only look at the LH? No. So, why would you want to use TSH to diagnose hypothyroidism? It is much better to look at the actual hormone. Hollowell *et al* looked at the current range for TSH and found within the range of normal .4-5.5, the mean was 1.4. Therefore, if you want to find out whether or not a patient has hypothyroidism, the best thing to do is test their T3 level. So, free T3 should be in the upper third of the reference range (3.5 – 4.2 ng/dl). If you do want to test for TSH it should be less than 1.9. What if a patient has no symptoms, but their free T3 is less than optimal? I would still recommend treating the patient, probably with a low dose to get their free T3 up to the optimal level. What if a patient has symptoms, but their free T3 is within the optimal range? Again, I would treat the patient, probably with a low dose. It is important to consider symptoms – not just numbers. Of, course it is also important to ensure that the patient does not become clinically hyperthyroid, the aim is to make the patient feel better.

Thyroid replacement therapy is a combination of T3 and T4. Armour thyroid contains 39 micrograms of T4 and 9 micrograms of T3. Of course, you can use a compounded equivalent instead. The short half-life of T3 makes it difficult to use T3 alone. Some people do it, but it is hard because if they miss a day, they are in trouble. The typical dose ranges between 1 grain and 4 grains. I would recommend giving patients 1 or 2 grains of Armour thyroid initially, and titrating the dose based upon symptom improvement and free T3 level. Sometimes patients will need large doses. That does not mean to say that you are doing anything wrong, as long as you are following the patient closely.

Is T3 plus T4 better than T4 alone? Yes. Patients say they feel better when using a combination of T3 and T4. Does thyroid replacement cause atrial fibrillation? No. We are not making people hyperthyroid. Does it cause osteoporosis? No.

It is important to educate your patients about the signs and symptoms of too much thyroid, for example palpitations, tachycardia, being too hot, sweating, and etc... And to tell them that they need to stop taking their medication and make an appointment to see you if that should happen.

FEMALE HORMONES

There is a delicate balance between estrogen and progesterone, sometimes antagonistic and sometimes complementary. In this paper we are going to consider the estrogens, progesterone, and testosterone, and their antagonistic relationship.

When talking about estrogen and progesterone replacement, the one study that comes to mind is the Women's Health Initiative (WHI) Study. However, there were so many things wrong with the WHI. The major mistake in the design of the WHI was the decision to use Provera and Premarin – neither of which are bioidentical hormones.

Progesterone

Symptoms of progesterone deficiency include: anxiety, agitation, irritability, anger, aggressiveness, weight gain, water retention, bloating, headache, achy joints, swollen or tender breasts, spotting or breakthrough bleeding, mood swings, and insomnia.

In women who are still having menstrual cycles it is best to look at progesterone levels on day 21 of their cycle. So, in serum the optimal level of progesterone at day 21 of the cycle is between 13 and 23 ng/ml. In saliva the optimal level in premenopausal women at day 21 of the cycle is approximately 300 pg/ml.

If you determine that a woman does indeed have deficient levels of progesterone, how much should you give her? A typical dose of oral bioidentical progesterone is somewhere between 50 mg and 200 mg, taken at bedtime. Gambacciani evaluated the effects of oral progesterone on sleep. Oral bioidentical progesterone can be of great help to women suffering from insomnia. You just have to be careful with the dose and titrate it until you get it right. The right dose will enable the patient to sleep well through the night without waking up in the morning feeling groggy. If the patient is not having any problems sleeping, they may be better off using transdermal progesterone (50 -100 mg) instead.

If the patient is premenopausal, you should go with her cycle and prescribe progesterone for days 14 through to the start of her menses. If the patient says she feels much better when taking progesterone, you could give her say 50 mg for days 1 to 14, 100 mg for days 14 to start of menses.

What about menopausal women? Continuous or cycling, which is best? There have not really been any head-to-head studies comparing the long-term outcome of taking progesterone each day with cycling treatment. There are a lot of reasons why it makes sense to cycle, and I think that it is probably the better way to do it, until we know more; it is good to have a few days off, however you need to ensure that your patients know that they may or may not have periods.

Is there any controversy surrounding the use of supplementary progesterone? The only controversy is the use of Provera, and that it because Provera is made from synthetic progestin, and synthetic progestins are not progesterone. Fournier has researched this issue in depth with large numbers of women. Provera is an anti-progesterone – it blocks progesterone receptors and therefore does not act in the way that bioidentical progesterone would. Basically, synthetic progestins are more androgenic, they do not have the same diuretic effect that progesterone does, and they lack the beneficial effects of progesterone. If you look at the follow-up of the WHI by Anderson, GL *et al*, where they looked at the arm of the study where the women had received Premarin alone, there was no increase in breast cancer. So, the big problem was the synthetic progestin. Amazingly, there are a lot of doctors that do not realize that synthetic progestins and progesterone are entirely different things.

Estrogen

When thinking about estrogen replacement it is important to remember that there are three estrogens: - estrone (E1), estradiol (E2), and estriol (E3). It is likely that a woman will already have more estrone than she needs. Estradiol is the effective estrogen, whilst estriol is a weak, cancer protective estrogen. Estradiol and estriol are the estrogens that need replacing. As we know, 17-beta estradiol is metabolized to either 16-hydroxyestrone or 2-hydroxyestradiol. 2-hydroxyestradiol is, in turn, metabolized to 2-methoxyestradiol by catechol methyltransferase (COMT). Catecholestradiols and methoxyestradiols help to protect against cardiovascular disease and cancer, thus, it is preferable that estradiol goes down the 2-hydroxyestradiol pathway. Is it possible to steer estradiol metabolism towards 2-hydroxyestradiol as opposed to 16-hydroxyestrone? Yes, indole-3-carbinol (I3C) or diindolylmethane (DIM) supplements, and eating certain cruciferous vegetables, especially broccoli sprouts can help to steer estradiol metabolism in the right direction.

Symptoms of estrogen deficiency include: hot flashes, night sweats, fatigue, poor memory and foggy thinking, low energy, depressed mood, decreased concentration, decreased sexual desire or libido, vaginal dryness, excessive daytime sleepiness, stress incontinence, urinary tract infections, osteoporosis, cardiovascular disease, and dementia.

Like progesterone, estrogen levels should be determined at day 21 of a women's cycle, if she is still menstruating. The optimal level of estradiol in serum on day 21 is approximately 150 ng/ml. The optimal level in saliva is 15 pg/ml. This is a better method of evaluating the effectiveness of transdermal estrogen treatment, which is the preferred mode of administration for estrogen. The optimal level of estradiol for menopausal women who are taking bioidentical estrogen via the transdermal route is 10-20 pg/ml.

The best form of estrogen replacement is bi-estrogen (bi-est), which contains both estriol and estradiol (80% estriol and 20% estradiol). A typical dose is between 1.25 and 5.0 mg/gm once per day or BID. For example, 1 gram of 80:20 bi-est 2.5 mg/gm is equivalent to 2.0 mg estriol and 0.5 mg of estradiol.

Symptoms of estrogen excess include: agitation, anxiety, weight gain, water retention, headaches, swollen or tender breasts, bloating, spotting or breakthrough bleeding, mood swings, poor sleep, achy joints, and excessive bleeding. Therefore it is important to be aware of the patient's symptoms and titrate the dose accordingly. Does a premenopausal woman actually need supplementary estrogen? She might or she might not, or she might just need progesterone. If in doubt start low with 1.25 mg/gm and she how she goes.

All women who are taking estrogen replacement therapy should have regular breast screening, an annual pap smear, and ultrasonagraphy of the breasts, ovaries, and uterus.

Does bioidentical estrogen increase the risk of breast cancer and cardiovascular disease? No, no, and no. Should you offer treatment on the basis of lab results or symptoms? The best idea is to look at both, but it is more important to treat clinical symptoms.

GROWTH HORMONE

If you are even considering prescribing growth hormone (GH) you need to be fully aware of the law surrounding its use. GH has unique legal status in that it has to be prescribed according to the directions of the Surgeon General. What does that mean? That means that GH can only be prescribed to adults for the treatment of adult GH deficiency. GH cannot be prescribed off label. Furthermore, GH must also be produced by an FDA-approved facility. So, if you have some compounded GH, you need to be 100% certain that it came from an FDA-approved facility. If you are in any doubt whatsoever it is better to err on the side of caution.

Symptoms of adult GH deficiency include: decreased quality of life, sarcopenia (loss of muscle mass), loss of exercise capacity, osteopenia (loss of bone), loss of strength, increased total and intra-abdominal fat, glucose intolerance, dyslipidemia, increased fragility of skin and blood vessels, decreased skin thickness, decreased muscle tone, decreased confidence and optimism, and decreased immune function.

When testing for GH deficiency you need to be looking at insulin-like growth factor-1 (IGF-1). After GH is secreted it migrates to the liver to produce IGF-1 – 60% of the effects that GH has on the body are exerted via IGF-1. For example, GH's anabolic effect upon muscle, bone, and cartilage, and its lipolytic effect on fat, are all mediated by IGF-1. Therefore IGF-1 is a useful measure of GH. Optimal IGF-1 levels are 350 in men and 290 in women. Low values of IGF-1 are associated with adult GH deficiency. However, a patient can have normal IGF-1 levels and be GH deficient. If a patient's IGF-1 level is less than 90 it is very likely that they would fail a stimulation test. So, you would have a good case for prescribing GH. What about if their IGF-1 levels 150-plus? If they also have a lot of symptoms you can probably make a good case for adult GH deficiency. If there IGF-1 is around the 300 mark and they aren't exhibiting many symptoms you will find it very difficult to make a case for adult GH deficiency. IGF-1 levels usually increase by 100 ng/dl per day if you are treating the patient with 0.33 mg GH. Random blood tests for GH are worthless, because GH only has a half-life of fifteen minutes. However, a 24-hour urine can be useful if the patient complies.

With regards to dosing, the best thing to do is start every patient off on 0.2 mg per day and see how they feel on that. If they do not present with any side effects, after a month of treatment, move them up to 0.4 mg per day, and gradually increase the dose until you achieve the desired IGF-1 level (290 in females and 350 in males) and clinical results. The average female dose is 0.6 mg/day, while the average male dose is 0.4 mg/day – women need higher doses than men in order to achieve the same clinical results. Elderly men often require less GH. Note: GH will not work in women taking oral estrogens (transdermal is okay).

In the past, patients were often given GH just two or three times a week. This is not good practice. The old way of doing it was not physiologic and was associated with a high incidence of side effects – both of which we do not want. Patients should be given GH everyday. Should you take GH at morning or at night? This is a matter of debate; roughly half of people think morning and the other half think night. You make GH during deep sleep so the morning supporters believe that taking GH in the morning will result in less suppression of nighttime secretion. While the night school of thought is that it is more physiologic to take GH at night because that is when you secrete it. So, it can be taken first thing in the morning or last thing at night before bed. Either way, GH should be avoided after meals when insulin levels are high.

The most common side-effects of GH are edema, arthralgia, and insulin resistance. Patients that are affected by edema or arthralgia are often being treated on a low-frequency, high-dose schedule. They are also associated with mg/kg doses instead of a gradually increasing dose. Both are reversible by simply decreasing the dose.

Another side-effect of GHRT is paresthesia. If a patient complains of paresthesia, or edema, or arthralgia, the best thing to do is stop their treatment for a few days, decrease the dose, and maybe treat them symptomatically with some NSAID's or mild diuretics. Potassium replacement can also help to ameliorate these symptoms. In rare cases, a patient cannot tolerate GH. If their arthralgia keeps coming back, GH is not for them and should be discontinued.

Does GH cause cancer? No. Why do people feel that GH might increase the risk of cancer? The answer is simple – because it does stimulate cellular replication. But does GH increase the risk of cancer? Vance *et al* concluded that there is *"No evidence that GHRT affects the risk of cancer or cardiovascular disease."* Meanwhile Molitch concluded: *"Although there has been some concern about an increased risk of cancer [with GH], reviews of existing, well-maintained databases of treated patients* have shown this theoretical risk to be nonexistent." Shalet *et al* concluded that there is "*No evidence of an increased risk of malignancy, recurrent or de novo.*" On the package insert on GH it says '*don't use in active malignancy'*. However, the Growth Hormone Research Society published a paper in the *Journal of Clinical Endocrinology* saying that there is no data to support this labeling, and that current knowledge does not warrant additional warning about cancer risk. They say that this line should be removed from the package insert because there is no evidence that GH increases cancer recurrence or *de novo* cancer or leukemia.

CORTISOL

Symptoms of cortisol deficiency include fatigue, anxiety, poor stress tolerance, feeling spacey or confused, depression, paranoia, irritability, and concentration problems. Adrenal fatigue is very prominent in our society and therefore it is a good idea to offer cortisol testing to patients with any symptoms.

The most commonly used test for cortisol is the morning cortisol test, however this test will only give you one data point, which is a problem become a patient's levels may be fine in the morning but may go awry later in the day. Therefore salivary testing is better as you can get the patient to take samples throughout the day, which will give you a much better picture of what is going on. Cortisol levels can be high, which is an indicator of stress, or low, which is an indicator of adrenal fatigue.

Treatment depends on whether a patient's cortisol levels are high or low. Patients with high cortisol levels should be encouraged to try and eliminate stress, follow a healthy lifestyle, and take up meditation. Patients with low cortisol levels need adrenal support. Do not be afraid of treating patients with bioidentical cortisol if they need it. If the patient has a hormone deficiency and has the symptoms of adrenal fatigue treat those with 5-30 mg (divided BID) compounded extended release bioidentical cortisol. That will help the patient tremendously. Do not treat them with corticosteroids.

CONCLUDING REMARKS

The first thing we should remember is that we should not be rushing to throw hormones at people. Hormone optimization is the finishing touch. A good physician should first consider the patient's lifestyle, including: nutrition, detoxification, exercise, stress reduction, antioxidants, and nutraceuticals. Of course, hormones should be used to treat a deficiency disease, and if hormone replacement is necessary it should be with bioidentical hormones titrated to youthful levels. Hormone optimization is an extremely powerful tool, however as we learned with the WHI Study, hormones need to be used properly in order to give us the desired results.

REFERENCES

Anderson, GL, Limacher M, Assaf AR, Bassford T, Beresford SA, Black H, et al. Effects of conjugated equine estrogen in postmenopausal women with hysterectomy: the Women's Health Initiative randomized controlled trial. *JAMA*. 2004;291:1701-1712.

Araujo AB, Handelsman DJ, McKinlay JB. Total testosterone as a predictor of mortality in men: results from the Massachusetts Male Aging Study. In: Proceedings of the Endocrine Society's 87th Annual Meeting; June 4-7, 2005; San Diego, Calif. Abstract P1-561.

Dimitrakakis C, Jones RA, Liu A, Bondy CA. Breast cancer incidence in postmenopausal women using testosterone in addition to usual hormone therapy. *Menopause*. 2004;11:531-535.

Fournier A, Berrino F, Clavel-Chapelon F. Unequal risks for breast cancer associated with different hormone replacement therapies: results from the E3N cohort study. *Breast Cancer Res Treat*. 2008;107:103-111. Epub 2007 Feb 27.

Gambacciani M, Ciaponi M, Cappagli B, Monteleone P, Benussi C, Bevilacqua G, Vacca F, Genazzani AR. Effects of low-dose, continuous combined hormone replacement therapy on sleep in symptomatic postmenopausal women. *Maturitas*. 2005;50:91-97.

Hollowell JG, Staehling NW, Flanders WD, Hannon WH, Gunter EW, Spencer CA, Braverman LE. Serum TSH, T(4), and thyroid antibodies in the United States population (1988 to 1994): National Health and Nutrition Examination Survey (NHANES III). *J Clin Endocrinol Metab*. 2002;87:489-499.

Kaczmarek A, Reczuch K, Majda J, Banasiak W, Ponikowski P. The association of lower testosterone level with coronary artery disease in postmenopausal women. *Int J Cardiol*. 2003;87:53-57.

Korenman SG, Morley JE, Mooradian AD, Davis SS, Kaiser FE, Silver AJ, Viosca SP, Garza D. Secondary hypogonadism in older men: its relation to impotence. *J Clin Endocrinol Metab.* 1990;71:963-969.

Molitch ME. Diagnosis of GH deficiency in adults--how good do the criteria need to be? *J Clin Endocrinol Metab.* 2002;87:473-476.

Morgentaler A. Testosterone and prostate cancer: an historical perspective on a modern myth. *Eur Urol.* 2006;50:935-939.

Oelkers W. Dehydroepiandrosterone for adrenal insufficiency. *N Engl J Med.* 1999;341:1073-1074.

Shalet SM, Brennan BM, Reddingius RE. Growth hormone therapy and malignancy. *Horm Res.* 1997;48 Suppl 4:29-32.

Vance ML, Mauras N. Growth hormone therapy in adults and children. *N Engl J Med.* 1999;341:1206-1216.

von Mühlen D, Laughlin GA, Kritz-Silverstein D, Barrett-Connor E. The Dehydroepiandrosterone And WellNess (DAWN) study: research design and methods. *Contemp Clin Trials.* 2007;28:153-168.

Zitzmann M, Nieschlag E. Hormone substitution in male hypogonadism. *Mol Cell Endocrinol.* 2000;161:73-88. Review.

ABOUT THE AUTHOR

As a pioneer in the field of anti-aging medicine, Dr. Ron Rothenberg was one of the first physicians to be recognized for his expertise to become fully board certified in the specialty. Dr. Rothenberg founded the California HealthSpan Institute in Encinitas, California in 1997 with a commitment to transforming our understanding of and finding treatment for aging as a disease. Dr. Rothenberg is dedicated to the belief that the process of aging can be slowed, stopped, or even reserved through existing medical and scientific interventions. Challenging traditional medicine's approach to treating the symptoms of aging, California HealthSpan's mission is to create a paradigm shift in the way we view medicine: treat the cause. He received his MD from Columbia University, College of Physicians and Surgeons in 1970. Dr. Rothenberg performed his residency at Los Angeles County-USC Medical Center and is also board certified in emergency medicine. He received academic appointment to the USCD School of Medicine Clinical Faculty in 1997 and was promoted to full Clinical Professor of Preventive and Family Medicine in 1989. In addition to his work in the field of anti-aging medicine, Dr. Rothenberg is an attending physician at Scripps Memorial Hospital in Encinitas, California. Dr. Rothenberg travels extensively to lecture on a variety of topics, which include anti-aging, preventive and regenerative medicine and is the author of the Amazon.com # 1 best seller *Forever Ageless, Advanced Edition*

Chapter 30
Training The Brain: A Review of Clinical Advancements That Reeducate the Central Nervous System To Feel Good
Dr. Ron Shane; Jodi Lasky, PA-C

ABSTRACT
Cognitive education or counseling is not prodigious enough to remodel the aberrantly allostatic central nervous system (CNS). This paper reviews the latest clinical medical advancements that reeducate the CNS to promote that cellular optimization and restorative homeostatic parameters such as the brain's reward system.

INTRODUCTION
Cognitive education or counseling is not prodigious enough to remodel the aberrantly allostatic central nervous system (CNS). Contemporary humans are going to have to partake in arduous programs, which will effusively modify their brain architecture and extracellular matrices to where homosapien motivation results in the release of endogenous ameliorative substrates that engender cellular optimization and restorative homeostatic parameters such as the brain's reward system. Exercise and emotional sustenance have been related to the expression of nitric oxide, IGF-1, BDGF, and other transforming growth factors. Thus, the ardent participation in a wide variety of bodily edifying activities will engender the expression of neurohormones, enzymes, cytokines and growth factors, which are associated with enhancing biochemical pathways that elicit positive CNS remodeling and overall salutary physiologic efficaciousness.

Man's style of living does not involve for the propensity of human phenotypes, a progression towards optimal morphological genesis. In the preceding twenty years, chronic CRF upregulation has been associated with the negative remodeling of many bodily axes. Medical practitioners are aware that their arsenal of pharmacological agents are not sufficient to therapeutically induce highly adaptive physiological remodeling in today's aberrant phenotype.

CLINICAL ADVANCEMENTS IN 2007
The authors attended the University of California San Diego's (UCSD) 2007 School of Medicine's six-day long Internal Medicine seminar and Pain Management Symposium. This program emphasized to clinicians that they must commence employing programs in their clinics, which are either complementary or integrative with traditional medical protocols to assuage today's lifestyle based epidemic pathogenesis.

Recently, Dr. Guarneri purported in her lecture to physicians that meditation, acupuncture, emotional touching, various kinds of exercise, Chi Gung, the movement arts and yoga m8ust be provided to their patients where health care professionals take on the responsibility to actively involve their clients in these medicinal strategies. The majority of the speakers at the April 2007 Pain Management Symposium regarded the integration of many edifying protocols as necessary for patients; however, physicians must find ways to increase the participation and compliance of their patients. Moreover, western medical practitioners are seeking strategies to treat today's pathogenic phenotype. It is necessary that other social institutions conjointly work with the medical community to facilitate the public's participation in those medicinal strategies, which can attenuate the body's maladaptive remodeling. Thus, today's western medical organizations have realized that man's lifestyle is eliciting pathologies, which are related to mind, body and environmental emotional factors.

Dr. Mayer argued in his 2007 lecture at UCSD's medical symposium that CRF dysregulation is responsible for chronic fatigue, syndrome X, certain kinds of psychiatric symptomatologies, IBS, fibromyalgia and other debilitating malaises. Moreover, the western medical community can't employ pharmacological agents or surgical interventions to rectify this kind of negative CNS pathogenesis. Today's population must adapt medicinal bodily strategies to upregulate heuristic enzymes and peptides, which will propitiously remodel man's allostatic CNS. The medical community is thoroughly cognizant as to what bodily/visceral protocols will make the human animal feel good as well as optimally physiological. Primatologists have written a plethora of papers, which demonstrate that higher primates employ sensuous strategies to euphorically evoke salubrious emotionality.

There have been numerous studies in rodents, which show that a mother licking her newborn pup will lead to the expression of auspicious peptides, which will then lead to the optimal neurogenesis of the CNS. Those pups, which were licked by their mothers will be emotionally edified as well as much more efficacious in terms of their ability to cope with stress, and are being more salutary in their overt and covert behaviors. Psychiatrists and psychologists have documented that humans don't have time for intimate social relationships with others. There is overwhelming empirical evidence that higher primates including homosapiens, must be amorously touched and stroked in order to release essential enzymes and peptides necessary for salutary CNS neurogenesis. Furthermore, sitting on a computer observing squalid pornographic images does not invigorate the CNS's pleasure system or lead to emotional salubrious remodeling.

The human organism's CNS allostatic aberrance as has been discussed in this review, impacts many other bodily physiological axes. Dr. Mayer further stated in his lecture that the concept of brain body separation is invalid and may be philosophically poignant, but has no physiological merit. CNS allostatic dysregulation has been overwhelmingly shown to be the etiological basis as previously mentioned for IBS, chronic fatigue syndrome, fibromyalgia, anxiety, for certain kinds of depression, migraines and other affective or mood disorders. Western society's current arsenal of medications is quite paltry in terms of treating these allostatic pathologies. In other words, these physiological symptomatologies are more suited for alternative and complementary medical protocols. Clinicians must reeducate their patient's neurobiological machinations. Surgical or pharmacological intervention has no real propitious benefit for CRF dysregulatory symptomatologies.

Taoist and yogic hierophants have argued that humans need to educate their psyche with medicinal strategies, which blithefully edifies the third chakra or lower dantien. Western physicians know that the gastrointestinal tract has trillions of neurons with similar neurotransmitter concentrations to that of the CNS. There is a very an essential relationship to the GI nervous system and the human brain. Moreover, many clinicians are asserting that there is a feed forward association from the GI tract to the body's CNS where human emotionality can be auspiciously regulated by the occult dynamics of this more simplistic nervous network. Motor movement activities like Chi gung, classical dance and the internal movement arts directly affects the physiology or molecular processes of the GI tract's nervous system, which then causes changes in the human brain. Research medical scientists have not been directly able to demonstrate the validity of this proposition, however, there have been studies which have shown that yoga, Tai chi or Chi gung will reduce lower back pain and other mind-body related pathologies. Stress, anxiety and hypertension can be efficaciously treated by these non-invasive modalities. It is estimated that four hundred thousand Americans die each year from inactivity, obesity or poor diet. It is projected that this figure will definitely increase in the ensuing years. Moreover, there needs to be some kind of adherence by today's population to integrated medicinal protocols, which will endogenously activate auspicious interleukins, cytokines and hedonic peptides of their GI nervous system in order to evoke salutary emotional signaling to the CNS. Indigenous humans participated in many movement activities, which positively aroused the body's GI nervous system and down regulated the CNS's sympathetic hypertonicity. In today's culture, there is no emphasis for humans to enact motor sequences that would optimize their body's molecular pathways, as well as to the salubriousness of the GI nervous system.

Medical clinicians know that there are no pharmacological substances, which will heuristically make humans feel good, but they understand that there are a plethora of bodily visceral activities, which will neurobiologically hedonically optimize the human brain. Many of today's medical conferences purport that exercise, a salubrious diet, caloric restriction, prolonged sexuality, emotional touching, play, creative activities and metabiological bodily activation will evoke the brain's endogenous enzymes and peptides responsible for heuristic pleasurable arousal. Medical science is evolving into an empirical discipline of bodily optimal emotionality. This scientific discipline must be the physic or compelling force to take the highly compromised co-morbid human phenotype to compliantly engage in complementary medicinal protocols in order to feel good or to be optimally physiological. This specie does not have to be allostatic or pathophysiological. This sophisticated organism has a choice as to how it will remodel.

The focus of this review was not to delineate the cultural factors or ideologies, which has lead to the skewed morassness of the human phenotype. Optimistically speaking there is a concerted effort in the medical community to work with patients to recontour their way of living as well as having them less dependent on pharmacological agents and surgical interventions. Moreover, the challenge for medical practitioners is more than transubstantiating their patient's ideologies. We have socially evolved to become a communal allostatic specie where the CNS is addicted to negative rewarding scenarios.

Clinicians must do more than inform their patients that they must make time for evocative play, exercise, emotionally edifying contact, metabiological activities and caloric restriction. Most patients concur with medical practitioners that these protocols are necessary for them; however, they are not compliant. For example, only eight percent of fitness club members actually utilize these facilities on a regular basis.

Highly trained medical practitioners are recognizing that modern humans have a bevy of energy blockages, which must be treated with alternative medicinal strategies. For example, Dr. Bonakdar, director of the pain management center at Scripps center for Integrative Medicine and Dr. Berkowicz from the Swedish Medical Center gave lectures at the 2007 Pain Management Symposium on the role of energy medicine or alternative medicinal protocols for the treatment of lifestyle induced morbidities. These medical practitioners spoke about chi channel perturbations and chakra blockages as the etiological basis of many pain symptomatologies and other physiological malaises. These clinicians purported that when the body is consumed by pathogenic energy obstructions this phenomenon causes a patient not to feel good, and can engender many other physiological morbidities. Ardent participation in alternative medicinal strategies can alleviate the body's energy aberrancies.

Dr. Berkowicz defines energy medicine as the "combining of rational knowledge with the intuitive understanding of the energy of the body and its environment". Furthermore, this physician stated that alternative medicinal modalities involve the concept that all earthly organisms are "surrounded by a sea of healing life force energies". Various cultures have referred to this metaphenomenon as ki, chi or prana. Dr. Berkowicz suggested that indigenous and eastern medical systems regard bodily malaise to be a result of chronic energy perturbation or chi flow constriction. Various cultures have evolved medicinal modalities, which treat and alleviate these kinds of pathogenic conditions. This was the focus of Dr. Bonakdar's lecture where he emphasized the importance of acupuncture for not only mitigating bodily energy obstructions, but also more importantly to reeducate the CNS and the GI nervous system. Dr. Devereaux who spoke about India's Ayurveda medicine concurred with the paradigm discussed by these other two clinicians.

Today's allostatic phenotype must not only engage in motor movement activities to optimize the body's cellular dynamics, but likewise pursue eastern and indigenous protocols to dramatically alleviate energy pathologies, which appear to engender emotional dyseuphoria. It has been discussed throughout this review that humans possess the volitional acumen to regulate their CNS's affective or mood state as well as the body's overall physiology. We can express morbid phenotypical remodeling or engender ameliorative CNS hedonic dynamics. Medical science's objective empirical veracity is now providing humans with sagacious lucidity where their consciousness in not besmirched by the enigmatic quagmire of philosophies or ideologies.

Humans can positively affect molecular pathways, which lead to highly adaptive CNS remodeling or they can invoke their body's deleterious cellular and morphological processes. It seems absurd that higher primates in the wild enjoy their CNS's pleasure network and are propitiously remodeled where as contemporary humans have fastidiously evolved maladaptive approach to brain hedonics and overall bodily optimal physiology. Today's medical clinician is extremely cognizant of this mendacious paradox, and they are trying to redress this ignominious scenario. Man's hyper upregulated allostatic brain can be remodeled to efficaciously feel good and experience edified bodily physiology. Western culture is not embracing the ineffable marvelment of other social medical paradigms in order for contemporary humans to achieve a more pleasurable emotional vibrancy.

Dr. Berkowicz purported that mind and body can be euphorically aroused and even ontologically actualized if humans are compliant to a lifestyle, which involves adherence and participation to a wide variety of medicinal protocols. Furthermore, she further suggested that contemporary humans are inundated with energy blockages, which can propitiously be treated with arcane medical strategies. Dr. Berkowicz stated that the body's profusive energy processes could be perturbed by either external or internal factors. She argues that "human beings are a network of complex energy fields interfacing with physical cellular processes... chakras modulate and transform human energies and they correspond to endocrine centers. Positive well-being decreases anxiety and improves immune function as well as overall emotional joyousness". Shakespeare writes the following: "Thy wit the ornament to shape and love misshapen in the conduct of both of them like powder in a skilless soldier's flask is set a fire by thy own ignorance". Humans possess the volition and the medical strategies to enhance the CNS's pleasure system as well as the body's salutary dynamics.

ABOUT THE AUTHORS

Currently Dr. Ron Shane is a research scholar at the University of California San Diego (UCSD) working in the field of neuroendocrinology and optimal physiology. He works as a medical consultant in Endocrinology, non surgical body sculpturing and skin rejuvenation in San Diego. Dr. Shane is a multi discpline PhD and doctor of oriental medicine and has completed post doctoral training in the disciplines of renaissance mysticism, neurobiology, psychiatry, neuroscience, internal medicine, oriental medicine and cross cultural shamanism. He is a certified master of Kundalini Yoga, an ITF international instructor and an expert sixth degree black belt in Tae Kwon Do; and is a core faculty member of the International Toaist University of Oriental Medicine. Dr. Shane is a former college strength and fitness coach and he has written many books and articles on martial arts, Taoism, Esoteric Yoga, Cross training regimes, Energy medicine, endocrinology, age management and cosmetic medicine, neuroscience, optimal health and oriental medicine. This master of health has focused his career on aesthetically and physiologically enhancing the body and essence of others. Dr. Shane regularly contributes feature articles to *Tae Kwon Do Times* and the American Academy of Anti-Aging Medicine's textbooks. Furthermore, he has given medical lectures throughout the country, has been involved in cosmetic dermatological laser research and is the producer and director of the Zen Beauty TV Program.

Jodi Lasky, PA-C is a Physician Assistant, Certified Life Coach, Certified Personal Trainer, Nutrition Consultant and ITF Tae Kwon Do Black Belt, and is a co-director of the Vitalique program, which is a comprehensive medical and training regime to induce overall bodily optimal health and well being. This super athletic woman has been a triathlete, gymnast, dancer, body builder and currently is an assistant instructor in the martial arts. She has developed psychological strategies to provide people with a greater sense of personal empowerment. Jodi has created with Dr. Shane, unique protocols which integrate weight training, dance exercises, yoga and other conditioning techniques to reshape and beautify the body. This expert in cosmetic procedures, sports medicine and orthopedics, has considerable knowledge in nutrition, energy work, as well as ways to motivate others to pleasurably lose weight. The focus of her work as a life coach is to motivate, encourage and provide others with an enhanced sense of optimal wellness and beauty. She is also a viable aesthetic and beauty practitioner treating patients with laser therapies, fillers and Botox® at a medical spa; has co-written many articles and books on medical and psychological optimal health, anti-aging, dermatological laser research, cosmetic enhancement, and the internal aspects of the martial arts; and is featured in the Zen Beauty TV Program and is pursuing a doctorate in oriental medicine.

Chapter 31
Cosmetic Medicine – 2008 Update:
A Review of Advancements in Aesthetics Protocols
Dr. Ron Shane; Jodi Lasky, PA-C

ABSTRACT

By 2025, 25% of Americans will be older than 65. The cosmetic medicine specialty is experiencing unprecedented growth. In 2006, Americans spent more than $12.1 billion on non-surgical (aesthetic) and surgical procedures ["Cosmetic Surgery National Data Bank: 2006 Statistics," American Society for Aesthetic Plastic Surgery (ASAPS)]. This aging demographic will continue to fuel the growth of the Cosmetic Medicine market, as Boomers seek ways to look, feel, and act younger and better. The intent of this review is to provide an overview of the available cosmetic protocols by surveying some of today's most popular aesthetic and surgical procedures, reporting on the latest technological advancements therein.

INTRODUCTION

Many patients are asking their primary care physicians about the vast array of aesthetic strategies. Thus, it is important to provide the plethora of clinicians with an essential understanding of appropriate and effective aesthetic protocols. Moreover, there is an ostensible degree of misunderstanding surrounding many cosmetic procedures in terms of their aesthetic and age management efficacy.

This paper is the result of information gathered by the authors' attendance at the 2008 American Society for Aesthetic Plastic Surgery (ASAPS) annual meeting. The exquisite presenters at this meeting were quite lucid and relatively objective on the divergent array of topics discussed at this meeting.

AESTHETICS ADVANCEMENTS IN 2008
Facial Concerns

Patients from the international community who are concerned about the aesthetic devastation of aging are seeking more non-invasive ways to combat the negative remodeling and molecular effects of this catabolic phenomenon. It is quite evident that some kinds of face-lifts can address facial sagging and in many instances, a decrement in facial volume. Dr. Victor Ross, a leading dermatological researcher stated at this conference that lasers couldn't enhance extensive deficiencies in facial volume nor provide deep tissue tightening. Dr. Bruce Connell the guru of facial plastic surgery, asserted that cosmetic surgery is currently the only way to elevate and plicate soft tissue aberrancies, which are associated with aging or facial sagging. He purported "a face-lift is not about tightening the skin, but rather is a non-tension based recontouring of the facial musculature". He further suggested that only 20% of board certified plastic surgeons are aesthetically prolific in terms of reducing the effects of aging as well as enhancing a patient's aesthetic appearance. Moreover, he purported when interviewed, that many plastic surgeons only memorize their way through medical training, and most likely do not have the necessary creative proficiency to be an exquisite practitioners. This world-renowned expert only trains medical clinicians who have finished their residency and are in private practice. Dr. Connell is not impressed by very popular seemingly non-invasive face-lift procedures; and he asserts that the MAC procedure is not capable of amelioratively treating sagging in the lower facial quadrants. He likewise cautions against very aggressive surgical protocols as not being very advantageous. This elite practitioner uses patient's youthful photographs as a blue print so that he can optimally reposition their soft tissues in order to generate youthful symmetry to the aging facial physiognomy.

The panel on facial plastic surgery, which evaluated the efficacy of aggressive surgical dissection unanimously agreed that less invasive or a more superficial plane of dissection has been shown to be far more beneficial to the patient. Dr. William Little stated that it was not necessary to be overly aggressive in terms of engendering an exquisite aesthetic outcome. All of the panelists lead by Dr. James Stuzin agreed that smaller scars and a more superficial plane of dissection leads to more rapid healing and less complications like hematomas and infections. Dr. Daniel Baker in his presentation commented on a ten-year study that demonstrated that a particular surgical approach did not produce any significant aesthetic improvements over any other. The study, which he referred to, had different surgeons employing distinctive facial surgical strategies on identical twins where then medical experts assessed the benefits over a ten-year period. Furthermore, he asserted that plastic surgeons are moving away from deep plane dissections, which were popular in the late 1990s. Dr. Baker is a leading proponent of the MAC face-lift, which involves a smaller incision, and there is a vertical elevation of a smaller portion of the facial flap. Dr. Paul Chasan who was not a presenter at this conference stated in his practice that this kind of face lift is only appropriate for certain kinds of patients who are usually younger with less lower facial laxity. Many other presenters suggested that this highly popular procedure does not address extensive sagging of the facial jowls as well as the neck. Thus, the minimally invasive face-lift appears to be only appropriate for certain phenotypes who don't present moderate to severe facial laxity or where there are not extensive volume deficiencies.

Many of the presenters implicitly stated that some patients before the age of fifty should undergo some kind of minimally invasive facial surgery. It has been empirically shown that those individuals who do undergo some kind of face-lift procedure will have a more youthful aesthetic appearance as they age. The hot topic panel created by Dr. Robert Singer asserted that lasers, fillers and botox do not replace the need for facial plastic surgery. Patients need to be educated by their primary care physician that if they desire to look more youthful for their age that there is not a non-invasive procedure in lieu of a facelift. A thorough volumization of an aging face, which appears to be deflated in many regions will cost between $5000-$8000 a year to maintain. Furthermore, a face lift by a superb practitioner will enhance overall facial volume, attenuate the furrows of the nasolabial folds, elevated mallor fat pads, and restore prominence to the cheeks usually without the need of prostheses.

In summary, patients under the age of 50 with facial sagging and volume loss should undergo some kind of mid face-lift to attenuate these aesthetic issues as the utilization of lasers and fillers is not the ideal aesthetic strategy. Conversely, the synergistic use of IPL treatments, fillers and ablative fractionated strategies are exquisite protocols for younger patients with lesser aesthetic devastation; and these cosmetic protocols can dramatically augment post-surgical face-lift procedures. Dr. Kurt Bivens a board certified plastic surgeon pointed out that patients who extensively exercise have an improved quality to their soft tissue in terms of its molecular dynamics. The mid face-lift is still the gold standard for facial rejuvenation in older phenotypes even though today's populous is fervently demanding non-invasive protocols.

Adiposity Concerns

It is now estimated that over 70% of the U.S. population is overweight and these individuals are seeking a variegated array of protocols, which don't involve caloric restriction or exercise to address their pathogenesis. Liposuction was originally employed for the reduction of adiposity in a particular bodily quadrant; however, it is now being utilized as a weight loss procedure where a patient can eliminate over 10 pounds of fat from his or her body per surgical session. Dr. Sharon Giese has been very successful in her practice in eliminating large amounts of subcutaneous fat from her patients who are 20 to 30 pounds overweight. Moreover, this panelist has also been able to motivate her patients to lose weight after undergoing a liposuction procedure. Thus, this surgeon is quite inspirational in terms of motivating her patients to lose weight, which enabled them to have an excellent overall aesthetic outcome.

Cynosure several years ago introduced a product, which is a laser guided lipolysis device for shearing membranes of adipose cells. In addition, this technology supposedly contracts the epidermal complex. The SmartLipo system has been FDA approved in terms of its safety in the U.S. for less than 2 years. This laser system only destroys adipose cells where some other protocol must be employed to retrieve the fatty emulsion. There are several methods, which are utilized by cosmetic practitioners to extract the fatty acid substrate. This particular laser strategy has captured the interest of the international public to where they believe that this cosmetic device can remove excessive bodily adiposity. Dr. Robert Singer, an elite member of ASAPS, and who created the hot topic session of this conference, presented a very revealing commentary on this popular liposuction procedure. He discussed studies pertaining to this protocol, which indicated that there was no empirical evidence of a sustained measurable skin tightening. Furthermore, Dr. Singer stated that SmartLipo was not as efficacious as traditional liposuction devices. Furthermore, he suggested that there needs to be more research on whether the 1064 or 1320 wavelength promotes significant skin tightening at the papillary dermis. Dr. Mitch Goldman, the author of the Laser Surgery Textbook, believes that the combination of two wavelengths will induce tissue tightening. The newest generation of Cynosure's SmartLipo laser system will combine both a 1064 and 1320 wavelength together for greater efficiency in terms of skin tightening.

This plastic surgeon suggested that this interesting technology might be nothing more than media sensationalism without any significant efficacy. Moreover, even though it induces thermal lysis in a small bodily area, the liquefied fat still must be aspirated in many instances with traditional liposuction cannulas. It appears from Dr. Singer's presentation as well as Dr. Adam's panel on SmartLipo that this technology can be likened to the "emperor's new clothes". For example, there is a surgical center in Fort Lauderdale, Florida where the owner who is not a physician is operating 5 SmartLipo machines, which he uses to attract patients into his medical practice. Several presenters from Dr. Adam's panels suggests that SmartLipo is not a very efficient strategy for Liposuction; to reiterate, there is no indication that this cosmetic procedure engenders any kind of significant skin tightening. However, some practitioners anecdotally speaking purport that they have seen definite skin tightening from this procedure. In general, the sales representatives from Cynosure state that this technology is only appropriate for the treatment of bodily regions where there is a slight degree of adiposity such as the triceps or the flanks and any other small pocket of adiposity. Is there any merit for a cosmetic medical practitioner to spend $130,000.00 on this machine? Several presenters purported that the SmartLipo will definitely bring patients into a medical practice; and non-surgically trained physicians can utilize this device as a way of procuring the lucrative benefits associated with cosmetic surgery.

There was considerable attention at this conference on fat grafting to the breasts as well as certain facial regions. Some practitioners are opting to transfer grafted fat to the breasts as a viable option to breast implants. Dr. Kotamo Yoshimuna from Japan discussed his successful results with fat grafting to the breast of very thin Asian women who were deficient in breast tissue. He was able to increase these women's breasts one-cup size. Moreover, there are many complications associated with this procedure such as adipose cell necrosis, calcification, cysts and infections. Some other presenters likewise demonstrated that autologous fat transfer works very well with breast implant augmentation in order to create a more pleasing outcome. Furthermore, it was asserted that fat grafting of the breast is still very unpredictable; and more research and refinement is necessary before this procedure becomes a viable option to implants for breast augmentation.

The hot topic expert panel found no merit for what was referred to as injection lipolysis commonly known as mesotherapy or liposdissolve. These procedures are usually executed by non-surgeons. It was suggested that even if the agents employed in these methodologies could only rupture the membranes of adipose cells, which has not yet been demonstrated, there still needs to be a secondary procedure to extract the fatty acid substrate. Macrophages could not effectively perform this physiological role. Injection lipolysis is not a benign procedure; and there are many anecdotal reports of problematic complications. Furthermore, there was some suggestion that the FDA will prevent licensed medical practitioners from performing this procedure on patients. If this pseudo form of lipolysis has any merit, it would be through the physiological actions of placebo. It was further stated that patients need to be informed of the side effects associated with mesotherapy and lipodissolve.

Facial Volume Concerns

There was some discussion whether fat grafting is comparable or as viable to fillers in terms of volumizing deficient facial regions. Most of the presenters stated that fat grafting is still problematic in the facial region, and it is patient specific in terms of obtaining a significant aesthetic improvement. Adipose cell necrosis is still a flagrant problem; and many aesthetic surgeons opt to place fat in deficient areas during a surgical procedure in order to enhance facial volume. However, the results are quite variable. Many cosmetic dermatologists are involved in autologous fat grafting for restoration of facial volume; and these practitioners anecdotally speaking oftentimes obtain only minimum aesthetic improvement as a result of this cosmetic procedure. Superb aesthetic results appear to be more of an anomaly.

Dr. Kotaro Yoshimuna gave a presentation at the hot topic session on the use of autologous adipose stem cells as a way of enhancing fat grafting primarily in the breasts. However, his novel procedure can also be employed in the face or other bodily areas. He demonstrated that nascent adipose stem cells as they differentiate provide as a function of paracrine and autocrine activity, an ameliorative array of growth factors to the surrounding tissue. Thus, this protocol improves the efficacy of fat grafting procedures. Dr. Yoshimuna refers to this fat grafting strategy as cell assisted lipo transfer. He purports that his methodology will certainly improve the survival of transferred adipose cells in terms of preventing atrophy or necrosis of grafted adipose tissue. Fat grafting in the older phenotype is usually necessary as these patients have depleted facial volume, and the use of stem cells could greatly improve the overall aesthetic outcome of this procedure.

Breast Concerns

There was extensive discussion at this conference on breast augmentation, reduction mammoplasty and mastopexy. Some of the highlights of these presentations are that cosmetic practitioners still prefer to place implants under the muscle as it provides a more naturalistic appearance resulting in less occurrence of breast ptosis and capsulation. In Dr. Thorne's panel presentation there was considerable discussion of a new silicone implant, which is comprised of a much firmer material and it is not a gel substance that can leak into the surrounding tissue if the implant should rupture. Moreover, it was stated that cosmetic surgeons are now using this implant in Canada. Allergan's innovative implant was shown to correct mild breast ptosis as a function of this prosthesis's ability to lift the nipple to ninety degrees. Dr. Paul Chasan a board certified plastic surgeon in La Jolla, CA took part in Allergan's FDA research study and he suggested that this silicone substance has a heavier feel to it and may not be as effective as purported by the manufacturer for actually correcting breast ptosis. Conversely, several of the panelists asserted that this implant would revolutionize breast augmentation procedures in the U.S. Dr. Goes from Brazil purported in his presentation on breast lifts, that he is obtaining remarkable results with a mesh support system, which he utilizes in his breast reduction surgeries. It appears that this protocol is effective and somewhat analogous to the internal bra, which likewise prevents breast ptosis. Both of these technologies mitigate the breast's dissent at the inferior pole maintaining the efficacy of the surgical lift.

There was a study presented by Dr. Grant Stevens and others showing in the rodent model that silicone reduces fibroblast proliferation; and thus, negatively affects tissue healing. Allergan's newest generation of silicone implants are not a gel like substance; and therefore, will not leak into the breast tissue and the systemic circulation if ruptured. In general, breast reduction surgeries with lifts, are being performed with smaller vertical and horizontal scars. Fat repositioning is still an essential facet of these procedures; oftentimes implants can augment the aesthetic outcome. The cosmetic results of these procedures were very positive and there was an implicit enthusiasm amongst the speakers to employ autologous fat recontouring whenever possible. Some of the presenters appear to be interested in using fat grafting in lieu of implants for breast augmentation surgeries.

Skin Rejuvenation

There was considerable discussion throughout the conference regarding all aspects of laser technologies for skin rejuvenation. Moreover, the various panelists from the hot topic session all agreed that lasers are not yet capable of deep skin tightening. Furthermore, they concurred that Thermage and other such technologies cannot reliably induce any kind of significant facial tightening. Thus, cosmetic clinicians should not be promising their patients that minimally invasive laser technologies can attenuate facial laxity. Dr. Dibernando's panel likewise expressed these sentiments. To reiterate again, the traditional mid face-lift is still the gold standard, and is the most efficacious protocol for inducing facial tightening and engendering volume.

All of the laser companies have FDA clearance for some form of fractionated laser treatment. There was a consensus of agreement amongst the various panelists that fractionated ablative laser technologies are far superior to non-ablative fractionated protocols. Thus, the field of laser technology is moving away from non-ablative fractionated systems to either Erbium or CO2 ablative fractionated strategies. Reliant was the first laser company to create fractionated systems; and they are now solely focused on ablative fractionated technologies. All of the speakers at this conference from Dr. Victor Ross to Dr. Mark Rubin were excited about the prospect of ablative fractionated technologies. However, all of the panelists who discussed this topic stated that more research needs to be executed to truly ascertain the actual aesthetic proficiency of either Erbium or CO2 ablative fractionated laser technologies.

It was purported by many speakers at this meeting that cosmetic researchers are currently trying to determine whether ablative fractionated Erbium systems are as effective in terms of attenuation of rhytids to that of CO2. In other words, it is still not known how large the spot size should be, the depth of penetration, the concentration of ablative pores per pass; and most importantly, the intensity of the actual fluence. It may take at least 2 years to reliably answer these questions. Lumenis, Cutera, Palomar and Reliant are the laser companies actively competing for the ultimate ablative fractionated technology for the reduction of rhytids with less down time and odious side effects. It is not clear as to what treatment protocol will produce the most viable aesthetic outcome. It may be most judicious to wait to purchase a $130,000.00 laser system until there are studies to support what is the optimal technology for ablative fractionated treatment of facial rhytids. Currently, the leading dermatological researchers in the field do not know how to answer this question. Dr. Mitch Goldman asserts that CO_2 fractionated ablative technology will provide patients with stellar results as compared to Erbium lasers. Furthermore, at least 4 sessions are needed for non-ablative fractionated technologies to have any kind of aesthetic effects and those lasers are unpopular and not recommended by board certified plastic surgeons.

There are some anecdotal reports of hypopigmentation and languid healing with some of the newest ablative CO_2 fractionated technologies, which Dr. Goldman strongly disputes. Some dermatological clinical researchers are suggesting that high fluence and deep penetration is necessary to reduce facial rhytids. However, recently Dr. Victor Ross completed a study in which he was able to obtain excellent cosmetic results comparable to employing a CO_2 fractionated ablative technologies with Palomar's 2940 ablative fractionated Erbium system. This technology will afford the aesthetic practitioner with a relatively minimally invasive laser technology for ablating the facial epidermal surface as well as a significant reduction of rhytids for younger patients who are not candidates for a face-lift as well as for older clients who have undergo an invasive facial surgical procedure.

It was likewise pointed out that recent advances in IPL technologies have made these systems excellent for reducing brown skin lesions, redness as well as overall dyschromia. Lumenis, Palomar and Cutera have the most outstanding IPL technologies and they have a less likelihood of complications. Furthermore, all of these companies also produce excellent hair removal systems. Thus, those physicians who are not board certified plastic surgeons, but who are actively engaged in less invasive cosmetic procedures can most effectively treat their patients with the following laser technologies: IPL system, hair removal lasers and some kind of Erbium or CO_2 ablative fractionated technology. It is most beneficial for a practitioner to purchase one platform, which can be utilized with a divergent array of hand pieces. It is estimated for less than $200,000.00 a cosmetic clinician can have hair removal, IPL, fractionated ablative technologies and vascular treatment protocols. Cynosure still makes the most exquisite Alexandrian laser system for the removal of various kinds of brown lesions and the Varilite technology is also superb for the removal of superficial veins and lentiginous lesions. Moreover, Cutera, Palomar, Lumenis and Cynosure have excellent hand pieces for the treatment of superficial vascular aberrations. Currently, all of these laser companies have technologies, which are excellent for improving facial pigment, removing brown lesions as well as epidermal discoloration, and the elimination of superficial veins; and it appears that the ablative fractionated technologies will mollify facial rhytids. Conversely, to reiterate, there is not any laser technology, which can reliably engender facial volume, attenuate facial laxity, significantly induce collagen genesis or engender facial tightening. There wasn't much discussion at this conference regarding the treatment of the sun-damaged torso.

In summary, it will be soon known whether Erbium fractionated ablative technologies can attenuate/remove facial rhytids as well as CO_2 systems. Ablative CO_2 fractionated lasers are more invasive and require a much longer recovery time compared to the Erbium system. There are anecdotal reports that non-ablative fractionated systems are excellent for acne and other scars, but are not effective for wrinkle reduction; and it takes many treatments to obtain any kind of aesthetic result. Many of the leading laser manufacturers have viable strategies for the treatment of vascular lesions; and the aberration may return. There are anecdotal reports that IPL treatment of a sun-damaged torso will allay uneven pigmentation, lentigines, red lesions, and dyschromia. Thus, all of these dermatological conditions can be treated on the torso with today's high-powered IPL systems. Many of these laser hair removal and IPL systems likewise have hand pieces for vascular lesions. Those medical practices that are primarily based on cosmetic protocols will also have technologies like Cynosure's Alexandrian laser, which is exquisite for alleviating all types of brown lesions or the Varilite laser. Moreover, it was mentioned at this conference that cosmetic practitioners are also addressing rhytids on the torso with either an Erbium, ablative fractionated laser or a more aggressive CO_2 system. The treatment of the lower torso requires more time to heal than that of the face; and adverse complications are more likely to occur in this region of the body. It was also discussed that some plastic surgeons are employing ablative fractionated technologies with a more superficial depth of penetration to treat the sun damage of the upper chest region. Furthermore, aesthetic practitioners traditionally use IPL systems to treat this area of the body.

Dr. Michael Kane and Dr. Steven Yoelin gave a 4-hour presentation as to how to rejuvenate a middle-aged face. Moreover, Dr. Kane emphatically stated that fillers and botox are appropriate for patients who do not have moderate to severe facial laxity. He further pointed out that those patients with moderate facial laxity and volume deficiency would be more appropriately served with some kind of mid face surgical procedure. To reiterate again, in the words of Dr. Connell, a MAC procedure or some other kind of less traditional face-lift will not attenuate laxity around the jowl line or neck. He feels that this procedure should not be utilized on older patients.

Both of these superb practitioners, Dr. Kane and Dr. Yoelin, used various hyaluronic acid products for distinctive areas of the face, which were considered to be off-label use. In general, Juvederm and Juvederm Ultra Plus only have FDA approval to correct volume depletion in the nasolabial folds. Moreover, these excellent cosmetic practitioners had very different approaches to the injection of hyaluronic acid products in depleted facial regions. For example, Dr. Yoelin employed a retrograde approach and did not inject as deep as Dr. Kane. This practitioner when injecting deep furrows utilized more vector angles than Dr. Kane, and was able to treat his patient in less time. Dr. Yoelin's results were excellent as he treated an attractive 40-year-old woman who was a very lean fitness model a day before with botox around her crow's feet, glabella and frontalis. This woman was very tan and appeared to have had years of excessive sun exposure as well as a deficit of subcutaneous fat in her face as a result of having a very low body fat composition below 12%. However, she exhibited very slight facial laxity. Dr. Yoelin treated the loss of volume in her nasolabial folds and then proceeded to add filler around the zygomatic arch and mallor fat pads. This practitioner proceeded to place a hyaluronic acid product into the lower cheek area and then corrected the laxity around her facial jaw line with a heavier hyaluronic acid product. This woman's upper lip was more enhanced than her lower lip. This practitioner stated that he always treats a woman's lower lip when plumping up the volume in the upper lip. Lastly, he placed a hyaluronic acid filler lateral to her marionette lines. This medical practitioner used nearly 8 syringes to thoroughly volumize her face. This would have cost a patient nearly $4000.00; and in the lower portions of her face, hyaluronic acid products are more quickly metabolized, and will last only about 6 months. A cosmetic practitioner would have to replace the loss of volume in those areas costing a patient several thousands of dollars. Dr. Yoelin purported hyaluronic acid products will last in the upper mid face region about 10 months. This aesthetic practitioner stated that fat grafting to volume depleted facial regions is not as efficacious as hyaluronic acid fillers due to adipose cell necrosis, and also there can be cyst formation.

In general, the aesthetic outcome with fat grafting is not as ameliorative as compared to hyaluronic acid products. It will cost this 40-year-old woman to maintain her botox and hyaluronic acid products in multiple facial quadrants between $6000.00 and $8000.00 a year. This does not include the expense of facial skin care products and laser therapies which are needed to maintain the epidermal texture of her facial skin. Thus, a woman with considerable sun damage in her late thirties who is thin could be spending up to $10,000.00 a year to preserve her facial beauty. It may be more cost effective for a middle-aged woman to have a face-lift to ameliorate her facial volume and attenuate laxity.

Dr. Kane at the hot topic session asserted that botox does certainly enter the systemic circulation, and has been shown to cross the blood brain barrier. He further stated that botox does not engender negative physiological consequences in the periphery of the body nor in the central nervous system. Furthermore, this cosmetic practitioner asserted that botox is most effective primarily at the neuromuscular junction upon injection. He also stated that when botox crosses the blood brain barrier it is most likely very inert; and thus, would not induce neurophysiological side effects. Recently, there have been some studies reported by the media suggesting that botox does pejoratively impact the central nervous system. Consequently speaking, medical practitioners most likely should not inject more than 60 units per session in case there are aberrant side effects associated with the cosmetic use of botox.

There will soon be several new fillers that will be available to the U.S.; and they are as follows, a semi-permanent collagen substance lasting 6 months, as well as a hyaluronic acid filler with lidocaine, which can be used by medical practitioners in the ensuing weeks. Moreover, adding lidocaine to a filler should ease a patient's discomfort and may reduce the need for topical lidocaine as well as a dental block. Several presenters from Dr. Gold's panel discussed the fact that fillers are comprised of distinctive hyaluronic particles, which vary in size as well as they are linked in a divergent manner. For example, hyaluronic fillers which have smaller particles and will be easier to inject, whereas others have less viscosity and are more difficult to place in a facial area with depleted volume. Juvederm and Juvederm ultra plus were recommended as the most pragmatic fillers for the less experienced cosmetic practitioner.

It was further suggested that hyaluronidase could be used to allay any complications associated with hyaluronic acid products. Dr. Mark Rubin purported that a medical practitioner could also puncture the skin and extract the filler. Hyaluronic acid products have a lesser likelihood of inducing an allergic reaction, since their biochemical composition is endogenous to the human body. A presenter pointed out that world wide there are over one hundred fillers and only some of them have been approved to be used in the U.S. Moreover, more experienced practitioners like Dr. Kane and Dr. Yoelin stated that they employ a diverse array of fillers depending on the facial region and the depth of the rhytid or furrow. Furthermore, these practitioners utilized distinctive techniques for the placement of the filler as a function of a particular facial area. The appropriate placement of the filler can dramatically rejuvenate the face; however, this aesthetic protocol can be quite costly to the patient.

There was a panel discussion devoted to the efficacy of Palomar's ablative fractionated erbium laser for the treatment of periocular and perioral rhtytids. It was demonstrated by the presenter that this less invasive laser strategy could attenuate rhytids with a similar effectiveness to Reliant's CO_2 ablative fractionated system or Lumenis's Total FX with a minimal risk of side effects and less down time. Dr. Mitch Goldman, a world leading laser surgeon suggests that CO_2 ablative fractionated technologies have much better aesthetic efficacy than Erbium ablative fractionated laser systems. Furthermore, it was stated that the Palomar system might be able to mitigate smaller wrinkles on various bodily quadrants. Currently, there is not any well-established laser therapy to treat torso rhytids. The Lumenis Corporation is asserting that their Total FX (Active FX and Deep FX combined) can cosmetically allay torso rhytids; however, the healing time on these bodily areas are much longer than facial regions. Older patients are robustly seeking non-invasive treatments for sun damage on all aspects of their torso. IPL, Alexandrian and Ruby laser therapies can significantly treat dyschromia, red and brown lesions, and other surface aberrations, but won't allay rhytids and improve collagen or elastin deficiencies.

Dr. Mark Jewell's panel on lower torso contouring presented intriguing and dramatic aesthetic results. All of the presenters were combining extensive liposuction with their abdominoplasties. Most of their patients had lost over 80 pounds, however, there were a few women who they treated that had undergone multiple pregnancies. There were some cases that were presented by these elite plastic surgeons, where they extracted over 10 pounds of skin and dissected out many kilograms of adipose tissue. These practitioners were profoundly able to aesthetically sculpture the torsos of patients who pre-optively displayed a morbid excess of hanging skin and subcutaneous adiposity, which could not be remodeled through further dieting or exercise. Moreover, the scars were extensive as a result of these aesthetic procedures even though some of the practitioners utilized biologically engineered glue, which to some degree alleviated the need the for staples, and mitigated the likelihood of hypertrophic scarring. Dr. Jean Pascal a leading authority of thighplasty was able to recontour the thighs of patients who had lost an inordinate amount of body weight. His methodology involved aggressive liposuction of the inner thigh and the elimination of excessive skin. The scar extended vertically from the knee to the pubic area, however, his aesthetic results were exquisite. This elite practitioner initially performed abdominoplasty followed by an extensive cosmetic procedure on the upper and lower back as well as the buttock region. Lastly he treated the excess skin and adiposity of the thighs. Many plastic surgeons are treating patients who have lost over 150 pounds or more from Lap Band surgery. Some aesthetic practitioners are likewise removing excessive skin and adiposity around the arms, and then performing breast reductions and lifts. To reiterate, diet and exercise won't mitigate the hanging of excess skin and inordinate subcutaneous adiposity of Lap Band surgical patients. It is evident that those patients who have undergone multiple surgeries to achieve overall bodily recontouring must then strictly maintain a lifestyle that involves caloric restriction, stress reduction and exercise. Furthermore, it is likely that older extreme weight loss patients will also opt for lower face and neck liposuction with a face-lift.

CONCLUDING REMARKS

In summary, the international community of plastic surgeons are able to beautifully contour all aspects of the human body. These extensive surgeries will obviously become more popular as today's populous is chronically obese, and Lap Band surgeries are now exceedingly popular as they produce fewer side effects than other bariatric surgeries. Moreover, Dr. Wilson Matos and Dr. Ricardo Ribeiro discussed the many complications associated with lipoabdominoplasty. Ideally speaking it is preferable for patients to lower their BMIs through diet and exercise as much as possible so that their bodies can then be contoured with liposuction or cosmetic surgery if necessary. However, those patients who lose more than 100 pounds will most likely need a lipoabdominoplasty to allay the negative remodeling associated with chronic obesity. For most of these patients, hormonal monitoring, caloric restriction and a variegated array of exercise strategies after a lipoabdominoplasty will likewise afford them with an efficacious way of sustain and even improving their aesthetic appearance. ASAPS's 2008 Aesthetic meeting was well organized and highly informative covering all aspects of cosmetic enhancement and rejuvenation.

ABOUT THE AUTHORS

Currently Dr. Ron Shane is a research scholar at the University of California San Diego (UCSD) working in the field of neuroendocrinology and optimal physiology. He works as a medical consultant in Endocrinology, non surgical body sculpturing and skin rejuvenation in San Diego. Dr. Shane is a multi discpline PhD and doctor of oriental medicine and has completed post doctoral training in the disciplines of renaissance mysticism, neurobiology, psychiatry, neuroscience, internal medicine, oriental medicine and cross cultural shamanism. He is a certified master of Kundalini Yoga, an ITF international instructor and an expert sixth degree black belt in Tae Kwon Do; and is a core faculty member of the International Toaist University of Oriental Medicine. Dr. Shane is a former college strength and fitness coach and he has written many books and articles on martial arts, Taoism, Esoteric Yoga, Cross training regimes, Energy medicine, endocrinology, age management and cosmetic medicine, neuroscience, optimal health and oriental medicine. This master of health has focused his career on aesthetically and physiologically enhancing the body and essence of others. Dr. Shane regularly contributes feature articles to *Tae Kwon Do Times* and the American Academy of Anti-Aging Medicine's textbooks. Furthermore, he has given medical lectures throughout the country, has been involved in cosmetic dermatological laser research and is the producer and director of the Zen Beauty TV Program.

Jodi Lasky, PA-C is a Physician Assistant, Certified Life Coach, Certified Personal Trainer, Nutrition Consultant and ITF Tae Kwon Do Black Belt, and is a co-director of the Vitalique program, which is a comprehensive medical and training regime to induce overall bodily optimal health and well being. This super athletic woman has been a triathlete, gymnast, dancer, body builder and currently is an assistant instructor in the martial arts. She has developed psychological strategies to provide people with a greater sense of personal empowerment. Jodi has created with Dr. Shane, unique protocols which integrate weight training, dance exercises, yoga and other conditioning techniques to reshape and beautify the body. This expert in cosmetic procedures, sports medicine and orthopedics, has considerable knowledge in nutrition, energy work, as well as ways to motivate others to pleasurably lose weight. The focus of her work as a life coach is to motivate, encourage and provide others with an enhanced sense of optimal wellness and beauty. She is also a viable aesthetic and beauty practitioner treating patients with laser therapies, fillers and Botox® at a medical spa; has co-written many articles and books on medical and psychological optimal health, anti-aging, dermatological laser research, cosmetic enhancement, and the internal aspects of the martial arts; and is featured in the Zen Beauty TV Program and is pursuing a doctorate in oriental medicine.

Chapter 32
Prophylaxis of Atherosclerosis and Promotion of Well-Being in Patients with Metabolic Syndrome: A Phytotherapeutic Approach

Günter Siegel, M.D., Ph.D. [1]*; F. Sauer*[1]*; L. Ringstad*[2]*; M. Malmsten*[2]*;*
H.W. Hofer[3]*; S. Just*[4]*; P. Schäfer*[1]
[1]*Charité – Universitätsmedizin Berlin, Campus Benjamin Franklin,*
Institute of Physiology (Berlin, Germany)
[2]*Department of Physical Chemistry, Institute of Pharmacy,*
Uppsala University (Uppsala, Sweden)
[3]*Faculty of Biology, University of Konstanz (Konstanz, Germany)*
[4]*Heart Center Coswig, Department of Cardiac Surgery (Coswig, Germany)*

ABSTRACT

The prevention or deceleration of atherogenesis in the steadily increasing number of patients with metabolic syndrome is one of the most significant anti-aging objectives since this is a matter of avoidance of myocardial infarction, stroke, and Alzheimer's dementia. Oxidized LDL and Lp(a) particles are highly atherogenic, therefore phytopharmaca which counteract peroxidation of blood lipids via their ROS scavenger qualities may help us to approach this prophylactic aim. On this background, we investigated in a clinical trial the effect of Ginkgo biloba (EGb 761: Rökan® novo; Ginkgold®), the oxygen free radical scavenging properties of which are well-documented, on atherosclerotic nanoplaque formation in early-stage metabolic syndrome patients.

In a pilot study, we had reported on the beneficial effects of Ginkgo biloba (EGb 761) on atherosclerotic nanoplaque formation and size in cardiovascular high-risk patients who had undergone an aortocoronary bypass operation. Briefly, nanoplaque formation and size, the ratio oxLDL/LDL, and the highly atherothrombotic lipoprotein(a) concentration were substantially reduced, while superoxide dismutase (SOD) activity and the blood concentration of the vasodilating substances cAMP and cGMP were upregulated.[50, 63] Methodically, the very earliest stages of atherosclerotic plaque development were measured by applying a novel nanotechnologic bio-sensor utilizing ellipsometric techniques (patent EP 0 946 876).[60] This so-called nanoplaque formation is represented by the ternary aggregational complex of the HS-PG receptor, lipoprotein particles, and calcium ions. The model was validated in several clinical studies on cardiovascular high-risk patients introducing their native blood lipoprotein fractions. Since the atherosclerosis prophylactic and well-aging promotive impact of Ginkgo extract has been undoubtedly proven in this pilot study of cardiovascular high-risk patients, we wanted to confirm these beneficial effects through a second observational clinical trial. The measurable variables formerly used were additionally supplemented by a wide, novel biomarker spectrum, through which the latest parameters and markers of plaque stability and progression, oxidative stress, and inflammation were available.

In eleven patients with metabolic syndrome in the initial stage, the reduction of atherosclerotic nanoplaque formation amounted to $14.3 \pm 2.9\%$ ($p < 0.0077$) and of nanoplaque size to $23.4 \pm 3.7\%$ ($p < 0.0004$), respectively, after 2-months of treatment with Ginkgo biloba extract (EGb 761, 2 × 120 mg daily, Rökan® novo, Spitzner Arzneimittel, Ettlingen, Germany; Ginkgold®, Nature's Way, Springville, UT, USA). Additionally, superoxide dismutase (SOD) and glutathione peroxidase (GPx) activities were upregulated by $19.6 \pm 10.0\%$ ($p < 0.0785$) and $11.6 \pm 2.3\%$ ($p < 0.001$), respectively, the quotient oxLDL/LDL lowered by $21.0 \pm 4.3\%$ ($p < 0.002$), and lipoprotein(a) concentration decreased by $26.3 \pm 4.8\%$ ($p < 0.001$) in the patients' blood after the 2-month medication regimen. The concentration of the vasodilating substances cAMP and cGMP was augmented by $43.5 \pm 12.0\%$ ($p < 0.001$) and $32.9 \pm 10.4\%$ ($p < 0.001$), respectively. Surprisingly, we found a lowering of the serum Ca^{2+} concentration by $5.4 \pm 1.6\%$ ($p < 0.0076$) from 2.37 ± 0.03 to 2.24 ± 0.04 mmol/L ($p < 0.0069$). Apart from an additional vasodilatory effect, the lowered extracellular Ca^{2+} concentration affects nanoplaque formation restrictively, since this is a Ca^{2+} driven process. Furthermore, we could show a favourable development of the biomarkers 8-*iso*-PGF$_{2\alpha}$, oxLDL/LDL, SOD, GPx (oxidative stress), hs-CRP, MPO, TNFα, TGFβ1 (inflammatory status) and MMP-9 (plaque stability) which, for the lack of space, can be discussed only in part. The markers selected here are suited to provide a comprehensive risk profile for the prevention of atherosclerosis.[55]

Finally, a multimodal regression analysis reveals a basis for a mechanistic explanation of nanoplaque reduction under Ginkgo treatment. The atherosclerosis inhibiting effect is due to an attenuation of the risk factors oxLDL/LDL, Lp(a), and $[Ca^{2+}]_o$ as well as to a significant increase in the vasodilator cAMP and cGMP concentration. Thus, Ginkgo with its pleiotropic effects should be assigned a fixed rank among the anti-aging medical therapeutics as a prophylactic measure, especially in patients with early-stage metabolic syndrome.

Keywords: clinical trial; metabolic syndrome; ellipsometry; ginkgo biloba; lipoproteins; nanoplaque formation and size; oxidative stress

INTRODUCTION

In medicine, "screening" means to reach out actively to a certain segment of an apparently healthy population and recommend tests to detect the presence of a so-far undiagnosed disease at its earliest stage. This is in contrast to "preventing", or prophylaxis, by which we mean advocating precautionary measures/actions/tests/means to disclose factors that, if changed, may eventually prevent the disease.[69]

The term "metabolic syndrome" describes a cluster of cardiovascular risk factors that frequently appear together, these include abdominally accentuated obesity, impaired glucose tolerance, hypertension, and dyslipidaemia.[22,23,47,71] The metabolic syndrome is associated with an increased risk of developing diabetes and cardio-cerebro-vascular diseases.[23,31,42,46,57,59,67] Previous reports have suggested that young adults with metabolic syndrome may have increased subclinical atherosclerosis, indicated as increased intima media thickness,[73] coronary artery calcium score,[5,70] endothelial dysfunction,[14,41,50] and augmented acute-phase plasma protein hs-CRP.[35,55] The development of atherosclerosis in response to risk factor exposure begins in early life.[15] Therefore, diagnosing metabolic syndrome in young subjects may be helpful in identifying a population of risk for increased subclinical atherosclerosis.[40]

It has been known for some time that circulating free fatty acids and arterial hypertension favour atherogenesis as the pathophysiologic basis of cardio-cerebro-vascular diseases. For some years, an increasing central role as a risk factor has been allocated to the fatty tissue.[71] Fat secretes several adipokines which have a multifarious influence on the body's own metabolism. For example, adipokines can amplify insulin resistance of insulin-sensitive target tissues – a central problem in diabetes mellitus.

The tight pathophysiologic links between the individual injuries to health as well as the abound appearance of all these risk factors, especially among the population of the industrialized world, justify their assemblage as "metabolic syndrome". It is frequently criticized that this term describes rather a risk score than a medical diagnosis, as the notion 'syndrome' implies. In the medical workaday routine, however, this designation proved to be wise, since – in the presence of one of the risk factors – the physician is bound also to search for other components of the metabolic syndrome and to treat these if necessary. By this means it is assured that maximal risk reduction is attained for the incidence of cardio-cerebro-vascular diseases in the patient.

Today, decisive importance must be attached to the metabolic syndrome since it leads to increased morbidity and mortality – and thus to a decreased life expectancy – and to higher direct and indirect healthcare costs. According to the WHO, the increase in prevalence of the metabolic syndrome between 1985 and 2030 is estimated at 42% and is expected to rise further,[66] due to growing obesity among children and adolescents. Through the distinct increase in obesity in young people, it becomes even more evident that the metabolic syndrome can appear in all stages of life. Alarmingly, data from the NHANES study has revealed that the prevalence of the metabolic syndrome in 12 to 19-year olds in the US is 4.2%.[11] It is important to note that even moderate weight loss can decrease the rates of morbidity and healthcare costs.

Definition of the Metabolic Syndrome

Hanefeld and Leonhardt introduced the conception of the 'metabolic syndrome' into practice in 1981.[22,23] Internationally, it was designated as 'syndrome X' or 'insulin resistance syndrome'. Even though the notion of the metabolic syndrome has such a long tradition, an internationally accepted definition was only worked out in 1998.[2] Recognition of the metabolic syndrome is generally based on finding several well-recognized signs in clinical practice: abdominal obesity, elevated triglycerides, reduced high-density lipoprotein (HDL-C), raised blood pressure, and elevated fasting plasma glucose.

Operational definitions of metabolic syndrome have been proposed by the World Health Organization (WHO)[2] and the NCEPIIIATP.[19,20] More recently, the International Diabetes Fed-eration (IDF)[3] proposed a global definition that emphasized the importance of central adiposity (Fig. 1). These and other definitions reported in the literature include the same core criteria (central obesity, hyperglycemia, dyslipidemia, and high blood pressure), but differ in the cut-off points for individual criteria, in specific mandatory requirements (e.g., abdominal obesity or insulin resistance) and in the inclusion of additional factors (e.g., microalbuminuria). Hence, they identify broadly similar, but not identical, groups of individuals with metabolic syndrome.[17] Thus, we included patients into our study with at least two NCEPIIIATP/IDF criteria and two additional factors (smoking, all patients; Lp(a) > 30 mg/dL, 9 patients) fulfilled. Among all the criteria above mentioned, ATPIII is one of the most widely employed.[19, 20]

Definition of the metabolic syndrome according to NCEP$_{III}$ ATP (2001) and IDF (2005)

- Blood pressure ≥ 130/85 mmHg

- Fasting morning glucose ≥ 110 mg/dL (6.1 mmol/L)

- Triglyceride concentration ≥ 150 mg/dL

- HDL-Cholesterol: ♂ < 40 mg/dL; ♀ < 50 mg/dL

- Central Adipositas: BMI > 30 kg/m² or
  WC ♂ ≥ 102 cm; ♀ ≥ 88 cm

Additional inclusion criteria:

- Smoking (all patients)

- Lp(a) concentration > 30 mg/dL (9 patients)

Figure 1. Definition of the metabolic syndrome.[3, 19]
Additional inclusion criteria of the present clinical trial are defined.

STUDY DESIGN

The study design of our clinical trial as well as the interconnective network and historical development of pathophysiologic pathways culminating in cardio-cerebro-vascular events are illustrated in Fig. 2. Besides nanoplaque formation and size, a wide spectrum of parameters and markers of oxidative stress, plaque stability and progression, inflammation, lipid composition including Lp(a) and second messengers were measured. As markers of oxidative stress, the isoprostane 8-*iso*-PGF$_{2\alpha}$, the ratio of oxLDL/LDL, and the activity of superoxide dismutase (SOD) were determined. The inflammatory status was characterized by highly-sensitive CRP (hs-CRP), myeloperoxidase (MPO), tumor necrosis factor α (TNFα), and transforming growth factor β$_1$ (TGFβ$_1$). Furthermore, matrix metalloproteinase-9 (MMP-9) was measured as a relatively new marker to assess plaque stability. Lp(a) is placed at a prominent site in the midst of the network of oxidative stress and inflammation parameters. These markers were deliberately chosen because various correlations and mutual inductions during atherogenesis became apparent and contribute to the general view of a risk assessment. Besides rating the oxidative stress status by 8-*iso*-PGF$_{2\alpha}$, oxLDL/LDL ratio and SOD, MPO, and MMP-9 are correlated in their function to free radicals. MPO catalyzes hydrogen peroxide being formed upon 'detoxification' of superoxide anions by SOD, with chloride ions to hypochlorous acid (HOCl), which is a potent antibacterial agent.[75] Thus, MPO is part of the physiologic defence mechanism. Moreover, MPO contributes to the enzymatic modification of LDL particles in macrophages.[27] Coincidently, it is correlated to the formation of MMP-9. MMP-9 in patients suffering from an acute coronary syndrome seems to be directly correlated to hs-CRP.[35,43] This is an indication towards a close connection between inflammatory status and plaque stability.[26]

As mentioned, MPO and hs-CRP constitute important inflammation markers; MPO also modulates intravascular signalling cascades. It oxidizes NO after its endothelial transcytosis and has a leukocyte-activating and cytokinic effect. That is why MPO has recently been designated as a key protein for the establishment of a pro-inflammatory environment. Moreover, MPO is implicated in plaque stability via a direct correlation to MMP-9. A Chinese study demonstrates that the 'macrophage migration inhibiting factor' (MIF) plays an essential role in plaque stability through a direct stimulation of MMP-9-expression. On the other hand, oxLDL induces MIF expression via vascular endothelial cells. Thus, the circle is completed between ROS status and plaque stability.[30]

Pathophysiologic development of cardiovascular events starting from the
metabolic syndrome as a complex of multiple symptoms

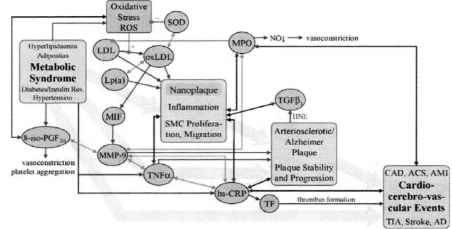

Figure 2. Starting from the metabolic syndrome as a complex of multiple symptoms, the pathophysiologic development of cardiovascular events is represented via atherogenic processes in their chronology (⊘). Furthermore, the essential biomarkers (→) are depicted as resultant products (→) and target quantities (→) of these pathologic processes in their cross-linkage and correlation (↔). ⁎ *Biomarker and measurable variable;* ▱ *Clinical pictures and sequelae;* ⁎ *Tissue factors and radical status; CAD, coronary artery disease; ACS, acute coronary syndrome; AMI, acute myocardial infarction; TIA, transitory ischemic attack; AD, Alzheimer dementia; ROS, radical oxygen species; MIF, macrophage migration inhibiting factor; TF, tissue factor.*

Recapitulating, it can be said that all markers discussed here are interlocked with each other. ROS status as well as inflammation and plaque stability are factors which must not be considered separately. The markers selected are therefore suited to provide a comprehensive risk profile for the prevention of atherosclerosis.

As mentioned, the present communication elucidates results from a clinical trial that confirmed the discovery of a further pleiotropic effect of Ginkgo biloba. This trial found that Ginkgo biloba is able to intervene in the process of plaque formation at the very earliest stages in atherogenesis before any cellular reactions have taken place (Fig. 2). Nanoplaque build-up and estimation of its size was pursued with ellipsometric techniques using an established molecular model for atherosclerosis,[60] which was tested in a nanotechnologic biosensor application with the lipid fractions of Ginkgo-treated metabolic syndrome patients. Since the initial lipid deposition steps in atherogenesis are surface-related phenomena at endothelial cells and vascular matrices, we carried out this investigation on the adsorption of lipoproteins in order to learn more about their interfacial behaviour. Hydrophobic silica surfaces were modified through adsorption of heparan sulfate proteoglycan (HS-PG), the latter substrate both mimicking the surface receptors exposed to lipoproteins in the bloodstream or on their paracellular pathway.[58,61] In order to obtain information of some biological relevance, an important aspect of the present investigation was to perform these experiments at close to *in vivo* conditions. In the present study, the results of a long-term intervention of Ginkgo, independent of any change in lipid concentrations, into atherosclerotic nanoplaque build-up using the plasma of eleven patients with early stage metabolic syndrome are discussed and mechanistically interpreted.

RESULTS AND DISCUSSION
Ginkgo Extract Reduces Nanoplaque Formation

In our atherosclerosis model, a hydrophobic methylated silica surface is coated by a monomolecular layer of isolated proteoheparan sulfate depositing through its transmembrane hydrophobic core domain (patent EP 0 946 876).[60] The glycosaminoglycan (GAG) side chains are stretched out into the blood substitute solution because of their negative fixed charges giving rise to electrostatic repulsion.[36,61,62] Lipoprotein particles or cations may interact with the GAG chains, because of their positive amino acid residues or simply their positive charges. Thus, the situation reflects physiological conditions, since, for example, in the endothelial cell membrane, the scenario differs only in one respect, that the short hydrophilic intracellular core domain is located in the cell interior. In this sense, the hydrophobic silica surface simulates the cell membrane overlaid with the glycocalyx quite perfectly.

Problem Formulation

- Is it possible in patients with early stage metabolic syndrome to reduce atherosclerotic nanoplaque formation with the special Ginkgo extract EGb 761?

- Is there a change in the preventive sense of SOD, GPx, oxLDL/LDL, TNFα, TGFβ_1, IL-6, Lp(a), cAMP, cGMP, and 8-*iso*-PGF$_{2\alpha}$ after a 2-month treatment with EGb 761?

- What are the underlying mechanisms?

Figure 3. Problem formulation.

With the present study we wanted to evaluate the applicability of the molecular model for nanoplaque formation in the clinical situation (Fig. 3). Thus a clinical trial investigating the effectiveness of Ginkgo extract on lipoprotein subfractions in patients with metabolic syndrome was instigated. The blood of the patients was taken before and after 2 months therapy with 2 x 120 mg Ginkgo daily (Fig. 4), and the *in vivo* concentration of the VLDL/IDL/LDL-fraction applied in our assay.[4,10] The atherosclerotic nanoplaque as represented by the ternary complex of the HS-PG receptor, lipoprotein particles, and calcium ions, was then pursued by increasing the Ca^{2+} concentration (Fig. 5). This ternary aggregational formation on endothelial cell membranes and vascular matrices may mimic the atherosclerotic "primary lesion" by causing endothelial dysfunction,[14] the very earliest stage of atherogenesis on a molecular level before any cellular reactivity.[59]

Study design

- **n = 11 Patients**
  Patients with an early stage metabolic syndrome

- **Therapy**
  2 x 120 mg special Gingko extract EGb 761 over 2 months
  No statins, no calcium antagonists, no nitrate compounds

- **Experimental Parameters**
  Nanoplaque formation and size (ellipsometry)
  Changes in blood lipid concentrations
  Activity of ROS scavenging enzymes and its consequences
  Concentration of vasoactive substances (cAMP, cGMP, 8-*iso*-PGF$_{2\alpha}$, $[Ca^{2+}]_o$)
  Concentration of biomarkers for oxidative stress, inflammatory status and plaque stability

Figure 4. Study design.

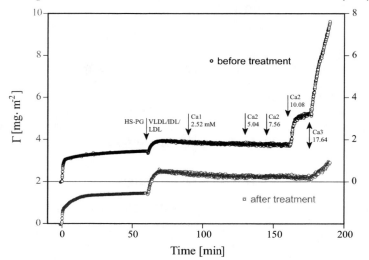

Figure 5. Total adsorbed amount versus time. At time zero, HS-PG (0.1 mg/mL) was adsorbed on hydrophobic silica from a Ca^{2+}-free Krebs solution. The first arrow indicates the addition of the plasma VLDL/IDL/LDL fraction at its in vivo concentration from a metabolic syndrome patient either untreated (o, black curve) or after 2 months treatment with daily 2 × 120 mg Ginkgo biloba extract (o, red curve). Total Ca^{2+} concentrations in solution are indicated at the arrows. The thick, solid lines were computed by an iterative parameter fit of the nonlinear allosteric-cooperative, simple saturative or exponential kinetics to the experimental points using an algorithm for least-squares estimates. The pH was 7.38 (o) and 7.20 (o), respectively.

Although there was no change in bulk lipid concentrations after Ginkgo medication, it is demonstrated in Figure 5 how nanoplaque generation can be reduced. The lipid docking mechanism to HS-PG changed after drug treatment, and the figure shows how the first gradual and then steep increase in nanoplaque formation was largely blocked by treatment with Ginkgo. Since nanoplaque formation is a Ca^{2+} driven process, a complete Ca^{2+} titration curve was measured. As one can easily see, the stepwise increase in adsorbed amount (nanoplaque build-up) upon Ca^{2+} additions of 10.08 and 17.64 mmol/L in the baseline measurement is strongly reduced after Ginkgo treatment. Calculating the percent reduction in nanoplaque formation and size at each Ca^{2+} concentration used, the mean value of all experimental points during the Ca^{2+} period in question was related to the mean value of all experimental points during the VLDL/IDL/LDL binding period ($[Ca^{2+}]$ = 0 mmol/L). The respective quotient for each Ca^{2+} period in the control curves was set to 100%.[59]

Moreover, Fig. 6 shows that beyond nanoplaque formation and deposition (A) also its dimensional build-up (B) is a Ca^{2+} driven process. Adsorbed layer thickness which is related to the molecular size of the ternary aggregational complexes did not markedly increase upon Ca1 addition, but prominently increased upon Ca2 additions, in complete accordance with former experiments in the absence of proteoglycan coating of the silica surface[62] and with light scattering experiments,[37] where the adsorbed amount and particle size, respectively, increased significantly with Ca2 incubation. The augmentation in adsorbed layer thickness with increasing Ca^{2+} concentration took a distinctly reduced course after 2 months of therapy as compared to the control curve. This applies particularly to Ca^{2+} concentrations up to 17.64 mmol/L.

These investigations with the atherogenic apoB100 lipoprotein fraction from 11 patients with metabolic syndrome emphasized that long-term treatment with Ginkgo can partly prevent both the formation and the size development of ternary nanoplaques, even at high Ca^{2+} concentrations. Figure 7 illustrates the extent of inhibition. There arose a similar curve profile for both the reduction in adsorbed amount and in adsorbed layer thickness of ternary nanoplaques dependent on the Ca^{2+} concentration used. The degree of inhibition varied between 14.3 and 54.1% for nanoplaque formation. Similar, but more prominent results were found for the reduction in nanoplaque size ranging between 23.4 and

71.1%. Thus, the special Ginkgo extract EGb 761 effectively diminished both atherosclerotic nanoplaque formation in metabolic syndrome patients and reduced nanoplaque size.

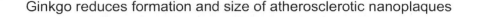

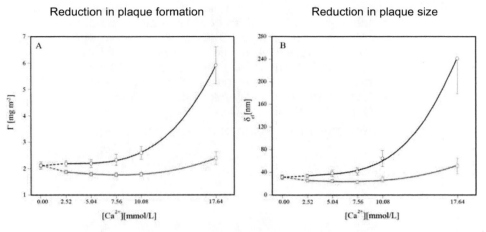

Figure 6. Total adsorbed amount (A) and adsorbed layer thickness (B) as derived from experiments as shown in Fig. 5, dependent on the Ca^{2+} concentration of the Krebs solutions. Adsorbed amounts and layer thicknesses were normalized to a common mean value of the VLDL/IDL/LDL incubation periods (zero Ca^{2+} concentration). Symbols as indicated in Fig. 5 (o,o) reflect the mean values of all experimental points during the Ca^{2+} period in question, averaged for 11 patients (A: $p < 0.0077, 0.0010, 0.0192, 0.0052, 0.0005$ for increasing Ca^{2+} concentrations; B: $p < 0.0004, 0.0188, 0.0149, 0.0181, 0.0138$ for increasing Ca^{2+} concentrations).

Ginkgo reduces formation and size of atherosclerotic nanoplaques

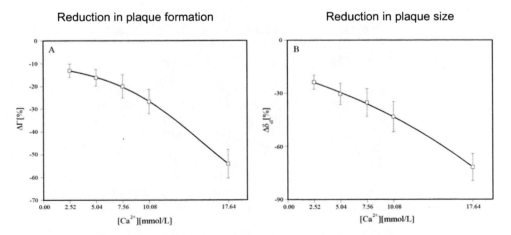

Figure 7. Reduction in Ca^{2+}-induced changes in adsorbed amount (A) and layer thickness (B) as derived from the curves in Fig. 6. The reductions upon application of the VLDL/IDL/LDL fractions taken from 11 patients treated with 2 × 120 mg/d Ginkgo biloba for a 2-month intake were calculated as a ratio to the control values of the untreated patients.

Mechanisms of Nanoplaque Reduction

Unlike statins, Ginkgo is neither an HMG-CoA reductase inhibitor nor a lipid-lowering drug. Therefore, it is not surprising that no correlations are seen between nanoplaque reduction on the one hand, and variations in the lipid fractions VLDL, IDL, and LDL applied in the experiment on the other hand. This result was to be expected. Since Ginkgo has been well known for a long time as an oxygen free radical scavenging substance with high antioxidative capacity[21, 25,64] as well as a potent vasodilator,[16, 29, 50] we determined superoxide dismutase (SOD) and glutathione peroxidase (GPx) activity, oxLDL/LDL ratio and cyclic nucleotide concentrations of cAMP and cGMP in the blood of the patients. In Fig. 8, the results for both the SOD and GPx activities and oxLDL/LDL ratios before and after a 2-month Ginkgo treatment are summarized. While the oxLDL/LDL quotient was reduced by 21.0% (p < 0.002), the SOD activity increased by 19.6% (p < 0.0785) and the GPx activity by 11.6% (p < 0.001) on average. Obviously, the reactive oxygen species (ROS) scavenging properties of Ginkgo diminished the share of oxidized LDL in total LDL cholesterol and in this way relieved cytosolic SOD and GPx of the free radical burden. Alternatively, a direct stimulation of SOD by Ginkgo has been described.[8, 44]

Mechanisms of action of the Ginkgo extract

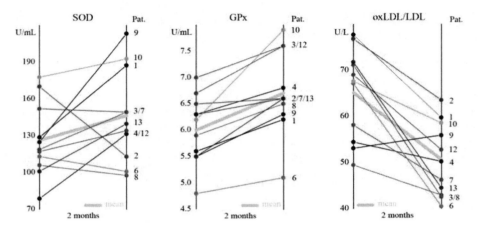

The Ginkgo special extract enhances the activity of free oxygen radical (e.g. O_2^-) scavenging enzymes and reduces the harmful oxidation of LDL-cholesterol.

Figure 8. Superoxide dismutase (SOD) and glutathione peroxidase (GPx) activity and oxLDL/LDL ratios in the blood of 11 metabolic syndrome patients before and after 2-months of Ginkgo therapy. Mean time courses are given by the thick grey lines.

As a powerful antioxidant, Ginkgo diminishes oxidative stress by its high content in flavonoid constituents.[7,33,49,74,79] These phenylbenzopyrones are free radical scavengers and thus decrease ROS.[45] Superoxide anion radicals generated in the respiratory chain and the uric acid cycle are dismuted by SOD to hydrogen peroxide, and one step further, by catalase and GPx to water and oxygen. Under physiological conditions, the conjugation of catalase to SOD ensures that as soon as a superoxide dismutation reaction occurs, the resultant H_2O_2 is removed by the immediate proximity of the catalase molecule.[39] Thus, catalase conjugated to SOD, and additionally the redox function of glutathione, minimize the conversion of hydrogen peroxide to hydroxyl radicals by the Fenton reaction. These highly aggressive and toxic hydroxyl radicals can attack lipids, proteins or DNA to acquire the missing electron (Fig. 9).

SOD and GPx upregulation reduces lipid/protein peroxidation

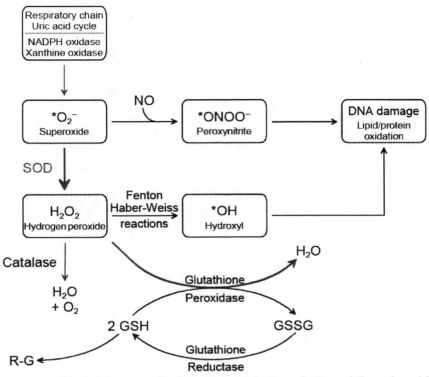

Figure 9. Production of free oxygen radicals in the respiratory chain and the uric acid cycle and their elimination and detoxification by superoxide dismutase (SOD), catalase and glutathione peroxidase. The SOD and GPx upregulation by Ginkgo extract attenuates the lipid/protein oxidation.

We have seen that the conversion of H_2O_2 to H_2O and O_2 is multiply safeguarded and normally not the rate limiting step. Under Ginkgo therapy, the SOD and GPx activities were upregulated, either because these enzymes were relieved through the radical scavenging properties of Ginkgo or directly stimulated by Ginkgo. Since in four patients the SOD activity was down-regulated (borderline significance for the average upregulation), one can speculate that the SOD could not cope with the burst of free oxygen radicals in these patients. This job, however, was completed by the following GPx, the activity of which increased in all patients (high significance for the average upregulation). In any case, the reaction

$^*O_2^- \rightarrow H_2O_2$ is strongly promoted, and the conversion under NO inward transfer from $^*O_2^- \rightarrow {}^*ONOO^-$ (peroxynitrite radical) largely ceases. Since catalase and glutathione peroxidase produce H_2O and O_2 from hydrogen peroxide, the $^*OH$ hydroxyl radical production is minimized. This effect is reflected by a decrease in the oxLDL/LDL ratio; the share of oxLDL generated through lipid peroxidation, in total LDL is diminished. This presumption is substantiated by the proof of a direct linear correlation between SOD, GPx and oxLDL/LDL.

There are several theories as to how oxLDL is created *in vivo*. In the blood plasma, there are many antioxidants, thus it is unlikely that an extended oxidation of LDL particles could take place. Moreover, endothelial cells of liver sinusoids and Kupffer cells, which are copiously occupied by scavenger receptors,[68] would immediately remove modified LDL from the circulation. Most probably, the oxidation occurs in the vascular wall itself, where microdomains – small spaces largely devoid of antioxidants – could develop.[76] There are also cells in the vascular wall that are able to cause an oxidation. Henriksen *et al* showed in 1981 that cultured endothelial cells can modify LDL,[24] and in the following years various working groups detected that smooth muscle cells and monocytes/macrophages can generate similar changes.[68] Finally, oxLDL promotes the build-up and progression of plaques.[51,52] The reduction of the oxLDL/LDL quotient observed under Ginkgo treatment is extremely important, because oxLDL leads preferably to the formation of unstable plaques via the induction of apoptosis.[18]

An increased LDL and Lp(a), arterial hypertension, diabetes mellitus, smoking, and lowered HDL, as well as genetic factors, are considered as the most essential risk factors in atherogenesis.[12,77] Analyzing the LDL subfractions in detail, we could confirm the pleiotropic Ginkgo effect of a marked Lp(a)-lowering, which we had unexpectedly detected in the first Ginkgo study in cardiovascular high-risk patients.[50] The Lp(a) concentration, which is known as a potent atherothrombotic risk factor,[34] was decreased by 26.3% (p < 0.001) falling from 50.8 to 39.5 mg/dL (p < 0.0005) (Fig. 10). Practically, Lp(a) cannot be influenced therapeutically.[53] The Lp(a) level is determined genetically to about 74%.[34,56] But this parameter, independent of the other lipid values, has an effect on the oxLDL level and vice versa. After a percutaneous intervention in the coronary arteries, both the oxLDL and Lp(a) concentration rose steeply for a few hours.[72] Also, with the intake of a low-fat, low/high-vegetable diet, oxLDL and Lp(a) changed concertedly.[65] The influence of Lp(a) on oxLDL is specially interesting, because Lp(a) showed no correlations to the other lipid parameters.[13] Thus, it should be realized that an outstanding correlation between circulating oxLDL and Lp(a) has been proven.[65] We found a statistically significant linear correlation between oxLDL/LDL and Lp(a) (r = -0.84; p < 0.0176).[55] A similar result was obtained by Witztum and coworkers:[72] oxLDL and Lp(a) are correlated to each other. The authors point out that in settings of enhanced oxidative stress and chronically elevated Lp(a) levels, the atherogenicity of Lp(a) may stem from its capacity as a carrier of proinflammatory oxidation byproducts. Only two patients of our clinical trial had a normal Lp(a) concentration of 5.3 and 22.5 mg/dL, whereas all other patients had highly pathobiochemic levels ranging from 31.2 to 83.1 mg/dL.

Mechanism of action of the Ginkgo extract

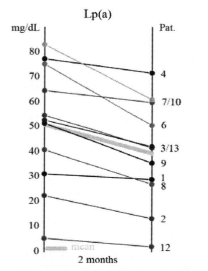

Ginkgo reduces lipoprotein(a) concentration, an important risk factor of atherothrombosis.

Figure 10. Lipoprotein(a) [Lp(a)] plasma concentrations in 11 patients with metabolic syndrome before and after a 2-month Ginkgo therapy. Mean time course is given by the thick grey line.

It is highly significant that Lp(a) lowering under Ginkgo therapy occurred not only in the patients with pathologically high Lp(a) concentrations but also in the two patients with normal values by on average 50.2%, that is much more than the medium reduction in all eleven patients. Although the plasma Lp(a) concentration is bound genetically, it is regulated via such mechanisms. As outlined, the decrease in Lp(a) was linearly correlated to the reduction in oxLDL/LDL by 21.0 ± 4.3% (p < 0.002) and IL-6 by 12.9 ± 7.0% (p < 0.0407) as well as an in-crease in TNFα by 68.5 ± 30.2% (p < 0.0076) and TGFβ$_1$ by 38.4 ± 11.8% (p < 0.0068) in the lower physiologic regulatory range.[46, 54] Therefore, the rise in TNFα and TGFβ$_1$ is not at all indicative of increasing inflammation as supported by the simultaneous decrease in IL-6.[46,78] Thus, the reduction in Lp(a) correlates with decreases in oxLDL/LDL[55,72] and IL-6[32] as well as with increases in TNFα and TGFβ$_1$.[46] Since the variation in plasma Lp(a) concentration is accounted for by inherited sequences within or closely linked to the apo(a) gene[34] and this gene has IL-6 responsive elements within its sequence,[46] a lowering of Lp(a) is explainable via down-regulation of IL-6.[55]

Blood Concentration of Vasoactive Substances

The results of the cyclic adenosine monophosphate (cAMP) and cyclic guanosine monophosphate (cGMP) measurements are depicted in Table 1. On average, the increase in cAMP amounted to $43.5 \pm 12.0\%$ ($p < 0.001$) rising from 40.3 ± 3.8 nmol/L to 54.5 ± 3.4 nmol/L ($p < 0.0002$). The augmentation of the cGMP concentration by $32.9 \pm 10.4\%$ ($p < 0.001$) was less pronounced compared to cAMP. The mean concentration increased from 8.5 ± 0.5 nmol/L to 10.9 ± 0.5 nmol/L ($p < 0.0016$). Both cyclic nucleotides are common regulators of ion channels and potent dilators of smooth muscle tissues.

Numerous clinical studies proved that Ginkgo extract has a marked vasodilating effect by improving the endothelium and smooth muscle function.[16,29,50] In pharmacologic investigations, a significant increase in smooth muscle cGMP concentration was measured, which can be explained by a stimulation of NO release from vascular endothelial cells.[28,29,48] After a 2-month EGb 761-intake we found the concentration of cAMP elevated by 43.5% and of cGMP by 32.9%, respectively. These enhancements even exceed the results of a Ginkgo therapy in cardiovascular high-risk patients.[50,63] They emphasize the membrane diffusibility for cyclic nucleotides,[6,9] which are even transported in the kidney.[1] This means that the strong rise in cyclic nucleotide concentrations in the blood of the patients reflects a similar augmentation within the cells. Such Ginkgo induced increases in cAMP and cGMP concentration could function both abluminally (providing vasodilatation) and luminally (reducing platelet aggregation, and platelet and leukocyte adhesion to vascular endothelial cells) to improve blood flow and tissue perfusion. Furthermore, the protection of NO against free radical attack (inhibition of peroxynitrite formation) can be added to the list of vasomotor actions of Ginkgo. Thus, the increase in cAMP and cGMP causes vasorelaxation, a beneficial effect in the metabolic syndrome patients, to remove their endothelial dysfunction.[14] Again, the cAMP increase was quite surprising for us. We assume that cAMP is augmented because in blood vessels, the NO release is generally combined with a corelease of PGI2. The latter would then increase the cAMP concentration.

As a biomarker of oxidative stress and a direct link between oxidative stress and in-flammation,[55] the isoprostane 8-*iso*-$PGF_{2\alpha}$ acts additionally as a potent vasoconstrictor and promoter of platelet aggregation, thus strongly supporting atherogenesis. Table 1 shows that Ginkgo treatment led to a reduction of the 8-*iso*-$PGF_{2\alpha}$ blood concentration by $24.5 \pm 14.5\%$ ($p < 0.084$) from 24.9 ± 4.6 nmol/L to 15.0 ± 2.0 nmol/L ($p < 0.0027$). This fall in vasoconstrictor 8-*iso*-$PGF_{2\alpha}$ significantly furthers cAMP/cGMP-induced vasodilatation. Moreover, this effect is supplementarily strengthened by changes in the serum Ca^{2+} concentration. Surprisingly, we found a lowering of the serum Ca^{2+} concentration by $5.4 \pm 1.6\%$ ($p < 0.0076$) from 2.37 ± 0.03 to 2.24 ± 0.04 mmol/L ($p < 0.0069$). Apart from an additional vasodilatory effect, the lowered extracellular Ca^{2+} concentration affects nanoplaque formation and size restrictively, since this is a Ca^{2+}-driven process directly proportional to the external Ca^{2+} concentration. Therefore, this modest decrease of $[Ca^{2+}]_o$ in the physiological range consequently impairs nanoplaque formation. As to a mechanistic explanation, we can only speculate at the moment. Because vascular tension is generally diminished through the vasorelaxing influences described above, the intracellular Ca^{2+} concentration in the vascular smooth muscle cells is very low on an average. In order to prevent the transmembrane Ca^{2+} gradient to become too significant, the kidneys seem to lower the blood Ca^{2+} concentration slightly. The question could be further clarified through intracellular recordings of the vascular smooth muscle membrane potential and measurements of the Ca^{2+} channel open probability.

Patient	cAMP [nmol/L]			cGMP [nmol/L]			8-iso-PGF$_{2\alpha}$ [nmol/L]			[Ca^{2+}]$_o$ [mmol/L]		
	before	after	change [%]	before	after	change [%]	before	after	change [%]	before	after	change [%]
1	17.8	43.7	+145.4	5.1	11.4	+123.3	30.2	28.4	-5.9	2.50	2.39	-4.4
2	33.5	57.2	+70.9	7.8	8.9	+14.5	29.4	14.5	-50.8	2.39	2.39	0.0
3	36.1	38.6	+7.1	8.1	9.6	+18.7	15.2	11.9	-21.6	2.33	2.27	-2.6
4	29.6	46.2	+56.3	8.1	10.4	+27.9	19.7	16.3	-17.3	2.25	2.27	+1.1
6	31.7	41.9	+32.2	10.4	12.0	+15.8	10.8	10.3	-5.0	2.39	2.36	-1.3
7	55.3	69.2	+25.2	9.6	12.9	+35.2	14.8	12.5	-15.7	2.42	2.17	-10.3
8	61.7	62.8	+1.9	9.9	12.1	+22.4	22.8	9.4	-59.0	2.43	2.09	-14.0
9	42.4	48.3	+14.0	7.6	9.9	+30.6	32.8	8.0	-75.5	2.27	2.13	-6.2
10	42.8	66.0	+54.2	7.8	12.9	+65.7	60.2	15.2	-74.7	2.57	2.25	-12.5
12	41.8	57.2	+36.7	11.0	11.1	+0.8	(68.8)			2.28	2.25	-1.3
13	50.8	68.4	+34.6	8.0	8.6	+7.6	12.9	23.4	+80.9	2.23	2.05	-8.1
Mean (11)	40.3	54.5	+43.5	8.5	10.9	+32.9	24.9	15.0	-24.5	2.37	2.24	-5.4
± SEM	3.8	3.4	12.0	0.5	0.5	10.4	4.6	2.0	14.5	0.03	0.04	1.6
Median			+34.6			+22.4			-19.5			-4.4
p	<0.0002		<0.001	<0.0016		<0.001	<0.0027*		<0.084	<0.0069		<0.0076

*Exact Wilcoxon signed-rank test

Table 1. cAMP, cGMP, 8-iso-PGF$_{2\alpha}$ and [Ca^{2+}]$_o$ blood concentrations in 11 patients with metabolic syndrome before and after 2-months of Ginkgo therapy.

Mechanisms of Nanoplaque Reduction

Because a 2-month intake of Ginkgo extract significantly reduced both the oxLDL/LDL ratio and the Lp(a) concentration and increased the cGMP concentration in the blood of the patients, we strived to unveil a potential relationship between these changes and the nanoplaque changes, and to disclose a mechanistic explanation for the latter. We found that the decrease in nanoplaque formation is correlated not only to changes in the oxLDL/LDL quotient but also to the Lp(a) concentration before treatment. Lowering in nanoplaque build-up is large in case of a strong reduction of the oxLDL/LDL ratio and a high concentration of Lp(a) before therapy.[50] Finally, a multiple correlation between nanoplaque reduction and the three risk factors high oxLDL/LDL, high Lp(a) and low cGMP reveals an estimate of their relative contribution to changes in nanoplaque formation (Fig. 11). In normal blood Ca^{2+} concentration of 2.52 mmol/L, reductions of oxLDL/LDL are to 34.7%, of Lp(a) to 43.3%, and of cGMP to 22.0% instrumental in nanoplaque diminution.

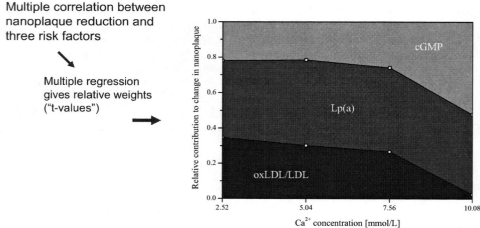

Figure 11. Relative contribution of the three risk factors oxLDL/LDL, Lp(a) and cGMP to changes in nanoplaque formation in dependence on the Ca^{2+} concentration. Performing multiple correlations over all Ca^{2+} concentrations by combining all three risk factors yields partly significant results and a trend of relative contributions (t-values) with consistent image.

Under mechanistic aspects it is therefore clear, that the reduction of the atherogenic risk factors oxLDL/LDL and Lp(a) mutually correlated to each other, had quite a predominating influence (78%) on nanoplaque reduction in normal Ca^{2+} blood substitute solution (Fig. 11). The multiple regression also demonstrates that in high Ca^{2+} concentrations the share in nanoplaque reduction is strongly shifted to the side of the blood cGMP and Lp(a) concentration (97.8%). This means that vascular and fatty effects share their influence on nanoplaque reduction equally. The Ca^{2+} concentration range applied in our experiments is justified, because counterion condensation of calcium up to a concentration of 25 mmol/L can appear in the immediate vicinity of the proteoglycan receptors with their highly negative charge density.[38] Also in the immediate proximity of the fully blown plaque, the extracellular Ca^{2+} concentration is so high that Ca^{2+} ions finally precipitate within the plaque after exceeding their solubility product.

Curative Effects of Ginkgo biloba

With respect to the numerous preventive Ginkgo effects described, it came to our mind to find out whether some of the inclusion criteria according to Fig. 1 were eventually not any longer fulfilled in the individual patients after the 2-month therapy, i.e. the pathological values returned to normal. Table 2 shows the result of the evaluations. Of the five pathologically changed inclusion criteria, one criterion each was normalized in four of the eleven patients, in one patient even two criteria. This obviously points to a curative effect of the Ginkgo therapy beyond all preventive measures. This success was not to be expected, however, it fully confirms the results of our Ginkgo study in cardiovascular high-risk patients.[50,55,63] It is important to note that the patients had not given up smoking during the therapy, did not lose weight (rather an increase) and were not provided with a special diet or physical exercises.

Reversal of risk factors in early stage metabolic syndrome patients

Patient	BP	TG	HDL-C	BMI/WC	Lp(a)
1	●		●	●	● ●
2		● ●	●	●	
3			●	●	●
4	●	●	● ●	●	●
6				●	●
7	●		●	●	●
8			●	● ●	● ●
9			●	●	●
10		●	●		●
12		●	●	●	●
13	● ●		●	●	●

Table 2. Reversal of risk factors in early stage metabolic syndrome patients. Black closed circles (●) indicate criteria for metabolic syndrome fulfilled in patients before Ginkgo medication, red closed circles (●) criteria no longer fulfilled in the same patients after 2-month Ginkgo treatment. In patient 8, WC was borderline positive before and borderline negative after Ginkgo medication. BP, blood pressure; TG, triglyceride concentration; HDL-C, high-density lipoprotein cholesterol; BMI, body mass index; WC, waist circumference; Lp(a), lipoprotein(a) concentration.

CONCLUDING REMARKS

According to these results and explanations, it is evident to compare the effects of the Ginkgo extract with those of statins.[63] Although, for example, the nanoplaque reduction can amount to 45-50% after a single dose application of fluvastatin without any lipid lowering[59] and is thus considerably stronger than Ginkgo, however both fluvastatin and other statin drugs are associated with a significantly higher risk of and wider spectrum of adverse side-effects.

In conclusion, even though this is a pilot study, we could measure remarkable effects in these early stage metabolic syndrome patients after 2-months of treatment with Ginkgo biloba (EGb 761) medication: atherosclerotic nanoplaque formation and size were diminished; the special extract did not change blood bulk lipid composition; the anti-atherosclerotic effect is due to an upregulation in the body's own radical scavenging enzymes and an attenuation of the risk factors oxLDL/LDL and Lp(a); Ginkgo strongly increased the concentration of the vasodilating nucleotides cAMP and cGMP thus removing endothelial dysfunction. Of course, further clinical studies are needed to corroborate these findings.

REFERENCES

1. Ahloulay M, Déchaux M, Laborde K, Bankir L. Influence of glucagon on GFR and on urea and electrolyte excretion: direct and indirect effects. *Am J Physiol.* 1995;269:F225-F235.
2. Alberti KGMM, Zimmet PZ. Definition, diagnosis and classification of diabetes mellitus and its complications. Part 1: diagnosis and classification of diabetes mellitus. Provisional report of a WHO consultation. *Diabet Med.* 1998;15:539-553.
3. Alberti KGMM, Zimmet P, Shaw J, for the IDF Epidemiology Task Force Consensus Group. The metabolic syndrome – a new worldwide definition. *Lancet.* 2005;366:1059-1062.
4. Anber V, Millar JS, McConnell M, Shepherd J, Packard CJ. Interaction of very-low-density, intermediate-density, and low-density lipoproteins with human arterial wall proteoglycans. *Arterioscler Thromb Vasc Biol.* 1997;17: 2507-2514.
5. Arad Y, Goodman KJ, Roth M, Newstein D, Guerci AD. Coronary calcification, coronary disease risk factors, C-reactive protein, and atherosclerotic cardiovascular disease events: the St. Francis Heart Study. *J Am Coll Cardiol.* 2005;46:158-165.
6. Baumann R, Blass C, Gotz R, Dragon S. Ontogeny of catecholamine and adenosine receptor-mediated cAMP signaling of embryonic red blood cells: role of cGMP-inhibited phosphodiesterase 3 and hemoglobin. *Blood.* 1999; 94:4314-4320.
7. Bonorden WR, Pariza MW. Antioxidant nutrients and protection from free radicals. *Nutr Toxicol.* 1994;2:19-47.
8. Bridi R, Crossetti FP, Steffen VM, Henriques AT. The antioxidant activity of standardized extract of *Ginkgo biloba* (EGb 761) in rats. *Phytother Res.* 2001;15:449-451.
9. Broadus AE, Northcutt RC, Hardman JG, Sutherland EW, Liddle GW. Effects of glucagon on adenosine 3'-5'-monophosphate and guanosine 3'-5'-monophosphate in human plasma and urine. *J Clin Invest.* 1970;49:2237-2245.
10. Camejo G, Hurt-Camejo E, Wiklund O, Bondjers G. Association of apo B lipoproteins with arterial proteoglycans: Pathological significance and molecular basis. *Atherosclerosis.* 1998;139:205-222.
11. Cook S, Weitzman M, Auinger P, Nguyen M, Dietz WH. Prevalence of a metabolic syndrome phenotype in adolescents. Findings from the third National Health and Nutrition Examination Survey, 1988-1994. *Arch Pediatr Adolesc Med.* 2003;157:821-827.
12. Danesh J, Collins R, Peto R. Lipoprotein(a) and coronary heart disease: meta-analysis of prospective studies. *Circulation.* 2000;102:1082-1085.
13. Dangas G, Ambrose J, D'Agate D, Shao J, Chockalingham S, Levine D, Smith D. Correlation of serum lipoprotein(a) with the angiographic and clinical presentation of coronary artery disease. *Am J Cardiol.* 1999;83: 583-585.
14. Davignon J, Ganz P. Role of endothelial dysfunction in atherosclerosis. *Circulation.* 2004;109:III-27-III-32.
15. Davis PH, Dawson JD, Riley WA, Lauer RM. Carotid intimal-medial thickness is related to cardiovascular risk factors measured from childhood through middle age: The Muscatine Study. *Circulation.* 2001;104:2815-2819.

16. Delaflotte S, Auguet M, DeFeudis FV, Baranes J, Clostre F, Drieu K, Braquet P. Endothelium-dependent relaxation of rabbit isolated aorta produced by carbachol and by Ginkgo biloba extract. *Biomed Biochim Acta*. 1984;43:212-216.

17. Ford ES. Prevalence of the metabolic syndrome defined by the International Diabetes Federation among adults in the U.S. *Diabetes Care*. 2005;28:2745-2749.

18. Glass CK, Witztum JL. Atherosclerosis: The road ahead. *Cell*. 2001;104: 503-516.

19. Grundy SM, Becker D, Clark LT, Cooper RS, Denke MA, Howard WJ, Hunninghake DB, Illingworth DR, Luepker RV, McBride P, McKenney JM, Pasternak RC, Stone NJ, Van Horn L. Executive summary of the third report of the National Cholesterol Education Pro-gram (NCEP) expert panel on detection, evaluation, and treatment of high blood cholesterol in adults (Adult Treatment Panel III). *JAMA*. 2001;285:2486-2497.

20. Grundy SM, Cleeman JI, Daniels SR, Donato KA, Eckel RH, Franklin BA, Gordon DJ, Krauss RM, Savage PJ, Smith Jr SC, Spertus JA, Costa F. Diagnosis and management of the metabolic syndrome. An American Heart Association/National Heart, Lung, and Blood Institute Scientific Statement. *Circulation*. 2005;112:2735-2752.

21. Halliwell B. How to characterize a biological antioxidant. *Free Rad Res Commun*. 1990;9:1-32.

22. Hanefeld M, Leonhardt W. Das metabolische Syndrom. *Dtsch Gesundheitswesen*. 1981;36:545-551.

23. Hanefeld M, Metzler W, Köhler C, Schaper F. Das metabolische Syndrom: „common soil" für Diabetes und Atherosklerose. *Herz*. 2006;31:246-254.

24. Henriksen T, Mahoney E, Steinberg D. Enhanced macrophage degradation of low density lipoprotein previously incubated with cultured endothelial cells: Recognition by receptors for acetylated low density lipoprotein. *Proc Natl Acad Sci USA*. 1981;78:6499-6503.

25. Ilieva I, Ohgami K, Shiratori K, Koyama Y, Yoshida K, Kase S, Kitamei H, Takemoto Y, Yazawa K, Ohno S. The effects of Ginkgo biloba extract on lipopolysaccharide-induced inflammation in vitro and in vivo. *Exp Eye Res*. 2004;79:181-187.

26. Kameda K, Matsunaga T, Abe N, Hanada H, Ishizaka H, Ono H, Saitoh M, Fukui K, Fu-kuda I, Osanai T, Okumura K. Correlation of oxidative stress with activity of matrix metal-loproteinase in patients with coronary artery disease. Possible role for left ventricular re-modelling. *Eur Heart J*. 2003;24:2180-2185.

27. Klebanoff SJ. Myeloperoxidase: friend and foe. *J Leukoc Biol*. 2005;77:598-625.

28. Koch E, Chatterjee SS. Experimentelle Grundlagen für die therapeutische Anwendung von Ginkgoextrakt EGb 761. *Hämostaseologie*. 1993;13:11-27.

29. Koltermann A, Hartkorn A, Koch E, Fürst R, Vollmar AM, Zahler S. *Ginkgo biloba* extract EGb® 761 increases endothelial nitric oxide production *in vitro* and *in vivo*. *Cell Mol Life Sci*. 2007;64:1715-1722.

30. Kong Y-Z, Yu X, Tang J-J, Ouyang X, Huang X-R, Fingerle-Rowson G, Bacher M, Scher LA, Bucala R, Lan HY. Macrophage migration inhibitory factor induces MMP-9 expression: implications for destabilization of human atherosclerotic plaques. *Atherosclerosis*. 2005;178:207-215.

31. Lakka HM, Laaksonen DE, Lakka TA, Niskanen LK, Kumpusalo E, Tuomilehto J, Salonen JT. The metabolic syndrome and total and cardiovascular disease mortality in middle-aged men. *JAMA*. 2002;288:2709-2716.

32. Lippi G, Targher G, Guidi GC. Ginkgo biloba, inflammation and lipoprotein(a). *Atherosclerosis*. 2007;195:417-418.

33. Lotito SB, Actis-Goretta L, Renart ML, Caligiuri M, Rein D, Schmitz HH, Steinberg FM, Keen CL, Fraga CG. Influence of oligomer chain length on the antioxidant activity of pro-cyanidins. *Biochem Biophys Res Commun*. 2000;276:945-951.

34. Lusis AJ, Fogelman AM, Fonarow GC. Genetic basis of atherosclerosis: Part I: New genes and pathways. *Circulation*. 2004;110:1868-1873.

35. Lusis AJ, Fogelman AM, Fonarow GC. Genetic basis of atherosclerosis: Part II: Clinical implications. *Circulation*. 2004;110:2066-2071.

36. Malmsten M, Claesson P, Siegel G. Forces between proteoheparan sulfate layers adsorbed at hydrophobic surfaces. *Langmuir*. 1994;10:1274-1280.

37. Malmsten M, Siegel G, Wood WG. Ellipsometry studies of lipoprotein adsorption. *J Colloid Interface Sci*. 2000;224:338-346.

38. Manning GS. Limiting laws and counterion condensation in polyelectrolyte solutions. II. Self-diffusion of the small ions. *J Chem Phys*. 1969;51:934-938.

39. Mao GD, Thomas PD, Lopaschuk GD, Poznansky MJ. Superoxide dismutase (SOD)-catalase conjugates. Role of hydrogen peroxide and the Fenton reaction in SOD toxicity. *J Biol Chem.* 1993;268:416-420.

40. Mattsson N, Rönnemaa T, Juonala M, Viikari JSA, Jokinen E, Hutri-Kähönen N, Kähönen M, Laitinen T, Raitakari OT. Arterial structure and function in young adults with the metabolic syndrome: the Cardiovascular Risk in Young Finns Study. *Eur Heart J.* 2008; 29:784-791.

41. Mullen MJ, Kharbanda RK, Cross J, Donald AE, Taylor M, Vallance P, Deanfield JE, MacAllister RJ. Heterogenous nature of flow-mediated dilatation in human conduit arteries in vivo: relevance to endothelial dysfunction in hypercholesterolemia. *Circ Res.* 2001;88:145-151.

42. Ninomiya JK, L'Italien G, Criqui MH, Whyte JL, Gamst A, Chen RS. Association of the metabolic syndrome with history of myocardial infarction and stroke in the Third National Health and Nutrition Examination Survey. *Circulation.* 2004;109:42-46.

43. Nomoto K, Oguchi S, Watanabe I, Kushiro T, Kanmatsuse K. Involvement of inflammation in acute coronary syndromes assessed by levels of high-sensitivity C-reactive protein, matrix metalloproteinase-9 and soluble vascular-cell adhesion molecule-1. *J Cardiol.* 2003;42:201-206.

44. Ozkur MK, Bozkurt MS, Balabanli B, Aricioglu A, Ilter N, Gürer MA, Inalöz HS. The effects of EGb 761 on lipid peroxide levels and superoxide dismutase activity in sunburn. *Photodermatol Photoimmunol Photomed.* 2002;18:117-120.

45. Pryor WA, Houk KN, Foote CS, Fukuto JM, Ignarro LJ, Squadrito GL, Davies KJA. Free radical biology and medicine: it's a gas, man! *Am J Physiol Regul Integr Comp Physiol.* 2006;291:R491-R511.

46. Ramharack A, Barkalow D, Spahr MA. Dominant negative effect of TGF-β1 and TNF-α on basal and IL-6–induced lipoprotein(a) and apolipoprotein(a) mRNA expression in primary monkey hepatocyte cultures. *Arterioscler Thromb Vasc Biol.* 1998;18:984-990.

47. Reaven GM. Banting lecture 1988. Role of insulin resistance in human disease. *Diabetes.* 1988;37:1595-1607.

48. Ren DC, Du G-H, Zhang JT. Protective effect of Ginkgo biloba extract on endothelial cell against damage induced by oxidative stress. *J Cardiovasc Pharmacol.* 2002;40:809-814.

49. Robak J, Gryglewski RJ. Flavonoids are scavengers of superoxide anions. *Biochem Pharmacol.* 1988;37:837-841.

50. Rodríguez M, Ringstad L, Schäfer P, Just S, Hofer HW, Malmsten M, Siegel G. Reduction of atherosclerotic nanoplaque formation and size by *Ginkgo biloba* (EGb 761) in cardiovascular high-risk patients. *Atherosclerosis.* 2007;192:438-444.

51. Ross R. The pathogenesis of atherosclerosis – an update. *N Engl J Med.* 1986;314:488-500.

52. Ross R. The pathogenesis of atherosclerosis: a perspective for the 1990s. *Nature.* 1993;362:801-809.

53. Sasaki S, Kuwahara N, Kunitomo, K, Harada S, Yamada T, Azuma A, Takeda K, Nakagawa M. Effects of atorvastatin on oxidized low-density lipoprotein, low-density lipoprotein subfraction distribution, and remnant lipoprotein in patients with mixed hyperlipoproteinemia. *Am J Cardiol.* 2002;89:386-389.

54. Satoh M, Shimoda Y, Maesawa C, Akatsu T, Ishikawa Y, Minami Y, Hiramori K, Nakamura M. Activated toll-like receptor 4 in monocytes is associated with heart failure after acute myocardial infarction. *Int J Cardiol.* 2006;109:226-234.

55. Schäfer P, Rodríguez M, Siegel G. Atherosclerosis, an inflammatory and fibroproliferative disease. A prophylactic phytochemical approach with *Ginkgo biloba* (EGb 761). *Atherosclerosis.* 2007;195:419-422.

56. Scholz M, Kraft HG, Lingenhel A, Delport R, Vorster E, Bickeböller H, Utermann G. Genetic control of lipoprotein(a) concentrations is different in Africans and Caucasians. *Eur J Hum Genet.* 1999;7:169-178.

57. Scuteri A, Morrell CH, Najjar SS, Lakatta EG. The metabolic syndrome in older individuals: Prevalence and prediction of cardiovascular events. *Diabetes Care.* 2005;28:882-887.

58. Siegel G, Abletshauser C, Malmsten M, Klüßendorf D. The acute effect of fluvastatin on lipoprotein deposition in a model substrate for ellipsometry studies at an endothelial membrane equivalent. *Desalination.* 2002;148: 407-414.

59. Siegel G, Abletshauser C, Malmsten M, Schmidt A, Winkler K. Reduction of arteriosclerotic nanoplaque formation and size by fluvastatin in a receptor-based biosensor model. *Cardiovasc Res.* 2003;58:696-705.
60. Siegel G, Malmsten M. Molecular model for athero/arteriosclerosis, patent EP 0 946 876; 2005.
61. Siegel G, Malmsten M, Klüßendorf D, Leonhardt W. Physicochemical binding properties of the proteoglycan receptor for serum lipoproteins. *Atherosclerosis.* 1999;144:59-67.
62. Siegel G, Malmsten M, Klüßendorf D, Michel F. A receptor-based biosensor for lipoprotein docking at the endothelial surface and vascular matrix. *Biosensors & Bioelectronics.* 2001;16:895-904.
63. Siegel G, Schäfer P, Rodríguez M, Weber T, Malmsten M. New developments in phytochemical nutrition for anti-aging: prevention of atherosclerosis. *Anti-Aging Therap.* 2007;IX:313-333.
64. Sies H. Oxidative stress: oxidants and antioxidants. *Exp Physiol.* 1997;82:291-295.
65. Silaste M-L, Rantala M, Alfthan G, Aro A, Witztum JL, Kesäniemi YA, Hörkkö S. Changes in dietary fat intake alter plasma levels of oxidized low-density lipoprotein and lipoprotein(a). *Arterioscler Thromb Vasc Biol.* 2004; 24:498-503.
66. Smyth S, Heron A. Diabetes and obesity: the twin epidemics. *Nature Med.* 2006;12:75-80.
67. Spagnoli LG, Bonanno E, Sangiorgi G, Mauriello A. Role of inflammation in atherosclerosis. *J Nucl Med.* 2007;48:1800-1815.
68. Steinberg D, Parthasarathy S, Carew T, Khoo J, Witztum J. Beyond cholesterol: modifications of low-density lipoprotein that increase its atherogenicity. *N Engl J Med.* 1989;320:915-924.
69. Stern S. Are we getting nearer to screening for atherosclerosis? *Circulation.* 2008;117:122-126.
70. Taylor AJ, Bindeman J, Feuerstein I, Cao F, Brazaitis M, O'Malley PG. Coronary calcium independently predicts incident premature coronary heart disease over measured cardio-vascular risk factors. Mean three-year outcomes in the Prospective Army Coronary Cal-cium (PACC) project. *J Am Coll Cardiol.* 2005;46:807-814.
71. Thalmann S, Meier CA. Local adipose tissue depots as cardiovascular risk factors. *Car-diovasc Res.* 2007;75:690-701.
72. Tsimikas S, Lau HK, Han K-R, Shortal B, Miller ER, Segev A, Curtiss LK, Witztum JL, Strauss BH. Percutaneous coronary intervention results in acute increases in oxidized phospholipids and lipoprotein(a): Short-term and long-term immunologic responses to oxidized low-density lipoprotein. *Circulation.* 2004;109:3164-3170.
73. Tzou WS, Douglas PS, Srinivasan SR, Bond MG, Tang R, Chen W, Berenson GS, Stein JH. Increased subclinical atherosclerosis in young adults with metabolic syndrome: the Bogalusa Heart Study. *J Am Coll Cardiol.* 2005;46:457-463.
74. van Acker SA, Tromp MN, Haenen GR, van der Vijgh WJ, Bast A. Flavonoids as scavengers of nitric oxide radical. *Biochem Biophys Res Commun.* 1995;214:755-759.
75. Weiss SJ. Tissue destruction by neutrophils. *N Engl J Med.* 1989;320:365-376.
76. Witztum J. The oxidation hypothesis of atherosclerosis. *Lancet.* 1994;344: 793-795.
77. Worthley S, Osende J, Helft G, Badimon J, Fuster V. Coronary artery disease: Pathogenesis and acute coronary syndromes. *Mt Sinai J Med.* 2001;68:167-181.
78. Yudkin JS, Kumari M, Humphries SE, Mohamed-Ali V. Inflammation, obesity, stress and coronary heart disease: is interleukin-6 the link? *Atherosclerosis.* 2000;148:209-214.
79. Zhou Y-H, Yu J-P, Liu Y-F, Teng X-J, Ming M, Lv P, An P, Liu S-Q, Yu H-G. Effects of *Ginkgo biloba* extract on inflammatory mediators (SOD, MDA, TNF-α, NF-κBp65, IL-6) in TNBS-induced colitis in rats. *Mediators Inflamm.* 2006;2006:1-9.

ABOUT THE AUTHOR

Primary author Dr. Günter Siegel is a cardiovascular researcher and Director of the Department of Neurophysiology at the Charité - Universitätsmedizin Berlin, Campus Benjamin Franklin, where he has taught for more than 30 years. In 1961, he commenced his study of physics in Munich. The following year, he began his study of medicine at Ruprecht-Karl University in Heidelberg, from which he was awarded his license to practice medicine and his doctorate of medicine.

Dr. Siegel's fields of research at the Charité involve membrane physiology of cardiovascular tissues, the reaction of blood vessels to a variety of pharmacologically active substances and the development of atherosclerosis.

His most recent research has focused on the role of ginkgo extract in preventing atherosclerotic nanoplaque formation (the very earliest stages in atherosclerotic plaque development). In 2004, Dr. Siegel conducted a landmark study in cardiovascular high-risk patients indicating that ginkgo can not only reduce the formation and size of atherosclerotic building blocks of nanoplaques, but can also diminish reactive oxygen species and increase vasodilating substances in the blood of the patients. This research applying a biosensor model is also highly significant because it provides scientists with an innovative research methodology with applications for testing of new drugs to combat atherosclerosis. He has recently finished a clinical trial in patients with metabolic syndrome which again confirms the impact of ginkgo biloba in the prophylaxis of atherosclerosis and promotion of well-aging.

Dr. Siegel has been awarded numerous prestigious commendations, including the Carl Friedrich award from Ruprecht-Karl University in Heidelberg in 1969; the Max Ratschow award from the German Angiology Society in 1984; an honorary certificate by the 2nd International Congress of Pathophysiology in 1994; and the Rudolf Schönheimer Medal from the German Arteriosclerosis Society in 2004.

Chapter 33
The Use of Adult Stem Cells and New Low-Molecular Weight Compounds for Regenerative Medicine and as Anti-Aging Agents

Shimon Slavin, M.D.; Aviv Gazit, Ph.D.
Department of Bone Marrow Transplantation & Cancer Immunotherapy,
Hadassah-Hebrew University Hospital (Jerusalem, Israel)

ABSTRACT

Over the years, there has been a constant increase in life expectancy; however, there has been no rise in maximum lifespan. Due to the aging process, trauma, and wear and tear, there is an increasing need for the development of new methods for tissue repair and regenerative medicine. The use of stem cells and experiments suggesting stem cell plasticity has created new hopes that regenerative medicine and life extension may become a clinical reality. As part of an intensive research program aimed at understanding the causes of aging, mutations in approximately 50 genes have been found to extend lifespan. Of these, the most universal is a mutation in the IGF1 gene, which produces a hormone important for growth and development. Genetic mutations that reduce IGF1 function have been found to lead to dramatic increases in lifespan, in nematodes.

With the goal in mind to develop low-molecular weight compounds with anti-aging properties, we have synthesized several low-molecular weight IGF1 inhibitors and investigated their effect on the extension of mean and maximum lifespan in lower organisms, namely *Caenorhabditis elegans* (*C. elegans*) nematodes and *Drosophila melanogaster* flies. We discovered compounds in six different intracellular signal transduction pathways (three of which are well established affecting genetically modified routes, and three of which are new) that produced between 30-60% mean lifespan extension in worms and nearly doubling of the maximum life span. Similar results were obtained in flies, but with somewhat of a lower lifespan extension capacity.

The aims of this paper are to discuss the potential of stem cells in regenerative medicine, and to consider how low-molecular weight molecules that block or enhance certain cell cycle pathways may provide us with a method of lifespan extension.

INTRODUCTION

Over the years, there has been a constant increase in life expectancy; however, there has been no rise in maximum lifespan. Due to the aging process, trauma, and wear and tear, there is an increasing need for the development of new methods for tissue repair and regenerative medicine. The use of stem cells and experiments suggesting stem cell plasticity has created new hopes that regenerative medicine and life extension may become a clinical reality. As part of an intensive research program aimed at understanding the causes of aging, mutations in approximately 50 genes have been found to extend lifespan. Of these, the most universal is a mutation in the IGF1 gene, which produces a hormone important for growth and development. Genetic mutations that reduce IGF1 function have been found to lead to dramatic increases in lifespan, in nematodes.

With the goal in mind to use low-molecular weight compounds with anti-aging properties, we have synthesized several low-molecular weight IGF1 inhibitors and investigated their effect on the extension of mean and maximum lifespan in lower organisms, namely *Caenorhabditis elegans* (*C. elegans*) nematodes and *Drosophila melanogaster* flies. We discovered compounds in six different intracellular signal transduction pathways (three of which are well established affecting genetically modified routes, and three of which are new) that produced between 30-60% mean lifespan extension in worms and nearly doubling of the maximum life span. Similar results were obtained in flies, but with somewhat of a lower lifespan extension capacity.

The aims of this paper are to discuss the potential of stem cells in regenerative medicine, and to consider how low-molecular weight molecules that block or enhance certain cell cycle pathways may provide us with a method of lifespan extension.

THE ROLE OF STEM CELLS IN REGENERATIVE MEDICINE

Over the last decade we have heard a lot of talk about stem cells. When we hear the media talk stem cells, they are usually referring to embryonic stem cells. There has been a lot of controversy surrounding the use of embryonic stem cells. This controversy is centered on the Evangelist belief that ensoulement occurs at the exact moment a sperm cell enters an egg cell. When scientists talk about embryonic stem cells, they are often talking about an eight cell embryo, which is only six or eight days old. According to the Jewish tradition, ensoulement occurs on day 40 of gestation, so Jewish people have no ethical problems with the use of embryonic stem cells. Similarly, Muslims believe that ensoulement occurs on day 120 of gestation, so there is no ethical problem with the use of embryonic stem cells in Islamic countries.

However, ethics are not the only problem surrounding the use of embryonic stem cells, there are many theoretical problems surrounding their use. For example, we do not yet know how to control their division and their differentiation, and therefore it is very dangerous to implant embryonic stem cells because they could lead to the development of a teratoma. There are also lots of immunological problems involved in their use, because the embryonic stem cells are going to be HLA different from their host, and therefore the host will attempt to reject the new cells. So, in order to use embryonic stem cells properly, we need to know how to control them properly and how to overcome the rejection barrier. So, there are many problems surrounding the use of embryonic stem cells, and therefore embryonic stem cell research is far behind clinical application. It is of course very exciting, and it has a lot of potential, but from a practical viewpoint embryonic stem cells will not be much use to us clinically for the next few years at least.

But what about adult stem cells? When we talk about adult stem cells we typically mean stem cells that are available after a person is born, for example stem cells can be obtained from bone. It is very popular now to obtain cord blood stem cells. This is done by collecting blood from the placenta and umbilical cord straight after the delivery of the baby. Cord blood contains enough stem cells for stem cell transplantation into an adult. Adult stem cells are now used on a routine medical basis.

Adult stem cells have two functions in life. One is to replicate themselves and the other is to create a lot of subsets, for example red blood cells, white blood cells, and platelets. Both of these functions are essential for life. Adult stem cell transplantation can be used to cure hundreds of different diseases, including leukemia, lymphoma, multiple myeloma, and some genetic diseases.

For the purpose of this paper, the most interesting cells that are derived from the hematopoietic cells in the bone marrow are mesenchymal stromal cells. These cells have been neglected and ignored for many years, however research has shown that they are multipotent cells that can create cartilage and bone, and can possibly create muscle and fat tissue. Some scientists believe that they can trans-differentiate into myocytes, pulmonary cells, and neural cells, however these claims are somewhat controversial.

Is it possible that a cell that is located inside the bone, whose major function is to create blood cells and immune system cells, can restore organ function? The simple answer is: Yes. The DNA inside the stem cell contains all of the genetic information that is needed to create every cell type. We have already established that we can produce bone, cartilage, and collagen from adult stem cells, and people are starting to reap the benefits of this technology. Regenerative medicine in terms of bone and cartilage is already here. So, now we know that this is possible there is no real reason why adult stem cells cannot be used to regenerate and rejuvenate organs, or treat Alzheimer's or Parkinson's disease etc.

We have published eight cases where patients with intractable congestive heart failure have been treated with stem cells. The cells were derived from their own bone marrow and injected into the coronary artery. Each patient who has undergone this procedure has showed improved heart function afterwards. It is likely that the injected cells have gone on to create new blood vessels and the physiological outcome of the procedure was similar to a bypass. So, we know that adult bone marrow cells can create new blood vessels. This means that adult stem cells may provide us with a method of repairing and restoring heart function. This may be of particular use in patients where it is technically difficult to insert a stent.

What about the central nervous system? Could adult stem cells be used to treat diseases such as Alzheimer's disease, amyotrophic lateral sclerosis (ALS), multiple sclerosis, and spinal injuries? Is it possible to restore nerve function with stem cell therapy today? Well, studies have shown that bone marrow-derived cells cultured under the right conditions acquire neuronal markers of neurons, axons, glial cells, and astrocytes. So, it has been shown that cells can transform or trans-differentiate into neuronal cells after both *in vitro* and *in vivo* treatment. Studies of animals with experimentally-induced brain injury have also shown that bone marrow-derived cells acquire neuronal markers both *in situ* and *ex vivo*. At present we don't know exactly how these function, but we know that they histologically and biochemically look like neurons, astrocytes, and glial cells.

We have treated several spinal injury patients with complete paralysis by injecting stem cells directly into the lesion. Some patients have seen some restored function. Of course we have to distinguish between wishful thinking and between real effects, but it has had positive results on some, but not all, patients. Obviously, this treatment is now under further investigation. We are also treating patients with ALS with stem cells injected into the spinal fluid to see if we can restore some neuron function, and more recently we have begun to give the same treatment to people with multiple sclerosis, with some early signs of success.

Therefore, whilst we are not able to claim any success using adult stem cells to treat diseases of the central nervous system, such as ALS, multiple sclerosis, Parkinson's or Alzheimer's disease, current research suggests that we may well be able to use bone marrow derived mesenchymal stromal cells to treat such diseases in the future.

USING LOW-MOLECULAR WEIGHT COMPOUNDS TO EXTEND LIFE

There are several basic principles that we need to consider when we think about the possibility of using low-molecular compounds to modify intracellular signal transduction pathways associated with the aging process.

The first and foremost is that the aging process is not a result of one pathway. The aging process is a multistep procedure, and therefore the senescence of individual cells and tissues will have to be dealt with by multiple agents that affect different pathways in the cells.

The second principle is that the aging process is not the same for all walks of life; therefore aging and lifespan are very complex to study. Some species survive only for a few minutes or a few days whereas others can survive for 200 years or more. So, the aging process is a very complex issue. However, there are some elements that are common in all species. Furthermore, the aging process is affected by genetics and some environmental factors. Sometimes, even in the same species with the same genetics, there are enormous variations; a good example of this is the bee. The queen bee has exactly the same genetics as the worker bees, however the lifespan of a queen been is 30-times that of the worker bee. Therefore, we can see that the genetics of aging is extremely accomplished.

Aging is very difficult to study in humans, dogs, or monkeys simply because of their long lifespan. However, we can use small animals as experimental models. The animal that is probably most often used in life extension studies is a worm known as *C. elegans*. *C. elegans* has a lifespan of exactly two weeks and therefore it is relatively quick and easy to determine if an experimental compound can extend its survival.

As we concluded above, the process of aging is extremely complex because there are a lot of genes that control the aging process. The most famous gene involved in the aging process one is the IGF-1 gene. Kenyon described a genetic defect in the IGF-1 gene of *C. elegans* that doubled the worms' lifespan. This discovery led us to consider whether or not it would be possible to extend lifespan by using low-molecular weight compounds to mimic the genetic defect of IGF-1, namely by inhibiting IGF-1.

The IGF-1 gene has been to shown to play a very important role in lifespan in many different species, including C. elegans, and *Drosophila melanogaster*. There have also been studies in mice. We have given mice our experimental IGF-1-inhibitors for as long as one year, without any problems. So, from the limited experience we have, these compounds appear to be relatively safe. We have designed several molecules that can induce IGF-1 inhibition and we think that one of them has the possibility to extend life. However, what we don't yet know is if it will extend the life of the entire individual, or just the life of certain cells. So, this compound may turn out to be the long searched for Fountain of Youth, or it may be used may be to prolong the survival of brain cells to prevent the senescence process of aging, likewise it may be found to prevent aging of the skin. So, we are already in possession of one group of potentially very important anti-aging molecules.

As we said, the aging process is a multistep procedure, and therefore the IGF-1 pathway is not the only pathway involved in aging. As we age the entire hormonal system undergoes dramatic changes, and research suggests that certain factors in the estrogen pathway may play a role in the aging process. Low-molecular weight molecules called aromatase inhibitors are routinely used in the treatment of women with breast cancer. These molecules work by inhibiting the action of the enzyme aromatase, which converts androgens into estrogen via a process known as aromatization. We have synthesized several aromatase inhibitors that are similar to the commonly used drugs Femara® and Arimidex® and we have evidenced that at least one of these compounds can extend the lifespan of C. elegans, *Drosophila melanogaster*, and mice. Thus, we have another potential agent that could be used to prolong life.

Another interesting pathway is the so-called c-Abl pathway. Werner syndrome is one of a number of very rare genetic diseases that causes premature aging. One of the pathological hallmarks of this disease is genomic instability of the chromosomes, and c-Abl phosphorylation seemingly plays a very important role in the induction of instability of chromosomes that leads to premature aging on the one hand and a high incidence of cancer on the other. This knowledge led us to question whether it may be possible to extend life by inhibiting c-Abl. The c-Abl pathway is well known, mainly because a c-Abl inhibitor called Gleevec® has been having a dramatic effect upon patients with chronic myelogenous leukemia. Because of the relationship between c-Abl and Werner syndrome we decided to study the potential efficacy of this molecule on the aging process, and whilst we have not yet concluded this study we are certain that the results will be positive.

Probably the most interesting compound that we have is a compound that amplifies the function of the enzyme telomerase. Every time a cell divides the chromosome gets shortened by 6 nucleotides, and therefore a cell cannot divide and multiply endlessly. Cells typically divide for up to 40 times and when the chromosome gets shortened to a critical length it will die. Chromosomal shortening is one of the most important factors that determine the lifespan of a cell. Now, if you could prevent this shortening process you could also prolong the lifespan of the cell. Telomerase is an enzyme that helps to prevent this shortening process by sticking back the pieces that are cut off the DNA after every cell division. We have now a small molecule that is capable of activating endogenous telomerase and therefore preventing the shortening of the telomeres. We think that this molecule is possibly the most exciting agent that we have in terms of extending the lifespan of cells and tissues, and certainly for preventing the aging process of the skin.

CONCLUDING REMARKS

In conclusion, aging is a very complex issue. Research suggests that adult stem cells will provide us with the ability to regenerate damaged organs and prevent the aging of organs in the not so distant future. Research also suggests that we may soon be able to slow the aging process and extend life with low-molecular weight compounds that affect intracellular signal transduction pathways linked to the aging process.

ABOUT THE AUTHORS

Dr. Shimon Slavin graduated from the Hadassah Hebrew University School of Medicine in Jerusalem, Israel, in 1967. He specialized in internal medicine and subsequently in clinical immunology at Stanford University, California, and the Bone Marrow Transplant Center at the Fred Hutchinson Cancer Research Center, Seattle. Dr Slavin serves on many editorial boards and national and international advisory boards. He is a member of the Executive Committee of the IBMTR and a member of the Immunotherapy Committees of the IBMTR and EBMT. Dr Slavin has authored more than 600 scientific publications and 4 books.

Dr. Aviv Gazit is a world-renowned biochemist working with Dr. Slavin with many past contributions in synthesis of tyrosine kinase inhibitors. At the present time Dr. Gazit is also heavily involved in synthesis of low molecular weight compounds with anti-aging properties.

Chapter 34
Avoiding Common Pitfalls, Mistakes, and 87% Failure
of Anti-Aging Saliva Hormone Testing

Dr. Paul Ling Tai, DPM, FACFS, ABPS
Department of Surgery, Oakwood Annapolis Hospital (Detroit, Michigan USA);
Professor, Department of Integrative Medicine,
New York College of Podiatric Medicine (New York, USA)

ABSTRACT

Saliva hormone testing is one of the most user-friendly, inexpensive, and accurate of all the hormone testing options currently available. However, samples are often taken, handled, and processed improperly, therefore significantly decreasing the accuracy of the results. This paper is concerned with the accuracy of saliva hormone testing and the aim of the paper is to discuss how the six most common mistakes associated with saliva hormone testing can be avoided.

INTRODUCTION

It is absolutely clear that the human body produces many different active and powerful hormones. These chemical messengers regulate virtually every body function, from the organization of thoughts and memory in our brain, to the beating of our hearts, to the production of energy in every cell of our body. In other words, hormones keep us healthy, young, full of energy, vitality, sharp and sexy.

Like a predictable mathematical graph, as we age, our glands produce less and less hormones, in turn, we become more fragile and weak, senile, and sick. Hormone deficiencies affect over 50 million women and over 40 million men in the USA alone. As physicians with special attention to anti-aging medicine, our therapeutic program generally starts with hormone testing of the patient to establish a baseline or check on follow up studies keeping track of dosage administration.

Saliva hormone testing is one of the most user-friendly, inexpensive, and accurate of all the hormone testing options currently available. However, samples are often taken, handled, and processed improperly, therefore significantly decreasing the accuracy of the results. This paper is concerned with the accuracy of saliva hormone testing and the aim of the paper is to discuss how the six most common mistakes associated with saliva hormone testing can be avoided.

MISTAKE #1: TIME OF SAMPLE COLLECTION

Keep in mind that there are predictable long-term hormone fluctuations. For example, testosterone levels are slightly higher in the summer than they are in the winter.

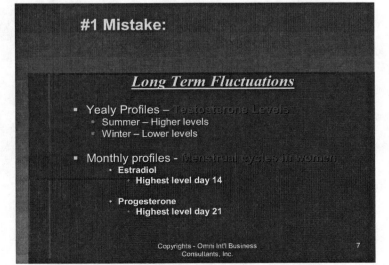

Figure 1. Long-term fluctuations in hormone levels can impact upon saliva testing.

Also keep in mind that during the menstrual cycle, estradiol peaks on day 14 and progesterone peaks on day 21. Therefore, interpretation of lab results must take into account the "Luteinizing Phase" and "Follicular Phase" of the menstrual cycle.

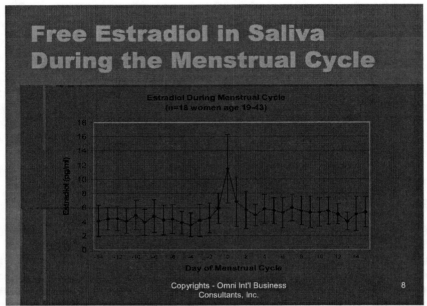

Figure 2. The level of free estradiol present in saliva peaks on day 14 of the menstrual cycle.

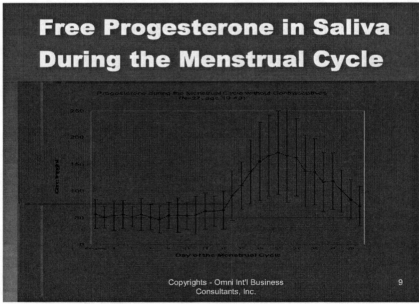

Figure 3. The level of free progesterone present in saliva peaks at day 21 of the menstrual cycle.

MISTAKE #2: SINGLE COLLECTION OR MULTIPLE COLLECTIONS

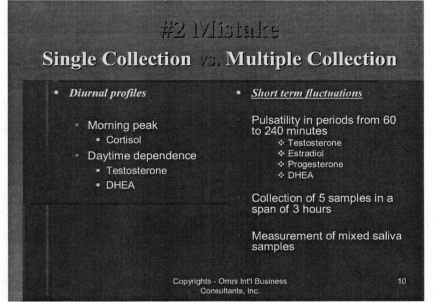

Figure 4. Multiple collection of saliva samples is needed to avoid the pitfalls of diurnal and short-term fluctuations that are associated with single collection.

Scientific evidence and our own laboratory data clearly shows a diurnal fluctuation with higher levels of DHEA and testosterone early in the morning, and diminishing levels towards the night, with a loss of as much as 25% to 50%.

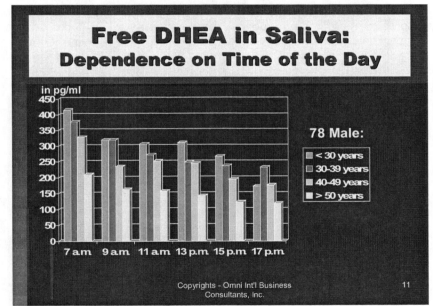

Figure 5. The level of free DHEA in saliva can fluctuate by as much as 25% to 50% depending upon the time of day.

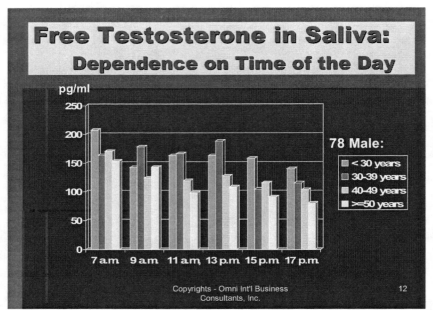

Figure 6. The level of free testosterone in saliva shows a significant diurnal fluctuation.

Our research data also reveals the presence of short-term fluctuations in hormone levels. It is important to bear in mind that hormones are not produced in a continuous stream, but are instead, produced in high levels of pulsatility ranging in periods of 60 minutes to 240 minutes for testosterone, progesterone, DHEA, and estradiol. The inter-hour highest level of hormone to the lowest level varies by approximately 300% - 500%.

In light of this new scientific evidence, a single sample of either blood or saliva is next to useless and is misleading as a diagnostic tool, and maybe worthless as a follow up or for dosage monitoring. Given that humans produce hormones throughout the day in spurts and fluctuations of 60-120 minutes intervals, the best approach to test the physiological hormone level is to average the hormone levels of 5 samples taken every 3 hours in a day. Our research data shows that such a collection procedure provides up to 90% accuracy.

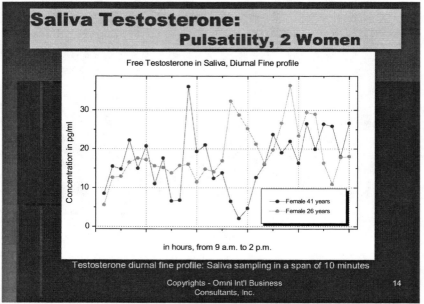

Figure 7. Short-term fluctuations of testosterone levels in saliva in women caused by hormone pulsatility.

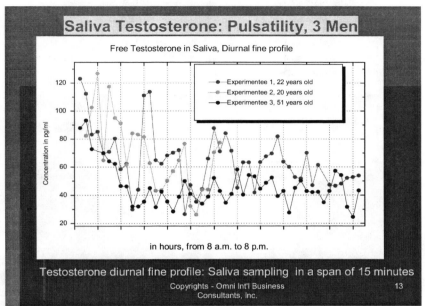

Figure 8. Short-term fluctuations of testosterone levels in saliva in men caused by hormone pulsatility.

MISTAKE #3: CORTISOL LEVELS STUDIES

Using blood tests to measure cortisol levels may give inaccurate and false reports on stress, chronic fatigue, and obesity; the venipuncture itself represents a severe stress factor to many patients and thus can result in false laboratory readings.

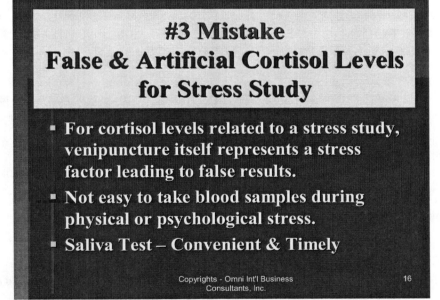

Figure 9. It is preferable to use saliva testing over blood testing for cortisol stress testing.

It is virtually impossible to get a correlation of blood sample cortisol levels to physical or psychological stress events because no one can predict when or where these stress events are going to happen, nor will someone be available to draw blood samples during the event. This is why saliva hormone testing for cortisol is so convenient and timely. All you have to do is spit. Additionally, there is a normal and important high cortisol level during the first hour of awakening; this very high level of cortisol is healthy, expected, and indeed necessary. If high levels of cortisol are not achieved in the first hour of awakening, possible adrenal fatigue and insufficiency should be suspected until confirmed or denied by the presence of symptoms. Cortisol levels rapidly drop off after two hours of awakening and drop to very low levels just before sleep.

If you have a patient with very high levels of cortisol throughout the day and evening, it is important to remember that the patient will be at increased risk of developing conditions such as metabolic syndrome (syndrome X), diabetes, and obesity.

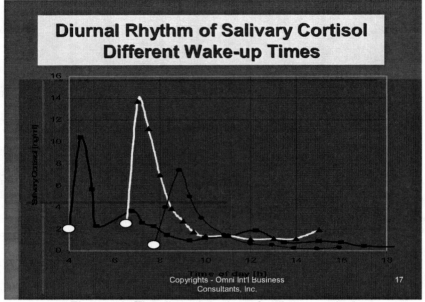

Figure 10. The diurnal rhythm of salivary cortisol.

MISTAKE #4: FOOD CONTAMINATION OF SALIVA SAMPLES CAUSES INACCURATE SALIVA HORMONE TEST RESULTS

In our laboratory, research data shows that food contamination, for example milk or cheese particulates, in saliva samples may change progesterone test results by over 100%. Therefore:
1. We advise patients to rinse their mouth to remove food particles from the tongue and teeth right after eating or drinking.
2. We recommend that patients do not eat or drink for at least one hour prior to collecting a saliva sample.
3. As an extra precaution, we recommend that patients rinse their mouth with clean water 15 minutes before a saliva sample collection.
4. We also advise patients not to eat red meat, milk, or milk products on the day of collecting saliva samples.

MISTAKE #5: SALIVA SAMPLE WITH BLOOD CONTAMINATION FROM GINGIVITIS OR BLEEDING GUMS YIELD ABNORMAL AND MISLEADING SALIVA HORMONE LEVELS.

Hormone levels in blood are over 100 times higher than levels of hormones in saliva. Therefore it stands to reason that even a small amount of blood contamination can change laboratory saliva hormone results drastically.

Research concluded in our laboratory revealed that the presence of blood visible to the naked eye in a saliva specimen is ground for rejection of the specimen. Our research showed that the naked eye can detect blood contamination of as little as 0.156%.

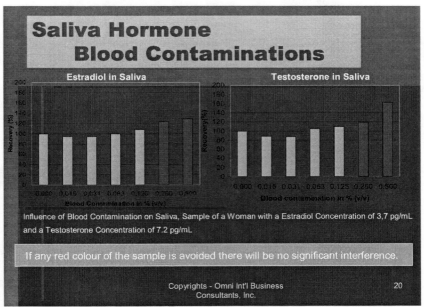

Figure 11. Mistake #5: Blood contamination of saliva samples.

Laboratory sampling of saliva specimens with blood contaminations of greater than 0.125% shows a misleading jump in 20% or greater than recorded hormones.

MISTAKE #6: COLLECTION CONTAINER MATERIAL MAYBE A SIGNIFICANT CAUSE OF MISLEADING AND ERRONEOUS SALIVA HORMONE RESULTS.

This step in the collection of saliva samples is often the first source of error. Our research shows that saliva hormones are small non-polar molecules (and therefore electrically charged particles), which tend to stick to plastic materials (which are also electrically charged). For example, Polyethylene is highly charged and therefore highly absorptive to progesterone, which is highly non-polar. Remember that polyethylene stoppers are also highly absorptive of hormones further compounding the problem.

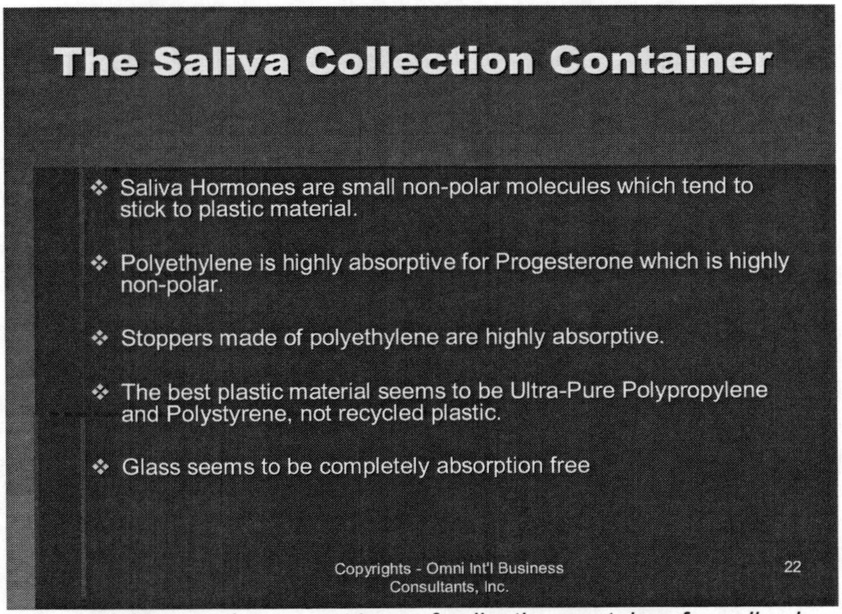

The Saliva Collection Container

❖ Saliva Hormones are small non-polar molecules which tend to stick to plastic material.

❖ Polyethylene is highly absorptive for Progesterone which is highly non-polar.

❖ Stoppers made of polyethylene are highly absorptive.

❖ The best plastic material seems to be Ultra-Pure Polypropylene and Polystyrene, not recycled plastic.

❖ Glass seems to be completely absorption free

Copyrights - Omni Int'l Business Consultants, Inc.   22

Figure 12. It is essential to use the correct type of collection container for saliva hormone testing.

Throughout our extensive research using labeled 3H progesterone, we were able to determine that the best plastic material is ultra pure polypropylene non-recycled plastic. We also found that polystyrene containers have the least absorbency of saliva hormones to the container wall during transportation and storage.

Just imagine, a sample of saliva hormone in a polyethylene container arriving at your laboratory destination containing only 13.5% of free progesterone remaining in the saliva sample – your patient effectively lost 86.5% of hormone bound to the sides of the container wall and stopper.

It is also important to remember not to use cotton salivettes to stimulate saliva production because they bind and therefore lower cortisol levels in the saliva sample.

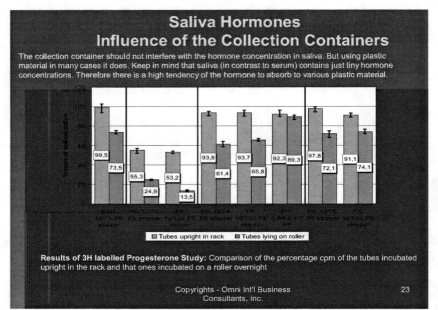

Figure 13. The influence of the sample collection container on saliva hormone levels.

CONCLUDING REMARKS

In summary:

1.   Take multiple samples
2.   Take 5 saliva samples every 3 hours throughout the day
3.   Avoid food contamination
4.   Discard any samples with blood contamination
5.   Do not use cotton salivettes
6.   Insist upon containers made with glass, polypropylene or polystyrene.

It is possible to keep errors to a minimum by avoiding the six common mistakes above. By taking these precautions and avoiding these six common errors the accuracy of your laboratory results may improve by more than 80%.

ABOUT THE AUTHOR

Dr. Paul Ling Tai is a trained Podiatric medical physician and Board certified surgeon with expertise in herbal compound engineering, research and development and nine (9) patents credited to his name.   In additional to his various capacities, Dr. Tai has served as Chairman of the Podiatric Physicians Continuing Education, as well as Chief Compliance Officer for the state of Michigan, supervising doctors.   He is also a professor in the New York College of Podiatric Medicine's Department of Integrative Medicine. Dr. Tai is the author of the best seller books *Cordyceps Miracles* and *8 Powerful Secrets to Antiaging*.

Chapter 35
Innovative Natural Anti-Wrinkle Plant Extract:
In Vitro and Controlled Clinical Studies

Paul Ling Tai, DPM, FACFS, ABPS
Department of Surgery, Oakwood Annapolis Hospital (Detroit, Michigan USA);
Professor, Department of Integrative Medicine,
New York College of Podiatric Medicine (New York, USA)

ABSTRACT

This paper presents a natural plant extract of Bamboo, Peapods, and Glucosamine (Complete Natural Plant Extract – CNPE) for its effect on skin cell renewal and collagen synthesis.

INTRODUCTION

Baby Boomers are now in their 6th decade of life. Notables like George W. Bush, Cher, Susanne Somers, and Bill Clinton are famous Baby Boomers. Every day, over 8,000 new baby boomers join the 80-million strong group, therefore making it the largest age segment of our population. What's more, Baby Boomers control over 70% of all spending. They are wealthy and demand a healthier lifestyle, with an emphasis on feeling better, living longer, and most of all – looking younger. This is demonstrated by the skyrocketing increase in plastic surgery, Botox, dermal fillers, mesotherapy, and a myriad of cosmetic enhancing procedures, in recent years.

This paper presents a natural plant extract of Bamboo, Peapods, and Glucosamine (Complete Natural Plant Extract – CNPE) for its effect on skin cell renewal and collagen synthesis.

PROCEDURE

- Peak cell growth
- Tritiated proline to culture
- Incubated for 24 Hours
- Add 10% TCA, heated 100°C for 30 minutes
- Total protein filtered 0.22um Millipore filters
- Filters dried and assayed tritium

RESULTS
Effects of CNPE on Collagen Synthesis

Results showed that Complete Natural Plant Extract (CNPE) is more effective at stimulating collagen synthesis than:

- Ascorbic Acid
- Retinoic Acid,
- Epidermal Growth Factor

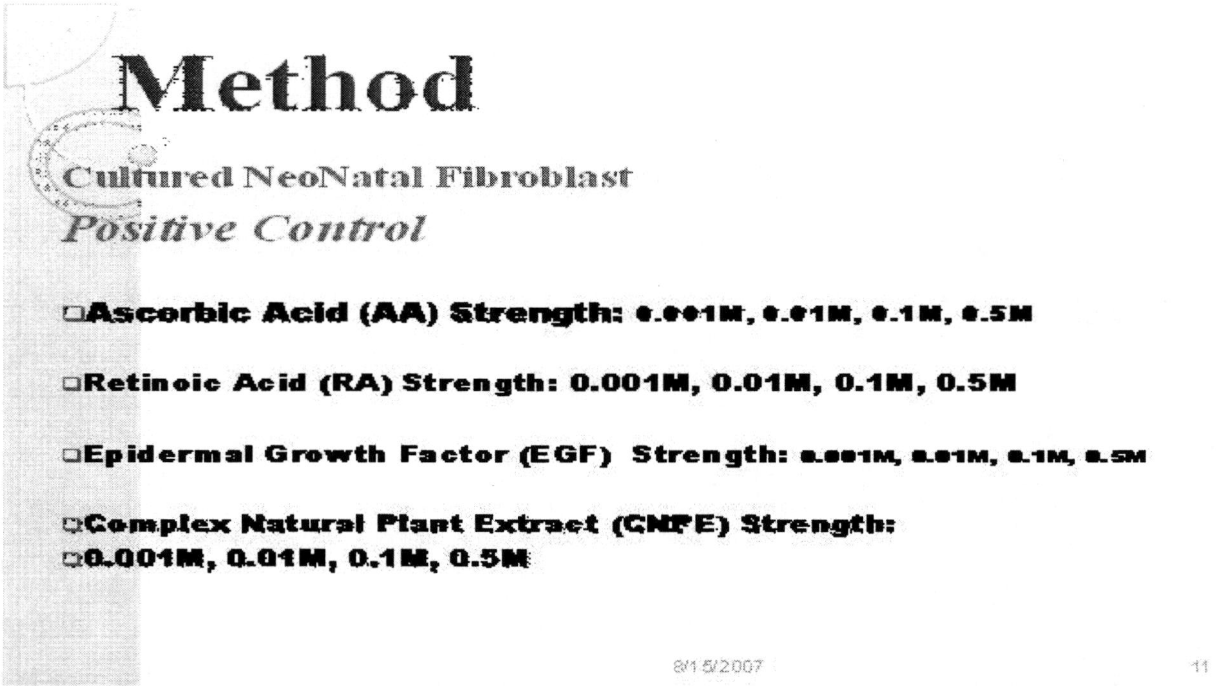

Method

Cultured NeoNatal Fibroblast
Positive Control

□Ascorbic Acid (AA) Strength: 0.001M, 0.01M, 0.1M, 0.5M

□Retinoic Acid (RA) Strength: 0.001M, 0.01M, 0.1M, 0.5M

□Epidermal Growth Factor (EGF) Strength: 0.001M, 0.01M, 0.1M, 0.5M

□Complex Natural Plant Extract (CNPE) Strength:
□0.001M, 0.01M, 0.1M, 0.5M

8/15/2007   11

Figure 1. In Vitro laboratory cell cultures of neonatal fibroblast measures collagen synthesis through assayed Tritiated Proline.

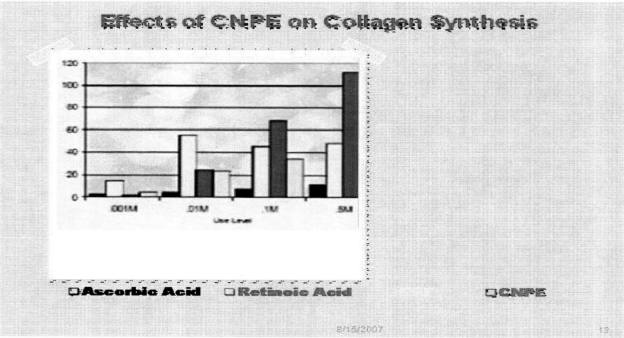

Figure 2. Effects of CNPE on Collagen Synthesis

Skin Exfoliation Test

In vivo skin exfoliation studies were performed and measured by photometer for light transmission and scattering of the light to assess the quantity of desquamated skin cells:

- D-Squame tape applied to skin test site
- Measure tape for light scattering with Custom Photometer
- Greater light scattering and less light transmission with greater number of skin cells on tape

Clinical Subjects:
- 20 Subjects
- Applied 3% of test material on ½ of the face
- Other ½ of the face used control gel (Carbopol)
- Total of 5 days treatment

Skin Exfoliation Test Results:
- Skin treated with CPNE had 84.7% increase of exfoliated cells
- Skin treated with control had 7.3% exfoliated cells

Results showed that CPNE increased exfoliation, improved skin cell turnover rate, increased cell renewal rate.

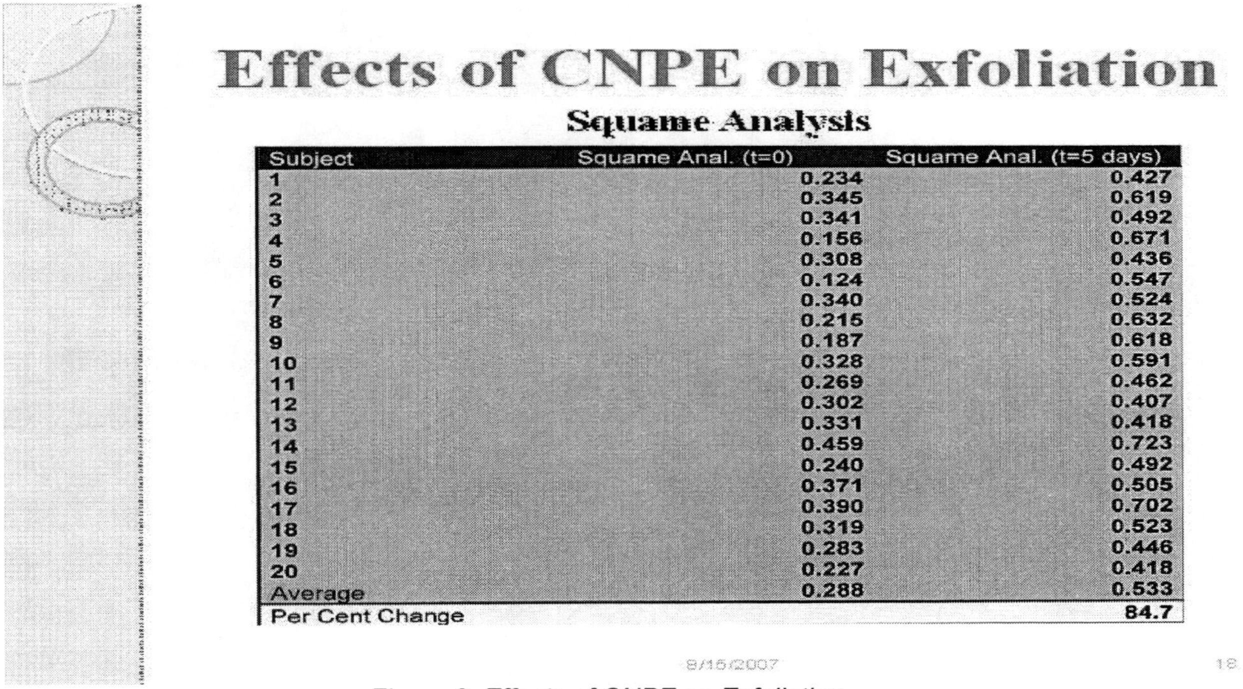

Effects of CNPE on Exfoliation
Squame Analysis

Subject	Squame Anal. (t=0)	Squame Anal. (t=5 days)
1	0.234	0.427
2	0.345	0.619
3	0.341	0.492
4	0.156	0.671
5	0.308	0.436
6	0.124	0.547
7	0.340	0.524
8	0.215	0.632
9	0.187	0.618
10	0.328	0.591
11	0.269	0.462
12	0.302	0.407
13	0.331	0.418
14	0.459	0.723
15	0.240	0.492
16	0.371	0.505
17	0.390	0.702
18	0.319	0.523
19	0.283	0.446
20	0.227	0.418
Average	0.288	0.533
Per Cent Change		84.7

8/15/2007   18

Figure 3. Effects of CNPE on Exfoliation

Effect of CPNE on Skin Wrinkles

Controlled clinical studies were performed on 20 female subjects with facial wrinkles with half of face treated using control gel and the other half face using CPNE for 4 weeks in order to determine the effect of CPNE on wrinkles and fine lines.

Clinical Protocol:
- 20 Females
- Aged 45-65 years old
- Scores greater than 10 on the Packman Wrinkle Scale

Method:

- Applied 3% of test material on ½ of the face
- Other ½ of the face used control gel (Carbopol)
- Application twice (2) daily
- Total of 4-weeks treatment

Results:

- Statistically significant and clinical skin improvement
- Reduce wrinkle analysis
- CPNE reduced line and wrinkle depth over 4 weeks
- Measured by Packman Wrinkle Scale
- Control Gel 4.7% Improvement

Effects of CNPE on Wrinkles
Skin Fine Lines & Image Analysis

Subject	SFL (t=0)	SFL (t=4wks)	IA (t=0)	IA (t=4wks)
1	23	17	10234	4754
2	31	16	13564	7645
3	19	8	14628	5215
4	21	11	15123	3218
5	19	7	16148	3361
6	19	12	12137	4681
7	24	11	10216	6789
8	23	13	10987	5811
9	25	11	11065	6432
10	22	11	15267	8435
11	17	11		
12	25	12		
13	17	11		
14	18	10		
15	23	14		
16	22	13		
17	16	9		
18	12	6		
19	17	9		
20	13	10		
Average	20.3	11.1	12936.9	5634.1
Per Cent Change	Not appl.	45.3		56.4

8/15/2007   27

Figure 4. Effect of CPNE on Wrinkles.

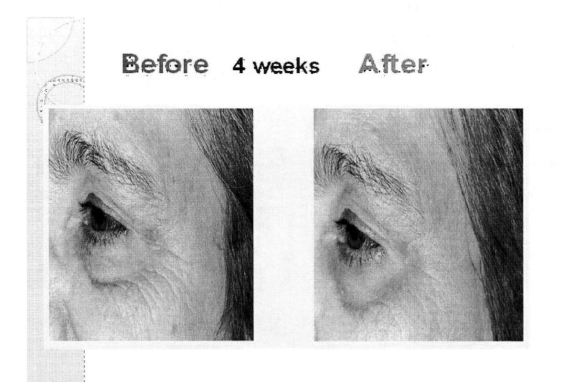

Before   4 weeks   After

Figure 5. Wrinkles before and after treatment with CPNE.

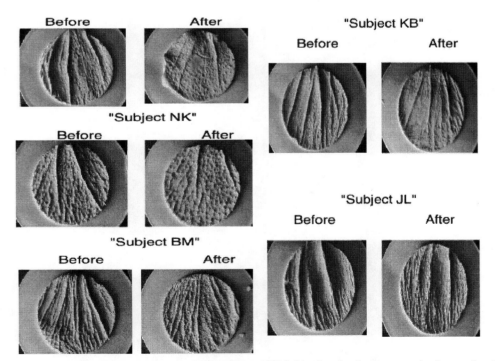

Figure 6. Before and after evaluation by Packman Wrinkle Scale. Image analysis, and wrinkle mold replica made for statistical and clinical quantitative and qualitative analysis.

CONCLUDING REMARKS

Treatment with CPNE increases collagen synthesis, improves skin cell turnover rate, increases cell renewal rate, and reduces line and wrinkle depth. Therefore regular treatment with CPNE will result in smoother and less wrinkled skin.

ABOUT THE AUTHOR

Dr. Paul Ling Tai is a trained Podiatric medical physician and Board certified surgeon with expertise in herbal compound engineering, research and development and nine (9) patents credited to his name. In additional to his various capacities, Dr. Tai has served as Chairman of the Podiatric Physicians Continuing Education, as well as Chief Compliance Officer for the state of Michigan, supervising doctors. He is also a professor in the New York College of Podiatric Medicine's Department of Integrative Medicine. Dr. Tai is the author of the best seller books *Cordyceps Miracles* and *8 Powerful Secrets to Antiaging*.

Chapter 36
Ribose in Chronic Fatigue Syndrome, Fatigue, Fibromyalgia, and Heart Disease
Jacob Teitelbaum M.D.
Medical Director, Fibromyalgia and Fatigue Centers

ABSTRACT

Mitochondrial dysfunction is thought to be an underlying or contributing cause of chronic fatigue syndrome (CFS) and fibromyalgia (FMS), and therefore we need to address whether anything can be done to make those cellular energy furnaces work better. This paper will discuss recent research showing that ribose, a key component of adenosine tri-phosphate (ATP), nicotinamide adenine dinucleotide (NADH), and other energy molecules that are critical to energy production resulted in an average 45% increase in energy after just 3-weeks of treatment. Ribose is also a key component of DNA and RNA and is deficient in energy depleted states. Because of this it is also very helpful in treating congestive heart failure (CHF) and other cardiac problems as well as generally improving athletic performance. Research on ribose in these areas will also be discussed.

INTRODUCTION

Mitochondrial dysfunction is thought to be an underlying or contributing cause of chronic fatigue syndrome (CFS) and fibromyalgia (FMS), and therefore we need to address whether anything can be done to make those cellular energy furnaces work better. This paper will discuss recent research showing that D-ribose, a key component of adenosine tri-phosphate (ATP), nicotinamide adenine dinucleotide (NADH), and other energy molecules that are critical to energy production, can help to improve mitochondrial energy production.

D-RIBOSE – THE NATURAL BODY ENERGIZER

When looking at energy production, it helps to look at the "energy molecules" such as adenosine tri-phosphate (ATP), nicotinamide adenine dinucleotide (NADH), and flavin adenine dinucleotide (FADH). These represent the energy currency in your body, and are like the paper that money is printed on. You can have all the fuel you want, but if it cannot be converted to these molecules, it is useless!

For years, I have talked about the importance of B vitamins, which are a key component of these molecules. These helped to a degree, but it was clear that a key component was missing. In looking at the biochemistry of these energy molecules, we see that they are also made of two other key components – adenine and ribose. Adenine is plentiful in the body, so we turned our attention to Ribose.

Ribose is made in the body via a slow, laborious process and cannot be found in food. CFS/FMS causes the body to dump other key energy molecules like acetyl-l-carnitine, and we subsequently found that the body does the same with ribose, thus making it hard to get the body's furnaces working again even after the other problems were treated. This discovery was akin to a "Eureka!" moment where things come together. Not having sufficient levels of ribose can be compared to trying to build a fire without kindling – nothing will happen. Therefore we wondered if giving ribose to people with CFS would jump-start their energy furnaces. The answer was a resounding yes!

Our recently published study of CFS/FMS patients treated with D-ribose showed an average 44.7% increase in energy after only 3-weeks (improvement began at 12 days), and an average overall improvement in quality of life of 30%. Furthermore, two thirds of the CFS/FMS patients felt they had improved.[1] Usually, a 10% improvement for a single nutrient is considered excellent. A 44.7% increase left us amazed, and I am now recommending ribose for all of my CFS/FMS patients, for athletes, and anyone with pain, fatigue, or heart problems.

Ribose recently became available (over the counter) to physicians, and is one of the few natural products actually starting with physicians and then moving out into health food stores. It is critical to use the proper dose for the first 3 weeks, which is 5 grams (5000 mg) three times a day. It can then be dropped to twice a day. I recommend the Corvalen form of ribose as it is the most researched and highest quality and is packaged with a 5 gm dosing scoop in it. One 280 gm container will be enough to tell you if it will work.

Corvalen M (which has ribose plus magnesium and malic acid) is also available, but the regular Corvalen is a better deal financially.

D-Ribose Accelerates Energy Recovery

D-ribose (referred to as ribose in this paper) is a simple, five-carbon sugar (known as a pentose by biochemists) that is found naturally in our bodies. However, ribose is not like any other sugar. Sugars we are all familiar with, such as table sugar (sucrose), corn sugar (glucose), milk sugar (lactose), honey (predominantly fructose), and others are used by the body as fuel. These sugars are consumed and, with the help of the oxygen we breathe, are "burned" by the body to recycle energy. Because they are used excessively, they can also be toxic. Ribose, on the other hand, is special. When we consume ribose, the body recognizes that it is different from other sugars and preserves it for the vital work of actually making the energy molecule ATP, which powers the heart, muscles, brain, and every other tissue in the body.

ATP is known as the energy currency of the cell because the amount of ATP we have in our tissues determines whether we will be fatigued, or will have the energy we need to live vital, active lives. Ribose provides the key building block of ATP, and the presence of ribose in the cell stimulates the metabolic pathway our bodies use to actually make this vital compound. Thus, if the cell does not have enough ribose, it cannot make ATP. So, when cells and tissues become energy starved, the availability of ribose is critical to energy recovery.

Normal, healthy heart and muscle tissue has the capacity to make all the ribose it needs. When normal tissue is stressed by overexertion, several days of rest will usually allow it to fully recover. The muscle may be sore during recovery, as we frequently see for the three or four days after a hard day of yard work or after a weekend pick up football game, but eventually energy levels will be restored and the soreness will disappear. But when the muscle is chronically stressed by disease or conditions that affect tissue energy metabolism, the cells and tissues simply cannot make enough ribose quickly enough in order to recover. Heart and muscle does not have the metabolic machinery needed to make ribose very efficiently. Therefore the result is chronic, persistent pain, stiffness, soreness, and overwhelming fatigue that may never go away.

The Link between Ribose, Energy, and Fatigue

Clinical and scientific research has repeatedly shown that giving ribose to energy deficient hearts and muscles stimulates energy recovery. One important study involved healthy athletes participating in high-intensity, endurance exercise over the course of one week. After exercise the energy level in the athletes' muscle was reduced by almost 30%. Giving 10-grams of ribose per day for three days following exercise restored muscle energy levels to normal, while treatment with placebo provided virtually no effect.[2] This study clearly showed that ribose stimulated the energy recovery pathways in the body, helping the muscle rebuild its energy supply quickly and completely. Even after three days of rest, muscle that was not treated with ribose remained energy starved and fatigued.

Two very interesting studies in animals showed how dramatic the effect of ribose could be on energy recovery in fatigued muscle. These studies were conducted by Dr. Ron Terjung, one of the top muscle physiologists in the United States. In their research, Dr. Terjung and his co-investigators found that ribose administration in fatigued muscle increased the rate of energy recovery by 340% to 430%, depending on which type of muscle was tested.[3] He also found that even very small amounts of ribose had the effect of helping the muscle cell preserve energy, a process known as energy salvage, and the higher the ribose dose, the more dramatic the effect on energy preservation.[4] Although this groundbreaking research was done in animals it was instrumental in defining the biochemistry and physiology associated with the use of ribose in overcoming heart and muscle fatigue. But most of us with CFS and FMS are neither top athletes nor animals, so the question remains: "How will ribose affect me?"

Research in ribose and CFS/FMS began with a case study that was published in the prestigious journal *Pharmacotherapy* in 2004.[5] This case study told the story of a veterinary surgeon diagnosed with FMS, who found herself becoming more and more fatigued, and her pain becoming so profound that she was finally unable to stand during surgery. As a result, she was forced to all but give up the practice she loved. Upon hearing that a clinical study on ribose in congestive heart failure (CHF) was underway in the university where she worked, she asked if she could try the ribose to see if it might help her overcome the mind-numbing fatigue she experienced from her disease. After three weeks of ribose therapy she was back in the operating room, practicing normally with no muscle pain or stiffness, and without the fatigue that had kept her bedridden for many months.

Being a veterinary surgeon, she was skeptical, not believing that a simple sugar could have such a dramatic effect on her condition. However, within two weeks of stopping the ribose therapy, she was out of the operating room again and back in bed. So, to again test the theory, she began ribose therapy a second time. The result was similar to her first experience, and she was back doing surgery in days. After yet a third round of stopping (with the return of symptoms) and starting (with the reduction of symptoms) the ribose therapy, she was convinced, and has been on ribose therapy since that time.

I found this report intriguing and decided to design the larger study in patients with FMS or CFS mentioned earlier. Along with two research collaborators, I recently published a scientific paper describing the results of this research.[1] The study we designed was intended to determine whether or not ribose would be effective in relieving the overwhelming fatigue, pain, soreness, and stiffness suffered by patients having this debilitating condition. Our study included 41 patients with a diagnosis of FMS or CFS who were given ribose at a dose of 5-grams three times per day for an average of three weeks. We found the ribose treatment led to significant improvement in energy levels, sleep patterns, mental clarity, pain intensity, and well being. Of the patients participating in the study, 65.7% experienced significant improvement while on ribose, with an average increase in energy of 44.7% and overall well being of 30% – remarkable results from a single nutrient! The only significant side effect was that 2 people felt too energized and hyperactive/anxious on the ribose. This is simply dealt with by lowering the dose and/or taking it with food.

Several of the patients participating in the study have contacted me regarding the relief they found with ribose therapy. Most importantly, they speak of the profound joy they feel when they are able to begin living normal, active lives after sometimes years of fatigue, pain, and suffering. Here is a sample of what one patient, Julie an elementary teacher, wrote: "*I had so much pain and fatigue I thought I was going to have to quit teaching. When I take [ribose], I feel like a huge weight is being lifted from my chest, and I'm ready to take on those kids again!*" The relief patients feel with ribose therapy is heartwarming, and goes directly to the dramatic impact ribose has on increasing energy, overcoming fatigue, enhancing exercise tolerance, and raising the patient's quality of life.

To further validate these findings, we are currently conducting a placebo controlled study, and hope to have the results published in the coming year [2009]. Interestingly, one of our study patients had an abnormal heart rhythm called atrial fibrillation. Ribose is outstanding in the treatment of heart disease as well, because it restores energy production in the heart muscle. Because of this, it was not surprising that this man's atrial fibrillation also went away on the ribose and he was able to stop his heart medications as well. Because of its importance and the research showing marked heart muscle dysfunction (because of low energy) in CFS, we will consider ribose and the heart in more detail.

Ribose and the Fatigue Associated with Heart Disease

Decades of research have shown that ribose has a profound effect on heart function in patients with CHF, coronary artery disease, and cardiomyopathy. Like the muscles in patients with FMS, sick hearts are energy starved.[6] This energy deprivation keeps the heart from relaxing between heartbeats, making it impossible for the heart to completely fill with blood (it surprisingly takes more energy for the heart muscle to relax than contract).[7] Because the heart does not fill completely, less blood is pumped to the body with each heartbeat. The heart then gets stiff and it strains to contract. Ultimately, the heart becomes enlarged, a condition known as hypertrophy, and it is unable to pump normally.

You can compare this to the effect of weight training on the muscles in the bicep of the upper arm. Over time, weight training against more and more weight makes the muscle larger and harder. Similarly, when the heart becomes stiff it is forced to contract against more and more pressure, making the heart muscle grow. While in the case of the bicep this may be a desirable outcome, in the heart it can be deadly. In contrast to the biceps muscle, hearts must remain supple so they can fill properly and empty fully with each contraction. If hearts cannot pump normal volumes of blood, muscles of the arms and legs and brain tissue become oxygen starved. The result is fatigue, pain on standing or walking, loss of interest in, or the ability to perform any physical activity, brain fog, and depression. In the end, the heart cannot pump enough blood to even supply itself with live-giving oxygen and a heart attack can be the result.

Using ribose to restore the energy level in the heart allows it to fully relax, fill, and empty completely to circulate blood to the outer reaches of the body.[8] Circulating more blood means muscles in the arms and legs, and the tissues of the brain, get the oxygen they need to function normally. This result was made evident in several important studies in patients with congestive heart failure and angina.

In one study conducted at the University of Bonn in Germany, patients with CHF were treated with either 10-grams of ribose or a sugar placebo every day for three weeks.[9] They were then tested for heart function, exercise tolerance (a measure of fatigue), and quality of life using a questionnaire designed for this purpose. In this study, ribose therapy had a significant effect on all measures of diastolic heart function, showing that increased energy in the heart allowed the heart to relax, fill, and pump more normally. Patients in the study were also much more tolerant to exercise when they were on ribose, and, through their responses to the questionnaire, showed they had a higher quality of life as a result.

Two additional studies went on to help explain how ribose therapy in CHF may affect fatigue and exercise tolerance.[10, 11] These studies showed that ribose treatment increased ventilatory and oxygen utilization efficiency, a medical way of saying that the patients were able to breathe better and use the oxygen they inhaled more efficiently. Improving the patient's ability to use oxygen means more oxygen is available to go into the blood and out to the tissues. Having more oxygen available allows the muscle to burn fuel more efficiently, helping it keep pace with its energy demand. The result is less fatigue, a greater ability to tolerate exercise, and a higher quality of life. An added benefit to improving ventilatory efficiency is that ventilatory efficiency is a dominant predictor of mortality in congestive heart failure. Increasing ventilatory efficiency with ribose therapy is, therefore, a direct correlate to prolonging life in this patient population.

CONCLUDING REMARKS

There are very few nutritional therapies that can legitimately boast of having such a profound of an effect on the tissues they target. None, other than ribose, can claim such an effect in cell or tissue energy metabolism. Ribose is a unique and powerful addition to our complement of metabolic therapies in that it is completely safe, proven by strong, well designed clinical and scientific evidence, natural, and fundamental to a vital metabolic process in the body.[12-16] Ribose regulates how much energy we have in our bodies, and for those suffering from fatigue, muscle soreness, stiffness, and a host of related medical complications, the relief found in energy restoration can be life changing. This is why I recommend that all CFS/FMS patients begin with D-ribose 5 grams (1 scoop of Corvalen) three times a day for 2-3 weeks then twice a day. It is critical to take the 3 scoops a day for the first few weeks to see the optimal effects. Many nutritional treatments take 6-12 weeks to start working, however most people feel the difference by the end of a single 280 gm container of D-ribose.

REFERENCES

References 17-38 are provided for those who wish to learn more about D-ribose.
1. Teitelbaum JE, St Cyr J, Johnson C. The use of D-ribose in chronic fatigue syndrome and fibromyalgia: a pilot study. *J Alternative and Complementary Medicine* 2006;12:857-862.
2. Hellsten Y, Skadgauge L, Bangsbo J. Effect of ribose supplementation on resynthesis of adenine nucleotides after intense intermittent training in humans. *American Journal of Physiology.* 2004;286:R182-R188.
3. Tullson PC, Terjung RL. Adenine nucleotide synthesis in exercising and endurance-trained skeletal muscle. *American Journal of Physiology.* 1991;261:C342-C347.
4. Brault JJ, Terjung RL. Purine salvage to adenine nucleotides in different skeletal muscle fiber types. *Journal of Applied Physiology.* 2001;91:231-238.
5. Gebhart B, JA Jorgenson. Benefit of ribose in a patient with fibromyalgia. *Pharmacotherapy.* 2004;24:1146-1648.
6. Ingwall JS. *ATP and the Heart.* Kluwer Academic Publishers, Boston, Massachusetts.
7. Reibel D, Rovetto M. Myocardial ATP Synthesis and Mechanical Function Following Oxygen Deficiency. *American Journal of Physiology.* 1978;234:H620-H624.
8. Zimmer HG, Ibel H, Suchner U. Ribose Intervention in the Cardiac Pentose Phosphate Pathway is Not Species-Specific. *Science* 1984; 223: 712-714.
9. Omran H, Illien S, MacCarter D, St Cyr JA, Luderitz B. D-Ribose improves diastolic function and quality of life in congestive heart failure patients: A prospective feasibility study. *European Journal of Heart Failure.* 2003;5:615-619.
10. Vijay N, MacCarter D, Washam M, St Cyr JA. Ventilatory efficiency improves with d-ribose in congestive Heart Failure patients. *Journal of Molecular and Cellular Cardiology.* 2005;38:820.
11. Carter O, MacCarter D, Mannebach S, Biskupiak J, Stoddard G, Gilbert EM, Munger MA. D-Ribose improves peak exercise capacity and ventilatory efficiency in heart failure patients. *Journal of the American College of Cardiology.* 2005;45(3 Suppl A):185A.

12. Griffiths JC, Borzelleca JF, St Cyr J. Lack of oral embryotoxicity/teratogenicity with D-ribose in Wistar rats. *Journal of Food and Chemical Toxicology.* 2007;45:388-395.

13. Griffiths JC, Borzelleca JF, St Cyr J. Sub-chronic (13-week) oral toxicity study with D-ribose in Wistar rats. *Journal of Food and Chemical Toxicology.* 2007:45:144-152.

14. Gross M, Dormann B, Zollner N. Ribose administration during exercise: effects on substrates and products of energy metabolism in healthy subjects and a patient with myoadenylate deaminase deficiency. *Klin Wochenschr.* 1991;69:151-155.

15. Wagner DR, Gresser U, Zollner N. Effects of oral ribose on muscle metabolism during bicycle ergometer in AMPD-deficient patients. *Annals of Nutrition and Metabolism.* 1991;35:297-302.

16. Gross M, Reiter S, Zollner N. Metabolism of D-ribose administered to healthy persons and to patients with myoadenylate deaminase deficiency. *Klin Wochenschr.* 1989;67:1205-1213.

17. Guymer EK, Clauw KJ. Treatment of fatigue in fibromyalgia. *Rheum Dis Clin North Am.* 2002;28:67-78.

18. Rooks DS, Silverman CB, Kantrowitz FG. The effects of progressive strength training and aerobic exercise on muscle strength and cardiovascular fitness in women with fibromyalgia: a pilot study. *Arthritis Rheum.* 2002;47:22-28.

19. Geenen R, Jacobs JW, Bijlsma JW. Evaluation and management of endocrine dysfunction in fibromyalgia. *Rheum Dis Clin North Am.* 2002;28:389-404.

20. Schachter CL, Busch AJ, Peloso PM, Shepard MS. Effects of short versus long bouts of aerobic exercise in sedentary women with fibromyalgia: a randomized controlled trial. *Phys Ther.* 2003;83:340-358.

21. Williamson DL, Gallagher PM, Goddard MP, Trappe SW. Effects of ribose supplementation on adenine nucleotide concentration in skeletal muscle following high-intensity exercise. *Med Sci Sport Exc.* 2001; 33(5 suppl).

22. Zollner N, Reiter S, Gross M, Pongratz D, Reimers CD, Gerbitz K, Paetzke I, Deufel T, Hubner G. Myoadenylate deaminase deficiency: successful symptomatic therapy by high dose oral administration of ribose. *Klin Wochenschr.* 1986;64:1281-1290.

23. Patton BM. Beneficial effect of D-ribose in patients with myoadenylate deaminase deficiency. *Lancet.* 1982;1701.

24. Salerno C, D'Eufermia P, Finocchiaro R, Celli M, Spalice A, Crifo C, Giardini O. Effect of D-ribose on purine synthesis and neurological symptoms in a patient with adenylsuccinase deficiency. *Biochim Biophys Acta.* 1999;1453:135-140.

25. Salerno C, Celli M, Finocchiaro R, D'Eufemia P, Iannetti P, Crifo C, Giardini O. Effect of D-ribose administration to a patient with inherited defect of adenylosuccinase. In: *Purine Metabolism in Man IX.* Plenum Press, New York, 1998.

26. Pauly D, Pepine C. D-Ribose as a supplement for cardiac energy metabolism. *J Cardiovasc Pharmacol Ther.* 2000;5:249-258.

27. Pauly D, Johnson C, St Cyr JA. The benefits of ribose in cardiovascular disease. *Med Hypoth.* 2003;60:149-151.

28. Pauly DF, Pepine CJ. Ischemic heart disease: Metabolic approaches to management. *Clin Cardiol.* 2004;27:439-441.

29. Dodd SL, Johnson CA, Fernholz K, St Cyr JA. The role of ribose in human skeletal muscle metabolism. *Med Hypoth.* 2004;62:819-824.

30. Zarzeczny R, Brault JJ, Abraham KA, Hancock CR, Terjung RL. Influence of ribose on adenine salvage after intense muscle contractions. *J Appl Physiol.* 2001;91:1775-1781.

31. Wallen JW, Belanger MP, Wittnich C. Preischemic administration of ribose to delay the onset of irreversible ischemic injury and improve function: studies in normal and hypertrophied hearts. *Can J Physiol Pharmacol.* 2003;81:40-47.

32. Wilson R, MacCarter D, St Cyr J. D-Ribose enhances the identification of hibernating myocardium. *Heart Drug.* 2003:3:61-62.

33. Van Gammeren D, Faulk D, Antonio J. The effects of four weeks of ribose supplementation on body composition and exercise performance in healthy, young male recreational bodybuilders: A double-blind, placebo-controlled trial. *Curr Ther Res.* 2002;63:486-495.

34. Sharma R, Munger M, Litwin S, Vardeny O, MacCarter D, St Cyr JA. D-Ribose improves Doppler TEI myocardial performance index and maximal exercise capacity in stage C heart failure. *J Mol Cell Cardiol.* 2005;38:853.

35. Pliml W, von Arnim T, Stablein A, Hofmann H, Zimmer HG, Erdmann E. Effects of ribose on exercise-induced ischaemia in stable coronary artery disease. *Lancet.* 1992;340:507-510.
36. Perkowski D, Wagner S, Marcus A, St Cyr JA. D-Ribose improves cardiac indices in patients undergoing "off" pump coronary arterial revascularization. *J Surg Res.* 2007;173:295.
37. Muller C, Zimmer H, Gross M, Gresser U, Brotsack I, Wehling M, Pliml W. Effect of ribose on cardiac adenine nucleotides in a donor model for heart transplantation. *Eur J Med Res.* 1998;3:554-558.
38. Grant GF, Gracey RW. Therapeutic nutraceutical treatments for osteoarthritis and ischemia. *Exp Opin Ther Patent*s. 2000;10: 1-10.

ABOUT THE AUTHOR

Dr. Jacob Teitelbaum is Medical Director of the Fibromyalgia and Fatigue Centers nationwide. He is senior author of the landmark studies "Effective Treatment of Chronic Fatigue Syndrome and Fibromyalgia – a Placebo-controlled Study" & "Effective Treatment of CFS & Fibromyalgia with D-Ribose". Dr. Teitlebaum is author of the best-selling books *From Fatigued to Fantastic!; Three Steps to Happiness! Healing through Joy;* and *Pain Free 1-2-3: A Proven Program to Get YOU Pain Free!*

Chapter 37
Reducing Cardio Metabolic Risk
Frederic J. Vagnini, M.D., FACS

ABSTRACT

Cardiovascular disease, namely high blood pressure, coronary atherosclerosis, and congestive heart failure, are the major cardiac problems both in this country and throughout the world today. These cardiovascular problems account for the high incidence of heart attack, stroke, and other circulatory problems, and heart disease continues to be the number one killer in the United States. Unfortunately, the statistics continue to rise in spite of the fact that many hi-tech advances have been made both in the pharmaceutical and surgical arenas, including powerful lipid-lowering drugs, robotic surgery, transplant surgery, and new innovations including gene therapy and stem cell therapy.

The present day treatment of heart disease is strictly reactive. In other words, patients are given pharmacologic therapy for cholesterol, blood pressure, triglycerides, or diabetes, whilst the underlying metabolic, genetic, and lifestyle problems are ignored. The aim of this paper is to show by addressing the problem of cardiometabolic risk and treatment of any underlying metabolic disorders it is possible to prevent and reverse heart disease, and also prevent other diseases such as diabetes and Alzheimer's disease.

INTRODUCTION

Cardiovascular disease, namely high blood pressure, coronary atherosclerosis, and congestive heart failure, are the major cardiac problems both in this country and throughout the world today. These cardiovascular problems account for the high incidence of heart attack, stroke, and other circulatory problems, and heart disease continues to be the number one killer in the United States. Unfortunately, the statistics continue to rise in spite of the fact that many hi-tech advances have been made both in the pharmaceutical and surgical arenas, including powerful lipid-lowering drugs, robotic surgery, transplant surgery, and new innovations including gene therapy and stem cell therapy.

The present day treatment of heart disease is strictly reactive. In other words, patients are given pharmacologic therapy for cholesterol, blood pressure, triglycerides, or diabetes, whilst the underlying metabolic, genetic, and lifestyle problems are ignored. The aim of this paper is to show by addressing the problem of cardiometabolic risk and treatment of any underlying metabolic disorders it is possible to prevent and reverse heart disease, and also prevent other diseases such as diabetes and Alzheimer's disease.

CARDIOMETABOLIC RISK

What does the term "cardiometabolic risk" mean? Cardiometabolic risk represents a group of modifiable risk factors that increases a person's chances of heart attack, stroke, diabetes, Alzheimer's disease, and some cancers. These risk factors include:

- Elevated blood pressure – remember, 135/85 is now classed as hypertension
- Intraabdominal adiposity (IAA) or visceral adiposity – defined as a waist circumference of 40" and above in men and 35" and above in women
- Low HDL-cholesterol
- Elevated LDL-cholesterol
- Elevated triglycerides
- Inflammatory markers
- Insulin resistance
- Smoking

Metabolic syndrome is a very important component of cardiometabolic risk. According to the Adult Treatment Panel of the National Cholesterol Education Program, the World Health Organization, the American Academy of Certified Endocrinologists, and the International Diabetes Foundation, metabolic syndrome is defined as:

- Elevated triglycerides
- Low HDL-cholesterol

- Elevated blood pressure
- Insulin resistance
- Two hour post glucose challenge >140
- Abdominal obesity (high waist circumference)
- High body mass index (BMI)
- Microalbuminuria

Metabolic syndrome is basically a genetic disorder complicated by poor lifestyle choices. The four most significant risk factors for metabolic syndrome are central obesity, hypertension, dyslipidemia, and abnormal glucose and insulin metabolism. What we are finding now is that people with metabolic syndrome often have low levels of HDL-cholesterol, low levels of testosterone, elevated uric acid levels, elevated homocysteine levels, and clotting abnormalities. Put together, all of these factors mean that a person with metabolic syndrome has an increased level of inflammation, and an increased risk of heart attack, stroke, Alzheimer's disease, certain cancers, and diabetes.

It is important to be aware that patients with one or two clinically evident cardiometabolic risk factors are likely to have more, and should therefore be evaluated for the full spectrum of cardiometabolic risk factors.

A number of physiologic pathways are involved in cardiometabolic risk, including: the endocrine system, intraabdominal adiposity (IAA) or visceral obesity (endocrine organ), renin-angiotensin system (RAS), immune system, dyslipidemia/atherogenesis, peroxisome proliferator-activated receptors (PPARs), and the endocannabinoid system.

Intraabdominal Adiposity is a Key Component of Cardiometabolic Risk

IAA is high-risk fat. IAA is now considered to be an endocrine organ in itself, and is associated with insulin resistance, elevated inflammatory markers, dyslipidemia, and hypertension. It is important to be aware that a person does not have to be obese to have IAA, it is possible for a person to be generally quite thin, but have a small amount of belly fat, which as we now know is very bioactive. Of course, if you see a patient like the one illustrated in Figure 1, it is obvious just by looking at them that their treatment is not going to be as simple as putting them on a diet. The man in Figure 1 clearly has a metabolic problem and low testosterone levels – he has the fat stomach, the gynecomastia, and very poor muscle tone.

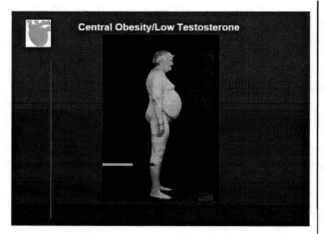

Figure 1. Illustration of a man with intraabdominal adiposity and low testosterone levels.

Why is IAA now classed as an endocrine organ in its own right? Because, it secretes a large number of very bioactive adipokines, including: leptin, tumor necrosis factor-alpha (TNF-α), interleukin-6 (IL-6), plasminogen activator inhibitor-1 (PAI1), adipsin, adiponectin, lipoprotein lipase, cholesterol ester transfer protein, apolipoprotein-E, angiotensisn, and resistin.

Adiponectin is secreted by fat. It is an adipose tissue-specific circulating protein, and is a key regulator of fat and metabolism. It is anti-atherogenic, anti-diabetic, and anti-inflammatory. IAA is associated with decreased levels of adiponectin, whilst a reduction in body weight is associated with increasing adiponectin levels. Decreased levels of adiponectin are associated with insulin resistance and increased levels of adiponectin are associated with improved insulin sensitivity. So, increased levels of adiponectin are desirable.

Pre-diabetes

If you really want to be a good anti-aging physician, you need to know how to treat diabetes correctly and you have to know how to identify pre-diabetes. Diabetics have a very short lifespan. The American Diabetes Association has now classified diabetes as both an endocrine disease and a cardiovascular disease.

An estimated 40-60 million US citizens have pre-diabetes. Pre-diabetes includes impaired fasting glucose (IFG) – a condition where blood glucose is above 90 but glucose tolerance is normal, and impaired glucose tolerance (IGT) – and is a significant risk factor for type 2 diabetes. Prior to developing type 2 diabetes, people almost always have pre-diabetes. Studies indicate that most people with pre-diabetes develop type 2 diabetes within 10 years. People with pre-diabetes and metabolic syndrome have an increased risk of atherosclerosis, heart attack, and stroke. Early recognition and treatment of pre-diabetes will allow the anti-aging physician to prevent the development of diabetes and its complications.

In a review article published in the *Lancet* in November 2006, Danaei *et al* concluded that higher than optimum blood glucose levels are responsible for 21% of deaths from ischemic heart disease and 13% of deaths from stroke worldwide. When added to deaths from diabetes, pre-diabetes becomes one of the top five causes of worldwide mortality, accounting for a staggering 3.16 million deaths per year.

If you have a patient with heart disease, take a look at their glucose levels. Many of them will have insulin resistance. They do not have to be obese. Take a look at their glucose. If you are in any doubt whatsoever, do an oral glucose tolerance test – not a fasting glucose test. Results of a study by Bartnik *et al* published very recently in January 2007 showed that patients with coronary heart disease need to have an oral glucose tolerance test instead of a fasting glucose, in order to accurately identify and classify impaired glucose regulation. Whilst fasting glucose will identify many cases of pre-diabetes, it will not identify all cases of pre-diabetes.

REDUCING CARDIOMETABOLIC RISK

Once you have established that a patient has IAA, metabolic syndrome, or pre-diabetes you need to do something about it. First and foremost you need to encourage them to lose weight, eat a healthy diet, and start exercising. Diet and exercise can be of great benefit, especially weightlifting. I get my patients to follow a program of resistance training and aerobic training, which helps to improve insulin sensitivity and reduce cardiovascular risk.

Then you need to start thinking about nurtraceuticals and pharmacological intervention. Many physicians would like to stay natural, but drug therapy is a must when you are dealing with sick cardiovascular patients, such as those with heart failure and postmyocardial infarction patients. Certainly, with diabetics you have got to use the full arsenal of drugs.

In order to reduce cardiometabolic risk we need to:
- Lower blood pressure
- Improve the lipid profile
- Reduce inflammation
- Increase immunity
- Reduce homocysteine levels
- Normalize hormone levels
- Improve gastrointestinal function
- Reduce bodyweight.

We are currently fighting a losing battle against obesity. In order to begin winning this battle we need to learn how to control appetite, improve glucose/insulin levels, block carbohydrates, decrease glycosolation, enhance thermogenesis, and increase energy. Most of all we need to begin targeting abdominal obesity (IAA).

Pharmacological Intervention

Glucophage (metformin) is a great drug; it helps to improve insulin sensitivity, decreases hepatic glucose production, and promotes weight loss. I use it extensively in my practice to treat obese people with high insulin levels and people with pre-diabetes. Glucophage is now being used in combination with other drugs, including thiazoladinediones (TZDs), for example Actos and Avandia.

TZDs work by activating peroxisome proliferator-activated receptors (PPARs), a group of receptor molecules inside the cell nucleus. Once activated the receptor migrates to the DNA and activates the transcription of a number of specific genes. TZDs are of great benefit to people with diabetes and metabolic syndrome because they improve insulin resistance, raise adiponectin levels, and lower levels of inflammatory cytokines such as IL-6. They also improve cardiovascular function by increasing nitric oxide (NO) bioavailability, decreasing the interaction between white blood cells and the endothelium, reducing vascular smooth muscle cell proliferation, and reducing cholesterol efflux from macrophages The downside to TZDs is that they can cause a patient to put on weight because they lower leptin levels (which increases appetite).

The endocannaboid system is a physiological system acting centrally and peripherally, which plays a key role in regulating body weight and metabolic processes. Research has shown that increased activity of the endocannabinoid system is associated with obesity, excessive food intake, and fat accumulation. Thus the endocannabinoid system represents a new target for pharmaceutical intervention.

Rimonabant is a selective CB1 cannabinoid receptor antagonist that has recently been approved in Europe. Rimonabant works by selectively blocking CB1 receptors both centrally and peripherally, which helps to normalize the overactivated endocannabinoid system. It has been shown to reduce all of the markers of metabolic syndrome – it reduces C-reactive protein levels, reduces IAA, improves dyslipidemia, and improves insulin resistance. Recent study results suggest that may also help to reduce hemoglobin A1c levels.

CONCLUDING REMARKS

It is extremely important for all anti-aging physicians to be able to easily recognize cardiometabolic risk factors. If a patient has two risk factors, or if they have abdominal obesity, the chances are that they are also going to have raised triglyceride levels, high blood pressure, and raised blood glucose levels, and should therefore be evaluated for the full spectrum of cardiometabolic risk factors.

Recognizing that a patient has metabolic syndrome or pre-diabetes and implementing an aggressive treatment protocol involving weight loss, improved diet, regular exercise, nutraceuticals, and, if necessary, pharmaceutical intervention, will help to significantly reduce their risk of heart attack, stroke, diabetes, Alzheimer's disease, and some forms of cancer.

REFERENCES

Bartnik M, Rydén L, Malmberg K, Ohrvik J, Pyörälä K, Standl E, Ferrari R, Simoons M, Soler-Soler J; Euro Heart Survey Investigators. Oral glucose tolerance test is needed for appropriate classification of glucose regulation in patients with coronary artery disease: a report from the Euro Heart Survey on Diabetes and the Heart. *Heart*. 2007;93:72-77. Epub 2006 Aug 11.

Danaei G, Lawes CM, Vander Hoorn S, Murray CJ, Ezzati M. Global and regional mortality from ischaemic heart disease and stroke attributable to higher-than-optimum blood glucose concentration: comparative risk assessment. *Lancet*. 2006;368:1651-1659. Review.

ABOUT THE AUTHOR

Dr. Frederic J. Vagnini is one of the most unique physicians in today's rapidly changing medical system. He embraces both traditional and holistic theories. Dr. Vagnini was graduated from Saint. Louis University School of Medicine where he received his Doctor of Medicine degree. He subsequently served in the United States Army as Lieutenant Colonel and entered into practice as a heart, blood vessel, and thoracic surgeon, which he continued for 20-plus years, and had, and continues to have a teaching appointment at Cornell where he is a Clinical Assistant Professor of Surgery. In more recent years, Dr. Vagnini has dedicated his practice to Clinical Nutrition and Preventive Medicine and the management of cardiovascular diseases, and he is presently Executive Medical Director for the Heart, Diabetes, and Weight Lss Centers of New York located in Westbury Long Island and in New York City.

Chapter 38
Two New Aspects of Astaxanthin for Human Health: Metabolic Syndrome and Eye Fatigue

Eiji Yamashita, Ph.D.
General Manager of Research & Development, Fuji Chemical Industry Co., Ltd.

ABSTRACT

Two new studies on natural astaxanthin, a carotenoid derived from the anti-aging microalgae *Haematococcus pluvialis,* revealed potential benefits for metabolic syndrome and eye fatigue. An animal study using metabolic syndrome model rats showed that 50mg/kg/day astaxanthin supplementation for 22 weeks significantly suppressed the development of metabolic syndrome by reducing blood pressure, fasting blood glucose level, and homeostasis index of insulin resistance, and improving insulin sensitivity. Astaxanthin administration also led to an improved adiponectin level, a significant increase in high-density lipoprotein cholesterol, and a significant decrease in plasma levels of triglycerides, and non-esterified fatty acids. Additionally, it showed significant effects on the white adipose tissue by decreasing the size of the fat cells. A double blind randomized placebo controlled human clinical study using visual display terminal (VDT) subjects (n=25 <treated> vs. 23 <placebo>) showed that 6mg/day astaxanthin supplementation for 4 weeks significantly improved visual accommodation during eye fatigue. The subjective questionnaire evaluating visual asthenopia revealed a marked reduction in "heavy head" claims. Other typical fatigue symptoms that showed improvements included "bleariness" and "stiff shoulders and back" in the treated group. Those findings suggest that astaxanthin is a promising natural candidate in lifestyle-related disease prevention and anti-fatigue, thus resulting in a decrease of medical expenses.

Keywords: ataxanthin, metabolic syndrome, eye fatigue, microalgae, *Haematococcus pluvialis*

INTRODUCTION

Astaxanthin is one of the most abundant carotenoids in nature, particularly in marine based life such as shrimps, crabs, salmon, and sea bream. In fact, it is one of the oldest carotenoids that was first isolated and identified from the lobster, *Astacus gammarus* in 1938.[1] Astaxanthin was first commercially used for pigmentation only in the aquaculture industry, that is until 1991 when biological activities – potent antioxidative properties and a physiological function as a vitamin A precursor in fish and mammals (rats) – were reported.[2, 3] It has also been reported that astaxanthin does not have any pro-oxidative properties, like β-carotene and lycopene,[4] and its potent antioxidative property is exhibited at the cell membrane.[5] Other studies suggest that astaxanthin may have anti-inflammatory[6, 7] and immunomodulatory[8] properties, and may also be useful for enhancing sport performance and endurance,[9] and limiting exercised-induced muscle damage.[10]

Synthetic astaxanthin has been available since 1984, but was limited to feed use. Nowadays, the research and demand for natural astaxanthin in human health applications are steadily growing. We have developed a mass production system to produce natural astaxanthin using the microalgae *Haematococcus pluvialis* (one of the major natural resources of astaxanthin), as we believe that astaxanthin can help to prevent lifestyle-related diseases and increase quality of life, and thus decrease medical expenses.

This purpose of this paper is to report our findings from two recent studies on astaxanthin – an animal study on the astaxanthin and metabolic syndrome, and a human study on astaxanthin and eye fatigue. The astaxanthin used in both studies is an extract from the microalgae.

ASTAXANTHIN AMELIORATES FEATURES OF METABOLIC SYNDROME IN RATS[11]

Metabolic syndrome is a worldwide-defined[12] lifestyle disease that is described as a clustering of multiple metabolic abnormalities and cardiovascular risk factors, including: hypertension, obesity, hyperlipidemia, and insulin resistance.[13] Metabolic syndrome has recently become a focus of a number of scientific studies aiming at its prevention and intervention.[14] We previously reported the antihypertensive effects[15-17] and action mechanisms[16] of astaxanthin in spontaneously hypertensive rats (SHR). In this study the effects of the astaxanthin on metabolic syndrome in SHR/NDmcr-cp (cp/cp), a model of metabolic syndrome (referred to as SHRcp) were investigated. This is the first study on the effects of carotenoids, including astaxanthin, on metabolic syndrome.

Methods

The animals were divided into three groups, a normal Wistar group and two SHRcp groups (6 rats/group), and were treated once daily for 22 weeks. The astaxanthin (AX) treated SHRcp group was administered daily AX [50 mg (83.8 mmol)/kg, intubation by p.o.], which was measured as 0.1 ml of the stock/100g bodyweight and diluted, for convenience and acceptability, by an equivalent volume of olive oil (OL) prior to administration. The other SHRcp-group and the Wistar group were adopted as control groups and were similarly treated with OL (1 ml/kg/day). All experimental procedures were performed in accordance with the standards established by the '*Guide for the Care and Use of Laboratory Animals at University of Toyama*'.

Body weight and food intake (FI) were measured daily during the experimental period. Blood pressure from the tail artery was indirectly measured once a week as previously reported[15] using tail-cuff apparatus (BP-98, Softron), which was controlled with a personal computer. Values are presented as the average of three independent measurements. Fasting blood glucose measurement was carried out at 0, 6, 12, and 18 weeks of treatment. Blood was withdrawn from the tail, and instantly tested using a blood glucose-measuring device – Antisense III (Horiba, Tokyo, Japan). Fasting insulin tolerance test was performed at 0, 30, 60, and 120 min after injection with insulin 1 ml/kg body weight (equivalent to 0.5 U/kg), i.p. Homeostasis model assessment of insulin resistance (HOMA-IR) was used to calculate the index of insulin resistance as [insulin (μU/ml) x glucose (mM)/ 22.5].[18] Blood insulin and adiponectin levels were measured using enzyme-linked immunosorbent assay kits (Morinaga Institute of Biological Science, Yokohama, Japan; and Otsuka Pharmaceuticals, Tokyo, Japan, respectively). Blood high-density lipoprotein (HDL)-cholesterol, free fatty acids (FFA), and triglyceride (TG) levels were determined by the HDL-cholesterol E, non-esterified fatty acid (NEFA) C-test, and TG L-type test (Wako, Osaka, Japan), respectively. To examine the size of white adipocytes, the number of adipocytes was counted in limited areas (capture size, 640 x 480 pixels, equivalent to 12,288 μm^2) of each stained specimen. The mean value of the adipocyte count was designated as an index of the cell size; as a larger number means a smaller size. Examination and photography of the slides was carried out using a light microscopy system (Olympus Provis AX80, Olympus Optical Co. Ltd., Tokyo). Calibration was carried out using a standard area of (1/20 x 1/20 mm) (Burker–Turk haemocytometer, JIS No. E3871, Kayagaki Irika Kogyo Co., LTD., Tokyo). Histological images were measured and analyzed blindly by two investigators using the UTHSCSA Image Tool for Windows, version 3.00 (San Antonio, Texas, USA). Statistical significance was determined by Student's t-test or Mann–Whitney Rank Sum Test for unpaired observations. One-way analysis of variance (ANOVA) was performed for multiple comparisons between groups. Differences with $p < 0.05$ were considered statistically significant.

Results

Effects of AX on blood pressure

In this study, AX showed a significant blood pressure-lowering effect on arterial blood pressure as shown in Figure 1. The body weight of AX-treated SHRcp did not significantly change, compared to the SHRcp-OL control group (data not shown). However, the SHRcp groups showed significantly higher body weight than the normal Wistar group, starting from 11 weeks of age (p<0.01), and exceeding a 100g difference from 22 weeks of age (p<0.001) (at the age of 25 weeks: Wistar, 420 ± 4 g; SHRcp, 534 ± 4 g). Similarly, no significant differences in daily FI were found among SHRcp groups, which also showed a higher FI than the Wistar group throughout the study (at 25 weeks: Wistar, 19 ± 0.4 g; SHRcp, 21 ± 0.7 g).

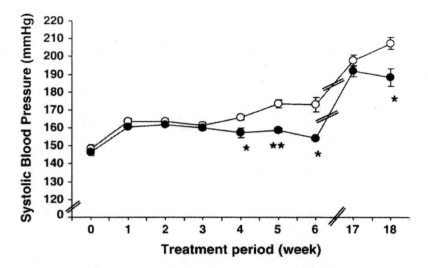

Fig. 1. Effects of oral administration of AX on systolic blood pressure in SHRcp. The animals received a control vehicle [OL (1 ml/kg/day), open circles], or AX [AX (50 mg/kg/day), closed circles] for an 18-week treatment period. Each data point represents the mean ± S.E.M. of 6 rats per group. *p<0.05; **p<0.01 vs. the control group (t-test).

Effect of AX on blood glucose level

The AX group showed a lower blood glucose level than the corresponding OL group (123.7 ± 0.3 and 154.7 ± 0.9 mg/dl, respectively). The effect was significant and comparable to the normal level in the Wistar group in the 18th week of treatment (Fig. 2).

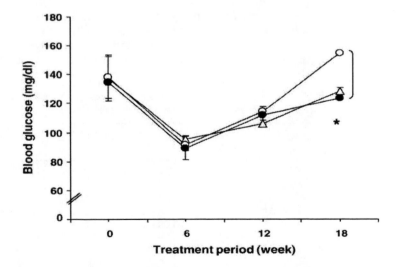

Fig. 2. Fasting blood glucose level in the AX-treated SHRcp group (closed circles), and the control OL-treated group: SHRcp (open circles), and Wistar (open triangles) rats. Data represent the mean ± S.E.M. (n = 5–6). *p<0.001 vs. the SHRcp control (t-test).

295

Effect of AX on insulin using insulin tolerance test

In insulin tolerance tests, 60 min after the insulin injection, the blood glucose level significantly dropped in the ASX group compared to the OL group. This effect was also maintained at 120 min (Fig. 3), indicating improved insulin sensitivity in SHRcp in the AX-treated group compared to the control group.

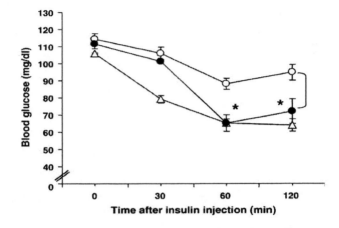

Fig. 3. Blood glucose level in the AX-treated SHRcp group (closed circles), and the control OL-treated group: SHRcp (open circles) and Wistar (open triangles) rats, at the insulin tolerance test. Data are the mean ± S.E.M. (*n* = 5–6). *p<0.05 *vs.* the control (*t*-test).

Time-course of the effects of AX on glucose metabolic parameters

During the 0–18 week-treatment period, fasting blood plasma of SHRcp showed lower levels of blood glucose and blood insulin in the AX group compared to the control OL group. The effect was significant on blood glucose after 18-week administration (Table 1). Plasma adiponectin level was higher in the AX group than in the control group, with a significant level in the 6th week (8.2 ± 0.1 and 5.9 ± 0.2 g/ml, respectively). The AX-treated group exhibited lower plasma levels of NEFA and TG than the control. The TG level was significantly lower for 6-week treatment (AX: 304.8 ± 10.6; OL: 414.8 ± 9.5 mg/dl).

Table 1. Time-course of the effects of AX on glucose metabolic parameters, measured from fasting blood plasma of SHRcp

Metabolic parameters	Treatment (week)	Wistar-OL	SHRcp-OL	SHRcp-AX
Blood glucose	0	137.0±15.1	138.3±4.8	135.0±2.1
(mg/dl)	6	95.3±2.4	91.7±4.3	89.3±8.2
	18	128.5±2.3	154.7±0.9	123.7±0.3*
Blood insulin	0	0.04±0.00	0.03±0.01	0.28±0.03
(ng/ml)	6	0.09±0.02	1.47±0.07	1.61±0.06
	18	0.19±0.03	1.78±0.04	1.63±0.07
HOMA-IR	0	0.28±0.04	0.23±0.09	2.23±0.15
	6	0.52±0.10	7.88±0.15	8.39±0.50
	18	1.18±0.09	16.15±0.30	11.87±0.50*
Adiponectin	0	4.81±0.28	7.38±0.27	7.08±0.43
(µg/ml)	6	4.44±0.59	5.91±0.16	8.21±0.14*
	18	4.87±0.29	5.18±0.15	5.84±0.29

HOMA-IR, homeostasis model assessment of insulin resistance.
Each value represents the mean±S.E.M. (*n* = 4).
*p<0.01 *vs.* the SHRcp control (*t*-test).

Effect of AX on lipid metabolic parameters, ex vivo

    After the treatment period, the non-fasting blood plasma in the AX-treated SHRcp group showed a significant increase in HDL-cholesterol level, compared to the control (77.77 ± 2.52 and 63.87 ± 2.32 mg/dl, respectively) (Fig. 4). It also exhibited a significantly lower level of NEFA compared to the corresponding control (0.71 ± 0.04 and 1.07 ± 0.07 mEq/l, respectively) (Fig. 5). The AX-treated group also exhibited a significant decrease in TG level compared to the OL group of SHRcp (360.8 ± 24.2 and 467.1 ± 11.8 mg/dl, respectively) (Fig. 6).

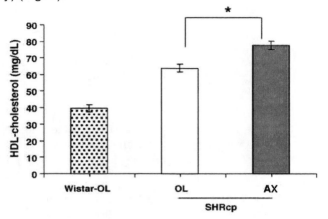

Fig. 4. HDL-cholesterol level in AX- and OL-treated SHRcp, *ex vivo*. Data are the mean ± S.E.M. (*n*=4–5). *p<0.01 *vs.* the control (*t*-test).

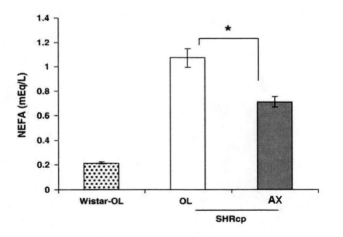

Fig. 5. NEFA level in AX- and OL-treated groups, *ex vivo*. Data represent the mean ± S.E.M. (*n*=4–5). *p<0.001 *vs.* the control (*t*-test).

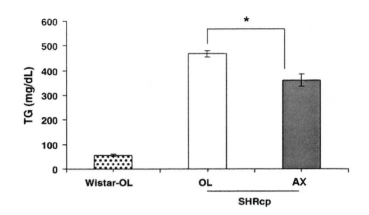

Fig. 6. TG level in AX- and OL-treated animals, *ex vivo.*
Data represent the mean ± S.E.M. (*n*=4).
*p<0.01 *vs.* the control (*t*-test).

Effect of AX on adipose tissue

In microscopic studies (Fig. 7), white adipose tissue of the AX-treated group showed large numbers and aggregates of small fat cells, clearly distinguished as discrete clusters or patches of cells. After treatment with AX for 22 weeks in SHRcp, the number of fat cells was significantly higher in the AX group than the control [SHRcp-AX group: 184 ± 3; SHRcp-OL: 140 ± 3 cells/12288µm^2 (mean ± S.E.M.), *n* = 5–6, p<0.01, *t*-test].

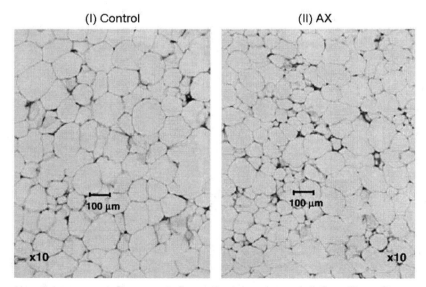

Fig. 7. Representative morphology of retroperitoneal white adipose tissue in control OL-treated (I) and AX-treated SHRcp (II).
Fat samples taken from a similar position as periperitoneal fat deposit were fixed, sectioned, and hematoxylin-eosin stained.

Discussion

In this study, AX significantly lowered the blood pressure, similar to our previous findings,[15, 16] and showed improving effects on glucose and lipid metabolic parameters. One of the most crucial findings was that AX significantly lowered the blood glucose level of SHRcp in insulin tolerance tests, suggesting that AX ameliorated insulin resistance and improved insulin sensitivity. The effect on insulin resistance was also significant, as shown by the HOMA-IR index, which is an indicator of insulin resistance, and closely correlated with insulin sensitivity.[18, 19] This is further supported by previous reports that AX (same material in this study) protects pancreatic β cells against glucose toxicity by preventing the progressive destruction of these cells in diabetic db/db mice.[20]

Another important finding is that AX showed an ameliorative and improving effect on lipid metabolic indices in SHRcp. AX significantly increased the HDL-cholesterol level in treated animals. It also significantly improved the levels of NEFA and TG, and the adiponectin marker. Lipid metabolic parameters have been widely described to play a crucial role in the development and progression of metabolic syndrome and its consequent sequelae. It is also worth mentioning that AX showed a significant effect on adipose tissue by inhibiting the proliferation of white adipose tissue, as indicated by the decreased size of adipocytes. The results showed a clear qualitative change reflected as an increase in cellularity as shown visually on the micrographs, where clusters of small adipocytes are clearly dispersed throughout the fat tissue. This adipogenic effect, which results in the generation of small fat cells, may explain the decrease in circulating FFA and the improvement in adiponectin and insulin resistance. These cellular effects are most likely attributed to regulatory factors, mainly peroxisome proliferator-activated receptors gamma (PPAR-γ), which are widely reported to reduce circulating levels of FFA and stimulate adipocyte differentiation, thus favoring the formation of smaller, more insulin-sensitive adipocytes.[21-23] This observed effect of AX on white adipose tissue may add further support to AX potential against metabolic syndrome. Considering the finding that AX did not show a significant effect on insulin level, it is unlikely that AX induces its effect on insulin resistance directly on the blood insulin level. It is widely accepted that, although insulin resistance leads to a decrease in glucose uptake, the relationship between glucose and insulin is quite complex and involves the interaction of many metabolic and regulatory factors.[24]

In conclusion, our results indicate that AX ameliorates insulin resistance by mechanisms involving the increase of glucose uptake, and by modulating the levels of circulating adiponectin and blood lipids. These findings suggest that AX is a promising natural candidate in lifestyle-related disease prevention. However, further studies on the molecular action mechanisms as well as clinical investigations are strongly recommended.

THE SUPPLEMENTATION EFFECT OF ASTAXANTHIN ON ACCOMMODATION AND ASTHENOPIA[25]

Along with the growth in the number of visual display terminal (VDT) workers, physical and mental fatigue suffered by individuals engaged in VDT work for long periods of time has become a major problem. In April 2002, Japan's Ministry of Health, Labor, and Welfare enacted new *Guidelines for Industrial Health Controls of VDT Operations*,[26] which describe in detail the standards for mitigating the physical and mental burdens on VDT workers. Occurrences of problems such as asthenopia, eye pain, eye dryness, stiff neck and shoulders, and headaches are cited as subjective symptoms of individuals engaged in VDT work, and asthenopia and its concurrent whole body symptoms have become problems. In addition to a survey to determine the presence of subjective symptoms, the ministry guidelines require ophthalmological examinations, including a visual acuity test, refractometry, eye position examination, and ocular accommodation examination, as items to be included in checkups of workers engaged in VDT work for 4 hours or more per day. A marked decrease in ocular accommodation has been reported to be a cause of asthenopia.[27] Treatments, such as vitamin B12 ophthalmic solutions, are being used to relieve asthenopia,[28] and there have recently been a number of trials of dietary supplements designed to prevent and mitigate asthenopia in VDT workers. We conducted a randomized double blind placebo controlled study to evaluate the effect on asthenopia of a dietary supplement containing astaxanthin (AX).

Subjects

The subjects were individuals chosen from among workers who regularly are engaged in VDT work and complained of asthenopia, and who satisfied the following selection criteria and did not fail the exclusion criteria.

1. Individuals who have engaged in VDT work for at least six hours per day for 1 year or longer and suffer from asthenopia on a daily basis.
2. As a rule, individuals whose amplitude of accommodation is lower than the amplitude of accommodation corresponding to their age (judged using near point ruler data).
3. As a rule, individuals whose corrected visual acuity for both eyes is 1.0 or higher, and who will not change the contact lens or glasses they use for correction during the study period.
4. As a rule, individuals ages 30 to 45 years old when they consent to participate in the study
5. Without regard to gender.
6. Individuals capable of observing the rules to be followed for the study and being tested and examined as set forth in the plan for the study.

Exclusion criteria

1. Individuals with an organic ophthalmopathy/ocular disease.
2. Individuals with an ametropia that is not being corrected appropriately.
3. Individuals with an ophthalmopathy thought to originate in a cause other than accommodative asthenopia, such as nervousness.
4. Individuals who are regularly taking medication (including ophthalmic preparations) or consuming products such as health foods thought to be effective against asthenopia (vitamin preparations, tonics containing taurine compounds, etc.).
5. Individuals with an allergy to medicine.
6. Individuals who are pregnant, breastfeeding, or might be pregnant.
7. Other individuals the governing investigator or the principal investigators find to be unsuitable.

Among the 86 individuals who visited the hospital for the screening examination, 25 individuals were evaluated to be unsuitable for the following reasons based on a clinical assessment, and were excluded;

*   Ametropia (−8.0 or higher diopter myopia. Or −1.5 or higher diopter astigmatism): 8 individuals.
*   Short VDT working hours: 3 individuals.
*   Age 50 or older: 4 individuals (including 2 with glaucoma).
*   Degree of asthenopia too small: 6 individuals (including 1 with an ametropia).
*   High value in hepatic function examination: 3 individuals.
*   Examination not possible because pupils would not dilate: 1 individual.

After excluding 2 individuals selected for the study because they did not visit the hospital for an examination before beginning supplementation, 59 individuals were ultimately included in the study.

A study review committee at Kyouryoukai Ichinomiya Nishi Hospital where the study was carried out verified the study presented no problems scientifically or ethically. The study was implemented with sufficient consideration of the subjects' human rights and in accordance with the spirit of the Declaration of Helsinki.

Methods

Materials

Soft capsules containing 3mg of AX and externally identical control placebo capsules that did not contain AX were used. Subject allocation to the AX supplemented group and the control group (placebo group) was performed to ensure uniformity between the two groups, based on amplitude of accommodation (D'ACOMO) values at the time of the screening examinations.

Dose and supplementation period

The AX 0mg group (control group) and the AX 6mg supplementation group (AX supplemented group) were compared in a double-blind study. The subjects took 2 capsules once each day after dinner for four weeks.

Test items and schedules

The test items and schedules are shown in Fig. 8.

	Observation period		Supplementation period	
	(2 weeks)		(4 weeks)	
	Week −2	Week 0	Week 2	Week 4
Test items				
Subject screening	●			
Allocation to groups		●		
Ophthalmologic examinations	●[1]	●[2]		●[3]
Subjective asthenopia evaluation	●	●	●	●
Blood biochemistry examinations	●			●
Blood chemistry examinations	●			●
Sphygmomanometry		●		
Interviews	●	●		●
Material intake circumstances		←———————————————→		
Subjective symptoms		←———————————————→		

1) Visual acuity testing, refractometry, amplitude of accommodation, slit-lamp examination, ophthalmoscopy
2) Visual acuity testing, amplitude of accommodation
3) Visual acuity testing, amplitude of accommodation, slit-lamp examination, ophthalmoscopy

Fig. 8. Test protocol

Ophthalmologic examinations

Because the majority of VDT workers who complain of asthenopia are thought to have accommodative asthenopia involving ciliary body function, during screening a visual acuity test, refractometry, slit-lamp examination, ophthalmoscopy, amplitude of accommodation examination, and an interview were conducted, and the presence or absence of muscular asthenopia (involving the extraocular muscles, such as squinting), symptomatic asthenopia (caused by an organic ophthalmopathy/ocular disease, such as glaucoma) and nervous asthenopia (caused by psychological factors, such as a nervous breakdown) was confirmed. Visual acuity testing and measurement of amplitude of accommodation were performed before supplementation (Week 0), and visual acuity testing, measurement of amplitude of accommodation, a slit-lamp examination and ophthalmoscopy were performed after supplementation for four weeks (Week 4). Measurements of amplitude of accommodation were made using a binocular opening constant point refraction near point ruler (D'ACOMO) manufactured by World Optical Corporation (WOC) and an infrared optometer (Accommodometer AA-2000) from Nidek Co., Ltd.

Subjective questionnaire

A subjective questionnaire was distributed before the study, in which subjects entered their subjective asthenopia evaluations, record of the material intake circumstances and subjective symptoms (adverse events) survey. The subjective asthenopia evaluation was completed by the subjects by entering checkmarks in the questionnaire before supplementation and after supplementation for two weeks and four weeks. The survey covered a total of 11 items as shown below, including items i) – vii) concerning the eyes and items viii) – xi) concerning physical condition, for which the subjects evaluated the level of their subjective symptoms at that time according to five levels: "No at all," "A little," "About half the time," "Somewhat frequently" and "Considerably."

i)   Tired eyes
ii)   Painful eyes
iii) Bleariness
iv)   Tearing eyes
v)   Red eyes
vi)   Seeing spots

301

Seeing double
viii) Stiff shoulders and back
ix) Easily irritated
x) Heavy head
xi) Headaches

Blood chemistry examination and blood biochemistry examination

Blood chemistry examination and blood biochemistry examination were performed before supplementation and after supplementation for four weeks. The following items were analyzed in the respective examinations.

- Blood chemistry examination; erythrocyte count, leukocyte count, hemoglobin content, hematocrit, MCV, MCH, MCHC, and blood platelet count.
- Blood biochemistry examination; total bilirubin, total protein, albumin, A/G ratio, AST, ALT, ALP, LDH, γ-GTP, CPK, total cholesterol, neutral fat, HDL cholesterol, arterial stiffness index, Na, K, Cl, Ca, Mg, urea nitrogen, creatinine, uric acid, fasting blood sugar level and HbA1c.

Sphygmomanometry

Blood pressure was measured before supplementation and after supplementation for four weeks.

Physician interviews

Examinations and interviews by a physician were performed when the subjects were selected, before supplementation, and after supplementation for four weeks. After supplementation for four weeks, the subjects also were surveyed concerning any adverse events.

Statistical analysis

For comparison of the data for the two groups, a test of homoscedasticity was performed using the F test, Student's t-test was performed to test assumption of homoscedasticity, and an Aspin-Welch t-test was performed to test assumption of heteroscedasticity. For time series data, a paired t-test was performed. For the asthenopia questionnaires and amplitude of accommodation data, a Mann-Whitney U test was performed on data between the groups. The time series data were analyzed using the Wilcoxon signed rank test. For data categorizing the rate of change in amplitude of accommodation, a chi-square test or Fisher's exact test was performed. The significance level was based on a degree of error of less than 5% ($p < 0.05$). The amplitude of accommodation and subjective asthenopia questionnaire data displayed a tendency to be less than 10% ($p < 0.10$).

Results

A total of 59 subjects were incorporated into the study, in a control group of 28 individuals and an AX supplemented group of 31 individuals. Of these, 5 individuals in the control group and 6 individuals in the AX supplemented group (including 1 individual who took only one capsule per day during the study period) who continually used an ophthalmic preparation during the study period were judged to be inappropriate for evaluating the effects of the materials, and were excluded from the evaluations of amplitude of accommodation and subjective asthenopia. Therefore a total of 48 individuals, including 23 in the control group and 25 in the AX supplemented group, were evaluated for effect, and a total of 59 individuals, including 28 in the control group and 31 in the AX supplemented group, were assessed for safety.

There were no differences between the two groups in age, gender (male/female ratio), height and weight. There were also no differences found between the two groups in systolic blood pressure and diastolic blood pressure before supplementation. No differences were found between the two groups in systolic blood pressure and diastolic blood pressure after supplementation as well, and no significant changes in blood pressure before and after supplementation were detected within the respective groups. Visual acuity was compared by converting uncorrected decimal visual acuity values to logMAR values. Although no significant change was shown within either group in the comparison before and after supplementation, in the comparison between the two groups, compared with the control group the AX supplemented group was significantly inferior both before and after ingestion. There was no difference between the two groups in the use of glasses and contact lens (data not shown).

Ophthalmologic Examinations

No abnormal findings were noted in either group by the slit-lamp examination and ophthalmoscopy performed before and after supplementation.

Table 2 shows the amplitude of accommodation measurement results. The measurements were taken by an orthoptist. For measuring instruments, D'ACOMO, which is used frequently by ophthalmologists to evaluate VDT fatigue and judge the suitability of contact lens and glasses, and Accommodometer AA-2000, which was used to verify the improvement effect of AX on amplitude of accommodation, were used. No difference was found between the two groups in amplitude of accommodation before supplementation using either measurement method. When the D'ACOMO was used, for the control group the value before supplementation was 4.16 ± 1.14 and 4.03 ± 1.12 after supplementation for four weeks. No significant difference was found before and after supplementation. For the AX supplemented group, on the other hand, the value before supplementation was 4.29 ± 1.11, and rose to 4.69 ± 1.17 after supplementation for four weeks, meaning a significant improvement in amplitude of accommodation was found before and after supplementation. In the comparison between the two groups as well, the AX supplemented group was significantly better compared with the control group. In the measurements using the AA-2000, there was no significant difference before and after supplementation in the control group, but a significant rise was found in the AX supplemented group. In the comparison between the two groups, the AX supplemented group tended to be superior compared with the control group.

Table 2. Amplitude of accommodation

Group	Placebo	Astaxanthin
D'ACOMO accommodation (D)		
Before supplementation	4.16 ± 1.14	4.29 ± 1.11
After supplementation	4.03 ± 1.12	4.69 ± 1.17*#
Magnitude of change	-0.13 ± 0.46	0.40 ± 0.74**
Rate of change (%)	-2.7 ± 10.0	11.1 ± 18.7**
AA-2000 accommodation (D)		
Before supplementation	4.22 ± 1.64	4.46 ± 1.73
After supplementation	4.01 ± 1.75	4.82 ± 1.54+#
Magnitude of change	-0.21 ± 0.59	0.36 ± 0.73**
Rate of change (%)	-6.0 ± 18.5	13.2 ± 23.5**

Each value shows mean ± standard deviation
*: $p < 0.05$, **: $p < 0.01$, Significant difference compared with placebo (t-test)
#: $p < 0.05$, Significant difference compared with before supplementation (paired t-test)
+: $p < 0.10$, Tendency compared with placebo (t-test)

As far as the magnitude of change of amplitude of accommodation before and after supplementation for each individual subject is concerned, in the measurements using the D'ACOMO the control group values were −0.13 ± 0.46 and those for the AX supplemented group were 0.40 ± 0.74, compared with the control group the magnitude of change of the AX supplemented group was significantly large. Similarly, in the measurements using the AA-2000, the magnitude of change of the AX supplemented group was significantly large. Moreover, the magnitude of change versus the values before supplementation was significantly better for the AX supplemented group compared with the control group.

The distribution of subjects by the extent to which amplitude of accommodation improved or changed (magnitude of change) compared with before supplementation was calculated from the D'ACOMO measurement results. In the AX supplemented group there were many subjects for whom amplitude of accommodation changed greatly, and compared with the control group the AX supplemented group was significantly better. The number of cases improved by 10% or more was 1 individual in the control group and 13 individuals in the AX supplemented group, and a significant difference between the two groups was found. Moreover, a similar result was obtained from the results of measurements using the AA-2000 (data not shown).

Subjective Asthenopia Evaluations

A subjective asthenopia evaluation was conducted by having the subjects check a questionnaire before supplementation and for both two and four weeks after supplementation (data not shown). The subjects evaluated the level of their subjective symptoms at the time of each assessment using a five-stage scale ranging from "0 – Not at all" to "5 – Considerably." As shown in Table 3, no differences were seen between the two groups in the level of each subjective symptom before supplementation. Compared with before supplementation, the subjective symptom items for which a significant difference was seen after supplementation (after supplementation for two weeks or four weeks) for the control group were the 7 items: "tired eyes," "painful eyes," "bleariness," "seeing double," "stiff shoulders and back," "easily irritated" and "headaches," while for the AX supplemented group, on the other hand, a difference was noted for the 7 items "tired eyes," "bleariness," "tearing eyes," "red eyes," "stiff shoulders and back," "heavy head" and "headaches." In a comparison between the two groups, after supplementation for four weeks the AX supplemented group was significantly better for the two items "bleariness" and "stiff shoulders and back," and an improvement tendency was seen for "heavy head."

Table 3. Subjective questionnaire

Group		Placebo					Astaxanthin				
		Level of symptom[1]					Level of symptom[1]				
		0	1	2	3	4	0	1	2	3	4
Tired eyes	Before supplementation	1	8	5	8	1	0	8	8	8	1
	After 4 weeks	3	10	6	3	1#	4	14	5	1	1##
Painful eyes	Before supplementation	10	7	6	0	0	15	4	5	1	0
	After 4 weeks	14	7	2	0	0#	17	7	0	1	0x
Bleariness	Before supplementation	2	11	7	3	0	7	9	6	3	0
	After 4 weeks	6	11	4	2	0#	15	7	1	2	0+##
Tearing eyes	Before supplementation	10	9	3	1	0	11	11	3	0	0
	After 4 weeks	15	5	2	1	0x	17	7	1	0	0#
Red eyes	Before supplementation	10	8	3	2	0	8	18	2	0	0
	After 4 weeks	11	10	1	1	0x	17	6	2	0	0##
Seeing spots	Before supplementation	8	10	4	1	0	10	11	2	2	0
	After 4 weeks	11	10	2	0	0x	15	6	4	0	0x
Seeing double	Before supplementation	14	4	4	1	0	12	8	3	2	0
	After 4 weeks	17	5	0	1	0#	15	6	3	1	0x
Stiff shoulders and back	Before supplementation	3	3	6	5	6	4	9	3	5	4
	After 4 weeks	3	6	9	5	0##	8	10	4	2	1+##
Easily irritated	Before supplementation	7	4	8	3	1	7	10	4	4	0
	After 4 weeks	9	7	4	3	0#	13	4	5	3	0x
Heavy head	Before supplementation	7	5	5	5	1	8	9	7	1	0
	After 4 weeks	9	7	2	4	1x	15	8	1	1	0+##
Headaches	Before supplementation	10	2	7	3	1	13	4	7	1	0
	After 4 weeks	13	4	3	2	1#	16	5	3	1	0x

1): 0 – Not at all, 1 – A little, 2 – About half the time, 3 – Somewhat frequently, 4 – Considerably
*: p<0.05 vs. placebo (Mann-Whitney's U test), #: p<0.05 & ##: p<0.01 vs. before supplementation (Wilcoxon signed rank test)
+: p<0.10, Tendency vs. placebo (Mann-Whitney's U test), x: p<0.10, Tendency vs. before supple. (Wilcoxon signed rank test)

Safety Evaluation

No significant differences or adverse events were detected between the treated and the placebo groups after four weeks of supplementation in the safety parameters analyzed (data not shown).

Discussion

Ocular accommodation measurements have been made in diagnoses of asthenopia,[29] and along with subjective symptoms the effects of vitamin B preparations on asthenopia have been evaluated using ocular accommodation.[28, 30, 31] Furthermore, in addition to subjective symptoms, an ophthalmologic examination including an ocular accommodation examination has been recommended in the Ministry of Health, Labor and Welfare's *Guidelines for Industrial Health Controls of VDT Operations*[26] as an examination to prevent worker health problems. The guidelines note that *"ocular accommodation decreases with age, but because a marked decrease is one cause of asthenopia, employers are to measure ocular accommodation before assigning workers to VDT work."* Based on the above guidelines, amplitude of accommodation was judged to be an important objective indicator for evaluations of asthenopia in the study.

For the measurements of amplitude of accommodation, the D'ACOMO which also is utilized for comparatively inexpensive VDT medical checkups was used for this study. Compared with the Ishihara-type near point ruler used in the past, with the D'ACOMO it is possible to take measurements under conditions most similar to natural sight, which is said to produce results with minimal variation as well as excellent reproducibility, and because operation is simple, measurements can be taken in a short time.[32-34] On the other hand, the Accommodometer AA-200 is a device that can measure amplitude of accommodation objectively. Therefore for this study, measurements were made simultaneously using both devices.

Consequently, significant improvements by AX supplementation were observed in ocular accommodation by objective instrumental measurement and in "bleariness" and "stiff shoulders and back" by subjective individual assessment for four weeks. It seems that muscular fatigue[9] in the ciliary body was ameliorated by increasing (normalizing) not just retinal, but, whole body blood flow[35, 36] and/or inhibiting the inflammation in the eyes.[7]

CONCLUDING REMARKS

The results of these two studies suggest that AX is a promising natural candidate for the prevention of lifestyle-related disease, such as metabolic syndrome, and eye fatigue, thus resulting in a decrease of medical expenses.

REFERENCES

1. Kuhn R, Sorensen NA. *Ber Deut Bot Ges*. 1938;71:1879.
2. Miki W. Biological functions and activities of animal carotenoids. *Pure & Appl. Chem.* 1991;63:141-146.
3. Matsuno T. Xanthophylls as precursors of retinoids. *Pure & Appl. Chem.* 1991;63:81-88.
4. Martin HD, Ruck C, Schmidt M, Sell S, Beutner S, Mayer B, Walsh R. Chemistry of carotenoid oxidation and free radical reactions. *Pure Appl.Chem.* 1999;71:2253-2262.
5. Goto S, Kogure K, Abe K, Kimata Y, Kitahama K, Yamashita E, Terada H. Efficient radical trapping at the surface and inside the phospholipid membrane is responsible for highly potent antiperoxidative activity of the carotenoid astaxanthin. *Biochim Biophys Acta*. 2001;1512:251-258.
6. Lee SJ, Bai SK, Lee KS, Namkoong S, Na HJ, Ha KS, Han JA, Yim SV, Chang K, Kwon YG, Lee SK, Kim YM. Astaxanthin inhibits nitric oxide production and inflammatory gene expression by suppressing I(kappa)B kinase-dependent NF-kappaB activation. *Mol Cells*. 2003;16:97-105.
7. Suzuki Y, Ohgami K, Shiratori K, Jin XH, Ilieva I, Koyama Y, Yazawa K, Yoshida K, Kase S, Ohno S. Suppressive effects of astaxanthin against rat endotoxin-induced uveitis by inhibiting the NF-kappaB signaling pathway. *Exp Eye Res*. 2006;82:275-281. Epub 2005 Aug 26.
8. Jyonouchi H, Zhang L, Tomita Y. Studies of immunomodulating actions of carotenoids. II. Astaxanthin enhances in vitro antibody production to T-dependent antigens without facilitating polyclonal B-cell activation. *Nutr Cancer*. 1993;19:269-280.
9. Sawaki K, Yoshigi H, Aoki K, Koikawa N, Azumane A, Kaneko K, Yamaguchi M. *Therap. & Med.* 2002;18:73-88.
10. Aoi W, Naito Y, Sakuma K, Kuchide M, Tokuda H, Maoka T, Toyokuni S, Oka S, Yasuhara M, Yoshikawa T. Astaxanthin limits exercise-induced skeletal and cardiac muscle damage in mice. *Antioxid Redox Signal*. 2003;5:139-144.
11. Hussein G, Nakagawa T, Goto H, Shimada Y, Matsumoto K, Sankawa U, Watanabe H. Astaxanthin ameliorates features of metabolic syndrome in SHR/NDmcr-cp. *Life Sci.* 2007;80:522-529.
12. WHO, Definition, Diagnosis and Classification of Diabetes Mellitus and its Complications: Report of a WHO Consultation, Geneva, Switzerland: Department of Noncommunicable Disease Surveillance. World Health Organization, 1999.
13. Eckel RH, Grundy SM, Zimmet PZ. The metabolic syndrome. *Lancet*. 2005;365:1415-1428.
14. Moller DE. New drug targets for type 2 diabetes and the metabolic syndrome. *Nature*. 2001;414:821-827.

15. Hussein G, Nakamura M, Zhao Q, Iguchi T, Goto H, Sankawa U, Watanabe H. Antihypertensive and neuroprotective effects of astaxanthin in experimental animals. *Biol Pharm Bull.* 2005;28:47-52.

16. Hussein G, Goto H, Oda S, Iguchi T, Sankawa U, Matsumoto K, Watanabe H. Antihypertensive potential and mechanism of action of astaxanthin: II. Vascular reactivity and hemorheology in spontaneously hypertensive rats. *Biol Pharm Bull.* 2005;28:967-971.

17. Hussein G, Goto H, Oda S, Sankawa U, Matsumoto K, Watanabe H. Antihypertensive potential and mechanism of action of astaxanthin: III. Antioxidant and histopathological effects in spontaneously hypertensive rats. *Biol Pharm Bull.* 2006;29:684-688.

18. Matthews DR, Hosker JP, Rudenski AS, Naylor BA, Treacher DF, Turner RC. Homeostasis model assessment: insulin resistance and beta-cell function from fasting plasma glucose and insulin concentrations in man. *Diabetologia.* 1985;28:412-419.

19. Pickavance LC, Tadayyon M, Widdowson PS, Buckingham RE, Wilding JP. Therapeutic index for rosiglitazone in dietary obese rats: separation of efficacy and haemodilution. *Br J Pharmacol.* 1999;128:1570-1576.

20. Naito Y, Uchiyama K, Aoi W, Hasegawa G, Nakamura N, Yoshida N, Maoka T, Takahashi J, Yoshikawa T. Prevention of diabetic nephropathy by treatment with astaxanthin in diabetic db/db mice. *Biofactors.* 2004;20:49-59.

21. Schoonjans K, Staels B, Auwerx J. The peroxisome proliferator activated receptors (PPARS) and their effects on lipid metabolism and adipocyte differentiation. *Biochim Biophys Acta.* 1996;1302:93-109.

22. Spiegelman BM. PPAR-gamma: adipogenic regulator and thiazolidinedione receptor. *Diabetes.* 1998;47:507-514.

23. Vázquez M, Silvestre JS, Prous JR. Experimental approaches to study PPAR gamma agonists as antidiabetic drugs. *Methods Find Exp Clin Pharmacol.* 2002;24:515-523.

24. Radziuk J. Insulin sensitivity and its measurement: structural commonalities among the methods. *J Clin Endocrinol Metab.* 2000;85:4426-4433. Review.

25. Nagaki Y, Mihara M, Tsukuhara H, Ohno S. *Therap. & Med.* 2006;22:41-54.

26. Ministry of Health, Labour and Welfare Labor Standards Bureau, Guidelines for Industrial Health Controls of VDT Operations, 2002.

27. Iwasaki T, Tawara A, Miyake N. [Reduction of asthenopia-related to accommodative relaxation] *Nippon Ganka Gakkai Zasshi.* 2003;107:257-264. [In Japanese.]

28. Yamachi R, Yamashita T, Kitano S. *Nippon Ganka Gakkai Zasshi.* 1978;32:1013-1025.

29. Nakamura Y. *J Eye.* 1997;14:1319-1326

30. Wakakura M, Kishida C, Ishikawa S. *Med Cons New-Remed.* 1989;26:1645-1653.

31. Irie L, Furuya H, Matsukuma K. *Med Cons New-Remed.* 2001;38:617-621.

32. Kubo T. *J. Jpn. Assoc. Cert. Orth.* 1989;17:71-74.

33. Kominai M, Uemura S, Nakagawa T. *J Jpn Soc Ophth.* 1990;11:137-141.

34. Nakagawa T, Uozato H. *Ophthalmology* 1991;33:591-594.

35. Nagaki Y, Mihara M, Takahashi J, Kitamura A, Yoshiharu H, Sugiura Y, Tsukuhara H. *Therap & Med.* 2005;21:537-542.

36. Miyawaki H, Takahashi J, Tsukuhara H, Takehara I. *J Clin Ther Med.* 2005;21:421-429.

ABOUT THE AUTHOR

Dr. Eiji Yamashita is the Global Research & Development Manager for Fuji Chemical Industry Co., Ltd. He completed a pre-doctoral fellowship at the University of Texas Health Science Center and received his Ph.D. from the University of Tokushima. Yamashita's research experience and scientific contributions span nearly 20 years in the study of carotenoids and antioxidants.

Chapter 39
Measurement of Free Steroid Hormone Levels in Anti-Aging Medicine: Techniques and Pitfalls

Dr. Wolfgang Ziemann
Biochemist, Demeditec Diagnostics GmbH

ABSTRACT

At present, the majority of steroid hormone determinations are conducted from serum samples, even if results in the low or very low concentration range are expected, for example, in elderly patients. This is a real challenge for any diagnostic laboratory. Another major problem associated with the measurement of free hormone levels from serum is the episodic secretion pattern of steroid hormones. It has been known since the 1980's that steroid secretion shows a significant episodic pattern in serum as well as in saliva. Nevertheless, most of the determinations are still made from just one serum sample. This results in non-reproducible results due to the biological CV. Moreover, the measurement of serum concentrations in the low concentration range is technically rather difficult, as it recently has been shown in the scientific literature. In general, serum measurements can only give the total steroid hormone concentration, whereas saliva testing results in the measurement of the free active hormone fraction. Therefore, salivary testing is a reliable alternative provided multiple sampling is done. We recommend that four of five samples should be obtained within 2 or 3 hours, and the successive measurement of one mixed sample. In contrast to this, steroid measurements in just one single saliva sample always will give arbitrary results.

The analytical sensitivity of current commercial saliva test kits allow for a reliable and reproducible measurement – even in the very low concentration range (below 1 pg/ml). Furthermore, these results represent the free hormone concentration, or the active hormone fraction. Therefore, saliva hormone measurements may well provide us with a better and more convenient alternative to serum testing for steroid determinations in anti-aging medicine in males and in females.

The aim of this paper is to discuss currently available analytical procedures used to measure steroid hormones in blood and saliva. All the major issue surrounding saliva sampling will be considered, including: interference in saliva sampling, the stability of saliva sampling, saliva sampling strategies, the physiology of steroid secretion, and laboratory aspects of saliva sampling.

INTRODUCTION

For almost a century various steroid hormone determinations have been performed from a variety of body fluids in the diagnostic laboratory to gather relevant information and assist clinicians in the diagnosis of various pathological conditions. Perhaps the most notable activity occurred in the 1960's when new analytical methods emerged that demonstrated superior analytical sensitivity at the low end of expected concentration ranges.

The concentration of the biologically active free fraction of steroid hormones in circulation is extremely low. Therefore it is important to use sensitive laboratory tests in order to quantify these low levels of analyte. Use of less sensitive lab tests may result in inaccurate assessment, which can, in turn, lead to the misinterpretation of a patient's condition. Unfortunately, there are still analytical methods in routine laboratory use that lack the appropriate analytical sensitivity. The aim of this paper is to discuss currently available analytical procedures used to measure steroid hormones in blood and saliva.

BLOOD, URINE AND SALIVA AS ANALYTICAL MATERIAL

Today, steroid hormone testing is primarily conducted from blood products (serum or plasma). The use of urine samples to measure steroid hormones is no longer common. For a urine sample to be useful, a 24-hour urine should be collected and tested. In fact, the 24-hour urinary excretion of conjugated steroids still gives a useful result correlating with free steroid activity. However, the collection process is not convenient for the patient and does not allow the clinician the possibility of establishing a profile of hormone activity (diurnal cycle) at strategic intervals throughout the day.

Steroid measurement in serum or plasma is by far more common than urine testing, although difficulties involved with blood testing have been documented, especially related to lower concentrations.

In 2003 Taieb et al[1] published a landmark study regarding the validity of the most common commercial methods used for the measurement of testosterone in serum. Remarkably, this study concluded that none of the ten commercial serum testing methods was found to be sufficiently reliable for measurement of low concentrations of testosterone (which are typically seen in children and women). Equally as notable, the editors of Clinical Chemistry, the journal in which the paper was published, commented that guessing would be just as accurate as a serum laboratory test for testosterone.[2] To extend this line of logic; guessing is fast, non-invasive, and inexpensive. Unfortunately, much like serum testing, it isn't very accurate. A number of other studies have produced similar results for estradiol and testosterone measurement in serum at low concentration levels.[3-5] These studies suggest that an additional extraction step would significantly improve the performance of commercial assays, thus suggesting that there is either a matrix effect or cross-reactivity to steroid conjugates (if not both) in commercial immunoassays for serum testing. Either possibility would result in inaccurate lab test results from serum samples.

In order to understand the basic differences in the measurement of steroid hormones in blood and saliva it is important to understand the different physiological forms of these hormones. Most of the steroid hormones in blood are tightly bound to special "carrier" proteins e.g. corticosteroid binding globulin (CBG), sex hormone binding globulin (SHBG), and others. This bound fraction represents between 95 and 99% of the total concentration of the hormone found in the human body. This bound hormone fraction has no hormonal activity within the human body, and its only function is to serve as a kind of biological reservoir. In contrast to this, hormone activity is exclusively based on the tiny fraction of 1-5% of the hormone that is not bound to a carrier protein, which is referred to as the free-fraction.

There are no reliable analytical methods available on the commercial market for the measurement of this free fraction in serum or plasma.[6] However, this free fraction can easily be measured in saliva, since only the free fraction of the analyte is found in saliva. Neither the carrier-protein bound steroid hormones nor the conjugates are found in saliva.

In order for a laboratory to assess hormone activity (free fraction) in serum it would be necessary to measure: (a) the total concentration of the bound and free steroid, and (b) the concentration of the binding (carrier) protein. Following these two lab tests, it would be necessary to apply a mathematical model to arrive at a theoretical estimate of the hormone activity (free fraction) in serum. This means that two laboratory measurements plus a mathematical formula would be necessary in order to yield one theoretical (indirect) estimate of the level of hormone activity.

Why is only the free steroid hormone fraction present in saliva? In the human body the blood supply and the salivary glands are separated by a porous membrane, this membrane allows small molecules to pass through it, provided that the molecules are non-polar in nature. Therefore very small and non-polar molecules can cross through this membrane by passive diffusion. This phenomenon applies to steroid hormones, which appear first in the blood supply in both the carrier-protein bound (inactive) form and the biologically active free fraction. The biologically active free fraction is capable of migrating through the salivary gland membrane, while the inactive carrier-protein bound fraction and the conjugated fraction are unable to do so. As a result, salivary assessment of steroid hormones provides a direct representation of biological activity and is therefore a valuable tool for clinical diagnostics.

Because a variety of conjugated molecules and polar molecules cannot migrate across the lipophilic salivary gland membrane there is no biochemical proof or reason that hormones such as DHEA-S, T3, or T4 will be found at physiological levels in saliva. The same is true for a variety of proteins such as luteinizing hormone (LH), follicle-stimulating hormone (FSH), prolactin, or thyroid stimulating hormone (TSH). Technically, if these hormones were available at physiological levels in saliva, then the lab assays are indeed capable of detecting them, but there is not much clinical value in doing so.[7-9] It is more likely that any level of these analytes (molecules) detected in saliva represents gingival or blood contamination in saliva, and is unfortunately not linked to physiological levels of analyte that can be used in clinical diagnostics.

As previously mentioned, there is no routine commercial method available for the measurement of the free steroid fraction in serum. There is only one reliable method available for research investigations and that is symmetric equilibrium dialysis. Symmetric equilibrium dialysis is currently the reference method for measuring free hormone fractions in serum samples.

Unfortunately, this reference method is very complex and expensive, and as a result it is not used in routine clinical diagnostics. However, the biological process by which the active free-fraction of steroid hormones in our bodies can pass from the blood supply through the membrane of the salivary gland and into the salivary gland represents a very similar "device" in our body. This "device" in our body mimics much the same function as the laboratory instrument that performs symmetric equilibrium dialysis. Measurement of the free-fraction steroid hormones in saliva follows the same principle as the reference method for serum testing.

Test methods for the detection and measurement of steroid hormones from saliva samples were first described in scientific publications in the 1980's, and have since been a subject of great debate in medical science. Saliva testing was not immediately popular in the clinical arena due to relatively large sample volume requirements, the need for extraction procedures in the testing labs, and the common use of radioimmunoassays to perform the lab tests. These features are not attractive to a medical diagnostic laboratory. Only at the very end of the last century were new saliva testing procedures developed. The newer procedures require small sample volumes and non-radioactive test reagents. These methods are still not commonly found in diagnostic laboratories although they are gaining in popularity.

A significant advantage of saliva testing over serum testing is that obtaining a saliva sample is a non-invasive procedure, whilst serum testing requires venipuncture. This is especially important when testing children, although many adults are uncomfortable with venipuncture sampling as well. In addition, saliva sampling can be done casually throughout the course of a day without the need for a clinic visit and phlebotomy (venipuncture) procedures. Multiple saliva samples can be collected easily within a short time span or over the course of a day, which is frequently desirable when assessing steroid hormones.

There is relative equilibrium between the concentration of steroid hormones found in blood and the concentration found in saliva. This equilibrium has been observed to adjust within 1 or 2 minutes of a fluctuation in steroid hormone concentration in blood. In general, the level of a steroid hormone in saliva is lower by a factor of 20 to 100, compared to the level of that same analyte in blood. This factor is influenced by many inputs and varies by different steroid hormone species. As shown by Vining et al,[10] there is a biphasic correlation changing the slope at the saturation point of the binding globulin. In case of abnormalities of the binding globulin (e.g. pregnancy or oral contraceptives) there is no correlation at all. As a result it is not possible to predict the salivary concentration of a steroid hormone by measuring the level in blood and applying an empirically derived correction factor. However there is good correlation between the free steroid hormone concentration in blood and the salivary steroid concentration. This supports the conclusion that salivary assessment of steroid hormones can be a valuable tool for measurement of steroid concentration in support of clinical diagnostics.

SALIVA SAMPLING

Saliva samples are easy to collect compared to blood samples. Sample collection does not require medical assistance, anxiety or significant discomfort to the patient. Even urine collection requires a place of privacy, which is not essential for a saliva sample. Saliva samples can be collected at home, while travelling, at work, or during physical exercise. As a result it has become possible to investigate new diagnostic strategies, which are not easily contemplated with blood samples.

Due to the extremely low steroid hormone concentrations in saliva there are special requirements for the selection of an appropriate sampling device. For analytes such as the steroid hormones that are expected to be present in a sample in the picogram concentration range, it is possible for several dynamic interactions to influence the analyte. One such interaction is non-specific adsorption of the analyte to certain materials, including many plastics that are commonly used for sample collection devices. This adsorption effect is important when collecting saliva, since saliva does not contain the rich protein concentrations found in blood.

Not all of the steroid hormones exhibit the same tendency for adsorption onto plastic surfaces. Progesterone, however, does demonstrate significant tendency for adsorption and this phenomenon can result in a significant loss of measurable progesterone in the saliva sample. Polyethylene (PE) plastics have a remarkable affinity for Progesterone, and as a consequence PE plastic should never be used for saliva sampling.

In the early days of steroid hormone testing, glass tubes were the preferred sampling devices, and to some extent this is still true today. In fact, glass tubes can be used as a reference for validation of a plastic device. As a note of caution, the stopper can be a weak point in the use of glass collection tubes. Typically, the liquid in a sample collection tube will come into contact with the stopper at some point in the process of shipping a sample to a testing laboratory. Because of this, the stopper must also be considered in adsorption validation studies. In many instances, stoppers for glass collection tubes are made of PE and these should be rejected for saliva sample containers. Moreover glass tubes are fragile and are not optimal for transporting samples or submitting to a laboratory by use of common carriers or the mail service.

Commercial saliva sampling devices called "Salivettes" are available on the market, which include a cotton or plastic roll. The roll is inserted in the mouth and held there until it has become saturated with saliva and then removed and placed inside the Salivette container. Studies have shown that these rolls can be the source of a variety of interaction effects with regard to the steroid hormones.[11, 12] Therefore the use of Salivettes is not recommended for collecting saliva samples for steroid hormone testing.

In summary, validation studies indicate that 2 ml snap-cap tubes made of ultra-pure polypropylene are the container of choice for collecting and submitting saliva samples for steroid hormone lab tests. These tubes come with an integral stopper attached to the tube. The capacity of these tubes is sufficient to accommodate a complete steroid hormone test profile in the laboratory, which can typically be completed with approximately 1 ml of saliva.

Interference in Saliva Testing

As with blood, saliva samples collected immediately after food intake may cause falsely elevated steroid hormone values. Therefore fasting is highly recommended. Specifically, meat and any milk products may have a strong impact on the measurement of salivary steroids and result in falsely elevated levels.

Many common medications and creams contain high concentrations of steroid hormones, and their use may result in remarkably elevated steroid hormone levels in saliva (or serum). In addition to resulting in elevated levels in serum and saliva, there is also the risk that a patient may inadvertently contaminate a saliva collection device by handling it after applying a cream containing steroid hormones. It is important for a patient using any topical creams to thoroughly wash their hands prior to touching and handling any saliva collection device.

Special care must be taken concerning blood contamination of saliva samples. As mentioned earlier, the concentration of steroid hormones in blood is between 20 and 100-fold higher than in saliva. Therefore any blood contamination will result in falsely elevated levels in saliva. All saliva samples should be checked for red coloration (evidence of blood contamination), by holding the sample in front of a sheet of white paper and inspecting for any slight indication of reddish tinge in the saliva. If the saliva in the sampling device shows any reddish tinge, then the sample should be discarded and another sample collected after rinsing both the mouth and the contaminated collection device with water. After waiting 10 minutes another saliva sample should be collected. If this sample still shows a reddish tinge then sampling should be done at another time when there is no bleeding in the mouth.

At certain times it is possible that production of saliva in the mouth is insufficient to collect a saliva sample. It is not recommended to chew anything to stimulate the flow of saliva, as pressure on the teeth from the chewing process will increase the gingiva in saliva and result in falsely elevated steroid measurements.[13]

Stability of Saliva Samples

It is common knowledge in laboratory medicine that serum and plasma samples are rather unstable. As a result, they must be refrigerated or kept cold during both transportation and storage. Saliva samples for steroid testing seem to be significantly more stable. If necessary, saliva samples may be stored at ambient temperature for several days. Saliva samples can be sent to a testing laboratory by routine mail service even in summer without special temperature protection. However, if refrigerator storage is easily available it is desirable, even though it is not required. Colder temperatures will always prevent or retard the growth of bacteria, which can potentially interfere with accurate lab testing. In contrast to serum or plasma samples, saliva samples may also be frozen and re-thawed repeatedly without causing problems. In fact, repeated freezing and thawing of saliva samples will result in lower viscosity, which is desirable in the testing laboratory.

Saliva Sampling Strategies

Optimal timing strategies for the collection of saliva samples will depend upon the diagnostic issue being investigated. Basically there are two strategies: measurement of the steroid hormone dynamics (fluctuation profile) or measurement of the average hormone level. For either scenario the sampling strategy must take into consideration that steroid hormone secretion will vary noticeably within any given timeframe. The dynamics of steroid hormone secretion demonstrates variability within:

- Daily timeframe
- Monthly timeframe
- Definable age categories
- Gender–specific categories

In addition to the categories listed above, it is possible to see additional episodic variation of steroid hormone secretion within a timeframe of between 1 and 3 hours. This episodic variation is seen in serum and plasma samples as well as in saliva. Therefore, lab testing done on a single sample of either blood or saliva is rarely optimal for establishing a diagnostic tool for the clinician to interpret accurately, because it does not account for the normal episodic variation or any of the time-related factors in the categories listed above. It is important to stress that the investigation of a single blood sample for the concentration of steroid hormones has the same inherent issue of reflecting only an arbitrary result.

Reliable lab test results can only be achieved if multiple sampling strategies are used at the time of collection. The only possible exception to this concept might be cortisol, which is the only steroid hormone that can yield clinically useful test results when one single sample is collected and tested. For any of the other steroid hormones, there is no logical alternative to multiple sampling in order to rule out episodic variation. It is unfortunate that the expense, difficulty, and level of discomfort associated with venipuncture and blood-drawing procedures have created an expectation at the clinic sites that one single blood sample is a suitable strategy for steroid hormone measurements. As a result, it is commonly thought that a single sample is appropriate for lab analysis, when the reality is that single sampling is a result of the degree of discomfort and difficulty related to multiple blood draws over a limited period of time. With the growing popularity of saliva sampling to test for steroid hormones it is now possible to collect the multiple samples that are needed to determine more accurate levels.

Physiology of Steroid Secretion

What causes the episodic pattern of steroid hormone secretion? The answer to this question can be found in the feedback mechanism that is a function of the hypothalamic/pituitary glands. These glands are a major part of the time-related control of physiological functions in humans (e.g. control of sleeping patterns). The secretion of hormones such as LH, FSH, or adrenocorticotropic hormone (ACTH) follows an episodic pattern with maximum secretion peaks every 1 to 3 hours. These hormone fluctuations also stimulate the target organs with fluctuating levels of intensity, and the efficiency of target organ stimulation is dependent upon the concentration of the pituitary hormones. Secondary steroid hormone secretion shows time patterns similar to the pituitary hormones.[14] Because steroid hormones are secreted in the free (unbound) form, the episodic secretion pattern is more exaggerated in saliva than it is in blood. This can be clearly seen in the steroid hormones testosterone, progesterone, estradiol, and DHEA. In cortisol it is not that obvious, mostly because the concentration of this steroid in saliva is relatively high. Salivary cortisol assessment will typically reveal a relatively (compared to serum) sharp morning peak followed by diminishing values during the day with lowest values at midnight. But there can be episodic concentration peaks during the day, possibly due to either psychological effects (stress) or food intake.

Measurement of average hormone concentrations (from multiple samples) is the most cost-effective strategy for steroid hormone testing in saliva, giving sufficiently reliable answers for routine steroid hormone testing. In most cases this strategy will provide useful information to the clinician. Because of the episodic secretion pattern it is recommended that multiple samples be collected over a timeframe of 2 or 3 hours beginning after a fasting period of at least 2 or 3 hours. The last meal prior to the collection period should not contain any food from animal origin, especially milk or meat-derived products. For reasons of convenience this collection period could be timed at best in the early morning before breakfast or just prior to a meal either in the late AM or in the PM hours before the evening meal. During the 2-hour timeframe for collecting saliva samples, they should be collected every 30 minutes. Modest variation in the collection timing will not be critical, and the collection timeframe can be extended up to 3 hours. It is only important that there is no food intake during this collection period. Drinking water is allowed and may even be necessary to create sufficient saliva flow.

Laboratory Aspects of Salivary Testing

Upon arrival in the testing lab, all saliva samples should be frozen, preferably overnight. The morning the samples are to be tested, they should be thawed and warmed to room temperature. Following this, the samples should be mixed and centrifuged. This should result in a clear supernatant. If the supernatant is not clear the freezing/thawing/centrifugation cycle should be repeated. After that a final visual check for any reddish color will be done to exclude samples with any sign of blood contamination. If measurement of the mean (average) steroid hormone level has been requested, the lab will need to mix equal aliquots from each of the series of saliva samples in a new collection container prior to testing.

It is important that the laboratory report format of any saliva test to the submitting clinician should also provide the reference ranges that have been established in that lab with the use of the test kits that are currently being used to test patient samples. Therefore it is also important for any testing laboratory to use carefully established reference ranges. For most of the steroid hormones these reference ranges should be specific for gender, age, and timing. It is expected that each test laboratory will generate their own reference ranges rather than relying on published data. If steroid concentrations are reported to the clinician together with reliable reference ranges then the interpretation of lab test results will be reliable and useful as a diagnostic tool.

CONCLUDING REMARKS

The most reliable methods for steroid hormone testing use saliva samples rather than serum samples. Significant advantages have been detailed in numerous scientific publications. It is clear that patients would benefit not only during the sample collection process but also from the improved diagnostic value of the more reliable and accurate laboratory test results derived from saliva samples. Clinicians would benefit from the superior diagnostic value of saliva measurements as well as from sample collection processes that do not depend on the presence (and cost) of a scheduled appointment with a licensed phlebotomist.

It is the author's belief that the time has come to collate existing published scientific information in order to critically review routine laboratory methods for steroid hormone testing as well as patient management/sampling strategies in the clinical setting. Clearly, in an environment where published information implies strongly that guessing would be more accurate than existing laboratory test methods for sera,[2] there is a need for laboratorians, scientists, and clinicians to understand as much as possible about existing alternatives rather than marching blindly forward doing exactly the same thing we did yesterday. There is also a need for continued research and discussion on this subject.

Finally, there exists a form of inertia provided by the manufacturers and the users (testing laboratories) of automated analytical systems for measuring steroid hormones in serum. These systems are one of the anchors for "*status quo*", representing developmental expense and commitment on the part of the manufacturers and hard-money commitment on the part of laboratories that are using them. The very definition of this equation stifles change. The manufacturers and users of these automated systems must be willing and able to speak to questions of whether or not the very samples they test are optimal or whether their recommended samples truly do not require preliminary extraction, as well as questions of their accuracy/reliability at low levels of concentration. Public health, individual patient health, laboratory science, and research-oriented biochemistry would all benefit as a result.

REFERENCES

1. Taieb J, Mathian B, Millot F, Patricot MC, Mathieu E, Queyrel N, Lacroix I, Somma-Delpero C, Boudou P. Testosterone measured by 10 immunoassays and by isotope-dilution gas chromatography-mass spectrometry in sera from 116 men, women, and children. *Clin Chem.* 2003;49:1381-1395.
2. Herold DA, Fitzgerald RL. Immunoassays for testosterone in women: better than a guess? *Clin Chem.* 2003;49:1250-1251.
3. Matsumoto AM, Bremner WJ. Serum testosterone assays--accuracy matters. *J Clin Endocrinol Metab.* 2004;89:520-524.
4. Wang C, Catlin DH, Demers LM, Starcevic B, Swerdloff RS. Measurement of total serum testosterone in adult men: comparison of current laboratory methods versus liquid chromatography-tandem mass spectrometry. *J Clin Endocrinol Metab.* 2004;89:534-543.

5. Stanczyk FZ, Cho MM, Endres DB, Morrison JL, Patel S, Paulson RJ. Limitations of direct estradiol and testosterone immunoassay kits. *Steroids*. 2003;68:1173-1178.
6. Rosner W. An extraordinarily inaccurate assay for free testosterone is still with us. *J Clin Endocrinol Metab*. 2001;86:2903.
7. Lac G, Lac N, Robert A. Steroid assays in saliva: a method to detect plasmatic contaminations. *Arch Int Physiol Biochim Biophys*. 1993;101:257-262.
8. Vining RF, McGinley RA. The measurement of hormones in saliva: possibilities and pitfalls. *J Steroid Biochem*. 1987;27:81-94.
9. Thijssen JH, Van Goozen SH, Van Engeland H, Matute LM, Blankenstein MA. None of four commercially available assays detects prolactin in human saliva. *Clin Chem*. 2000;46:1409-1410.
10. Vining RF, McGinley RA, Maksvytis JJ, Ho KY. Salivary cortisol: a better measure of adrenal cortical function than serum cortisol. *Ann Clin Biochem*. 1983;20:329-335.
11. Groschl M, Rauh M. Influence of commercial collection devices for saliva on the reliability of salivary steroids analysis. *Steroids*. 2006;71:1097-100.
12. Shirtcliff EA, Granger DA, Schwartz E, Curran MJ. Use of salivary biomarkers in biobehavioral research: cotton-based sample collection methods can interfere with salivary immunoassay results. *Psychoneuroendocrinology*. 2001;26:165-173.
13. Vining RF, McGinley RA, Symons RG. Hormones in saliva: mode of entry and consequent implications for clinical interpretation. *Clin Chem*. 1983;29:1752-1756.
14. West CD, Mahajan DK, Chavre VJ, Nabors CJ, Tyler FH. Simultaneous measurement of multiple plasma steroids by radioimmunoassay demonstrating episodic secretion. *J Clin Endocrinol Metab*. 1973;36:1230-1236.

ABOUT THE AUTHOR

Dr. Wolfgang Ziemann is a biochemist based in Germany. He is a well-known specialist for hormone testing in central Europe. After leaving the university in 1975 he joined a medical diagnostic lab and developed the first quantitative immunoassays for the measurement of steroids in serum using tritiated tracer and extraction with organic solvents. He has used such assays for 4 years in the medical testing lab. Then he switched to the professional industry for developing such immunoassays to be used in medical diagnostic testing labs world wide. The new assay techniques used for the development of routine steroid assays have been direct methods without extraction using Iodine-125 tracers. In 1995 he started the development and the production of steroid assays for salivary testing. At the beginning these have been chemiluminescence assays, later he switched to the ELISA technology. Currently he is building up a major commercial laboratory for saliva testing in Germany. He is fully dedicated to saliva testing of steroids covering the development and production of such testkits as well as the practical use in the diagnostic laboratory for routine patient care.

Protocol Chapter 1
The PATH to Life Extension Executive Health Program

Eric R. Braverman, M.D.
Director, PATH Research Foundation;
Director, Integrative Medicine Program, Cabrini Medical Center

CASE STUDY
36 y.o. female complains of fatigue, headache, night sweats, chest pain, frequent urination, sexual dysfunction, back pain, loss of balance, memory loss, anxiety, panic attacks, depression, and sleeping problems.

INVESTIGATIONS

Initial Survey:

- **Medical History**: past medical history (diseases, disorders, illnesses, surgeries, injuries), social history, current medical state (diseases, disorders, illnesses, symptoms, conditions, allergies), and family history.
- **Measurements**: height, weight, BMI, pulse, blood pressure, comprehensive physical exam.
- **Questionnaire:** (degree of) signs and symptoms, primary medical conditions, and questions.

Diagnostic Testing Based on Initial Survey:

- **Head-to-Toe Ultrasounds:** echocardiogram, carotid, transcranial, thyroid, pelvic, breast, abdominal, hepatic, and renal ultrasounds.
- **Vascular Studies:** ABI, bi-lateral digits, MVO
- **Bone Density:** Dual Energy X-ray Absorptiometry (DEXA), body fat/muscle composition
- **Nerve Conduction Velocity (NCV)**
- **Psychological Studies:** Millon, MBTI, MMSE, WMS III, GAMA, CNSVS, Y-Bocs
- **Brain Electrical Activity Mapping (BEAM):** VEP testing, AEP testing, extended EEG, quantitative EEG, TOVA
- **Nutritional:** Rainbow diet consultation and CES device demonstration and consultation.
- **PET-Whole Body** (outside facility)
- **Allergy Testing**
- **Urinalysis & Blood Draw:**

Anemia	Vitamin & Mineral	Diabetes	Urine	Immune	Health Scan I	Health Scan II	Thyroid
Ferritin (RIA)	Lead	Hemoglobin A1C	Urine Microalbumin	ESR	Chem screen	Free T3	T3
Vitamin B12	Cadmium	Insulin level	Urine Drug Screen 10 with confirm	CRP	RPR	Free T4	T3 uptake
RBC Folate	Aluminum	Erythropoietin		T-helper / T supp ratio	U/A		T4 total
	Mercury						Thyroid Auto-Abs

Osteoporosis	Cacitonin	Ionized calcium	Osteocalcin	Parathyroid hormone	Urine Telopeptides	Vitamin D,1,25 Dihydroxy	Vitamin D,25 hydroxy

Endocrine	LH	DHEA	TSH – 3rd gen	Estradiol – day of cycle____	Progesterone	Prolactin RIA	Testosterone (Free & Total)
	FSH	Fract. Estrogen (F)	Serum cortisol	Sex Hormone Bind. Globulin	DHEA-S	Pregnenolone	IGF-1, IGF-BP3
	DHT						

Lipid	Triglycerides	Cholesterol	HDL cholesterol	LDL cholesterol	Fibrinogen	Homocysteine

Hypertension	**GH**
CBC with diff	Leptin

TREATMENT PLAN
Brain Health
- CES device usage (45 minutes – 1 hour)
- Risperdal
- Klonopin
- Amino acid supplements (Brain Calm, Brain Energy, Brain Mood, Brain Memory).
- Consultation (to discuss how obesity can have an overall ill effect by impacting brain chemistry which affects pulmonary, cardiac, endocrine function, and brain health)
- Tenuate SR 75 mg
- Citrinate
- CLA with Rainbow diet
- Daily exercise regimen
- Food diary (for evaluation)
- Follow up with PATH Medical, PC nutritionist.
- Repeat body fat composition test in one year.
- Vitamin B_{12}
- Multivitamin
- MRI-Brain
- Tyramine diet
- Follow up with neurosurgeon and neurologist.

Cardiovascular
- Exercise regimen
- Perform thallium stress test
- Perform CT-angiogram
- Perform MRI/MRA of brain
- Perform MVO
- Nutritional supplements - Vitamin B complex, Omega-3 fish oil, Niacin, and Cholestene
- Ecotrin 81 mg
- Repeat ECG/Echocardiogram in one year and monitor
- Repeat carotid and transcranial ultrasounds in one year
- Repeat circulatory tests in one year
- Monitor inflammatory markers on blood tests
- Monitor for worsening of symptoms
- Monitor clotting factor blood tests
- Follow up with a cardiologist and a vascular specialist

Endocrine
- Perform glucose tolerance test
- Lantus, Vasotec, and Humalog
- Biotin 5 mg
- Chromium 500 mg
- Glucosynergy
- Pregnenolone
- Weight reduction and diet modification
- Monitor fasting glucose, insulin, HbA1C blood levels
- Monitor urinalysis/microalbumin levels
- Monitor sex hormone blood levels
- Follow up with endocrinologist and ophthalmologist recommended

Gastrointestinal/Genitourinary

- N-Acetylcysteine
- Alpha lipoic acid
- Repeat abdominal and renal ultrasound in one year
- Monitor liver and pancreatic function tests
- Monitor for worsening of symptoms
- Repeat and monitor urinalysis and kidney function blood tests
- Follow up with GI specialist
- Increase fluid intake

Hematological

- Repeat blood test
- Monitor heavy metal blood levels
- Monitor canned food intake
- Chelation therapy

Musculoskeletal

- Promote weight-bearing exercises
- Advise over-the-counter medication (Ibuprofen) for pain.
- Nutritional supplements – Osteo Pak
- Monitor Vitamin D/PTH/calcium/phosphorus/calcitonin/osteocalcin blood levels, urine telopeptides.
- Repeat bone density test in two years.
- Follow up with acupuncturist.

Dermatological

- Metrogel 1%
- Follow up with dermatologist

Physician assistants and doctors are to follow-up with patients once a week or every two weeks (via telephone consults or visits). During this time, patients must fill-out a Review of Systems check-in-sheet and mark down symptoms and/or concerns, as well as any questions regarding their health or treatment plan. This method ensures patient satisfaction and quality treatment.

ABOUT THE AUTHOR

Dr. Eric Braverman is the Director of The Place for Achieving Total Health (PATH Medical), with locations in New York, NY, Penndel, PA (metro-Philadelphia), and a national network of affiliated medical professionals. Dr. Braverman received his B.A. Summa Cum Laude from Brandeis University and his M.D. with honors from New York University Medical School, after which he performed post-graduate work in internal Medicine with Yale Medical School affiliate. Dr. Braverman is the author of five medical books, including the *PATH Wellness Manual*, which is a user's guide to alternative treatment. He has appeared on CNN (Larry King Live), PBS, AHN, MSNBC, Fox News Channel and local TV stations. Dr. Braverman has been quoted in the *New York Post, New York Times* and the *Wall Street Journal*.

Protocol Chapter 2
Protocols for Work-Up and Anti-Aging Treatment
for Photodamaged Skin

Madalene C.Y. Heng, M.D., FRACP, FACD
Clinical Professor of Medicine/Dermatology at UCLA School of Medicine

INTRODUCTION

Photoaging skin is characterized by cosmetic changes such as atrophy, pigmentation, and telangiectasia, as well as wrinkling and increased laxity of the skin. More importantly, photodamaged skin is associated with the development of skin cancers, such as basal cell carcinomas, squamous cell carcinomas, and malignant melanomas, which are preceded by premalignant lesions such as actinic keratoses, solar lentigenes, and premalignant lentigo maligna. Both the premalignant and malignant lesions are associated with DNA damage. While the premalignant lesions are associated with DNA damage in the promoter sequence, additional damage to the p53 suppressor gene transforms the cell into the malignant phenotype. DNA damage may occur as point mutations, or by the release of bipyrimidine photoproducts. Point mutations on the DNA are caused by both ultraviolet A (UVA) and ultraviolet B (UVB) exposure. These tend to be more easily repaired. However, bipyrimidine photoproducts from UVA exposure tend to convert to Dewar products, causing damage which is poorly repaired, and therefore highly mutagenic. While UVB is known to produce redness, burning and blistering, these rays (290-320 nm) do not penetrate much below the skin surface, and cause more damage to the keratinocytes than to basal cells and melanocytes. On the other hand, UVA penetrates down to the deep dermis, and is the major wavelength causing basal cell carcinomas, malignant melanomas and dermal changes associated with photoaging such as solar elastoses, telangiectasia, wrinkling, and sagging of the skin. While UVB rays are blocked by clothing and sunscreens, UVA rays are effectively blocked only by bone. For this reason, melanomas and basal cell carcinomas have been observed to develop in areas usually covered by clothing. In view of the lack of adequate protection against UVA exposure by current sunscreens, the use of alternative measures directed at antiphotocarcinogenesis is being explored. More recently, curcumin, the active ingredient in turmeric, has been shown to have anticarcinogenic properties, with the ability to selectively induce apoptosis in photodamaged cells, while leaving normal cells unaffected. We have observed improvement in premalignant lesions such as solar lentigenes, actinic keratoses, as well as erythema, pigmentation, telangiectasia, and wrinkling. However, the improvement, although lasting, is not immediate, but requires at least 6 months to a year or more to effect.

SUGGESTED PROTOCOLS

Initial Work-Up:

This includes a detailed past and family history of non-melanoma skin cancers (basal cell carcinomas, squamous cell carcinomas) and malignant melanomas (type, level, lymph node dissection etc). A positive family history of melanoma suggests that there may be a genetic predisposition, particularly if the patient is young or has multiple melanomas. It is believed that in some cases, there is a genetic defect in the DNA ligase, the enzyme that repairs DNA damage after UV exposure.

The history should include amount of sun exposure (work-related, golf, walking/running, swimming, fishing, surfing, sailing, and gardening), and the time of day of sun-exposure. Smoking is also a predisposing factor, as well as exposure to arsenic and radioactive products.

The patient should have a thorough total body skin check from the scalp to the toes to look for abnormalities such as premalignant lesions (solar lentigenes, dysplastic nevi, actinic keratoses), and malignant lesions (lentigo maligna, malignant melanoma, Bowen's disease (squamous cell carcinoma in situ), squamous cell carcinomas, and basal cell carcinomas.)

Skin Biopsies and Excisions:

The malignant lesions should be biopsied and removed/excised accordingly.

Photography

Premalignant lesions should be photographed for future monitoring. The patient should be followed up every 3 months and the same lesions/locations photographed using the same magnification and same lighting. Should these lesions fail to improve with the curcumin gel, they should be biopsied, and dealt with according to the biopsy results.

Curcumin Gel Therapy

(1) Photodamaged Skin, Pigmentation, Telangiectasia, Wrinkles:

After a morning shower, the skin is "pat-dried" with a towel. The product spreads more easily if the skin is slightly damp (but not wet). A dab of curcumin gel is transferred from the jar with a Q tip, spreading the curcumin gel all over the affected area with the fingers to cover as large an area as the gel will allow until the area feels dry. This ensures that only a thin layer of gel is applied to the skin. More gel may be applied as necessary. Do not double dip to avoid transferring the bacteria from the skin back into the jar. After use, close the lid tightly to avoid drying out of the product. Application of rubbing alcohol before the curcumin gel is not necessary.

Photographs with close-ups of the skin before treatment is started, with sequential photographs every three to six months during therapy, is recommended in order to detect subtle changes in skin wrinkling, telangiectasia, and pigmentation. The photographs should be with Polaroid film, complete with dates of exposure so that the "Before" and "After" photographs can also be assessed by the patient at the time of the visit.

(2) Actinic Keratoses:

Areas with multiple actinic keratoses are treated in the same way as for photodamaged skin by first applying a thin layer all over the affected area (face, forearms, hands etc...). If the keratosis has a thick scale, the thick scale will prevent the curcumin gel from penetrating the skin beneath the scale. To enhance the penetration of curcumin through the scale, pretreat the keratosis with a little alcohol. Then massage curcumin gel into the wet alcohol, which will then "drag" the curcumin gel through and under the scale.

(3) Solar Lentigenes and Premalignant melanomas:

Biopsies may first be performed to make sure that the lesion is not a lentigo maligna or a malignant melanoma. Curcumin gel should be applied over the lesion and the rest of the surrounding skin. After the curcumin gel is dry, apply a layer of sunscreen solely over the pigmented lesion. Photography is essential at 3 monthly intervals. Be prepared to perform surgery if the lesion enlarges or does not improve.

Sunscreens

Select a sunscreen with a higher SPF (sun protection factor) number i.e. 45 to 70. Make sure that the patient is not allergic to the sunscreen. The sunscreen should be applied above the curcumin gel layer if the patient plans to be exposed to sunlight.

For pigmentary lesions such as melasma and solar lentigenes, curcumin gel is first applied all over the face or hands/forearms. When the curcumin gel is dry, which should be almost immediate or shortly after application, sunscreens are applied to the areas of pigmentation, taking care to apply more sunscreens to the darker areas and less to the lighter areas, so that the dark areas will lighten more than the light areas.

ABOUT THE AUTHOR

Dr. Madalene Heng is Clinical Professor of Medicine/Dermatology at UCLA School of Medicine. From 1979 to 2003, she was Chief, Division of Dermatology, UCLA San Fernando Valley Medicine Program. She is currently practicing at the Centers for Family Health, Community Memorial Hospital, Ventura, California. Dr. Heng is a reviewer for the Journal of the American Academy of Dermatology, American Journal of Geriatric Medicine, British Journal of Dermatology, Lancet, London, and International Journal of Angiology. With more than 130 scientific publications, including 71 published peer-reviewed articles on topics such as phosphorylase kinase activity and psoriasis, pathophysiology of disease, and wound healing, Dr. Heng is able to link treatment of diseases to their etiology at the basic science level. Dr. Heng is the developer of curcumin gel (Psoria-Gold).

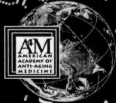

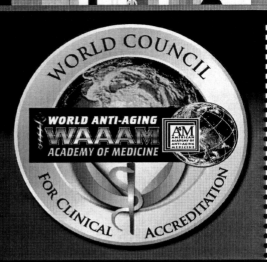

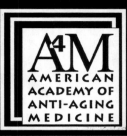
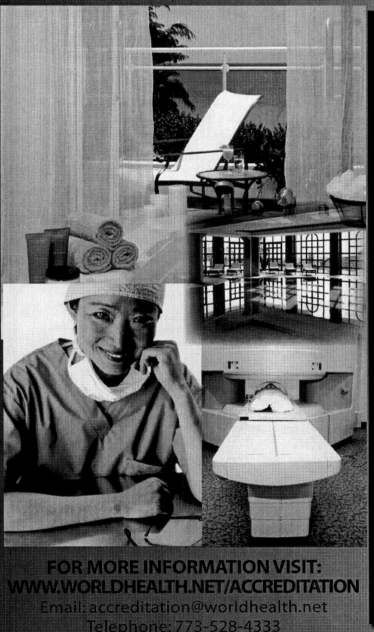
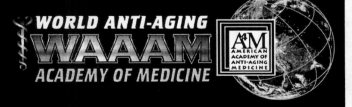

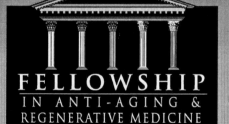
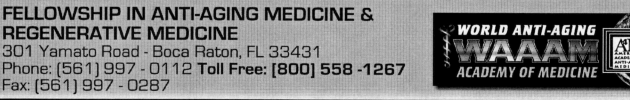

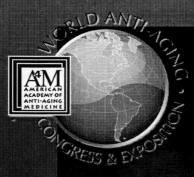
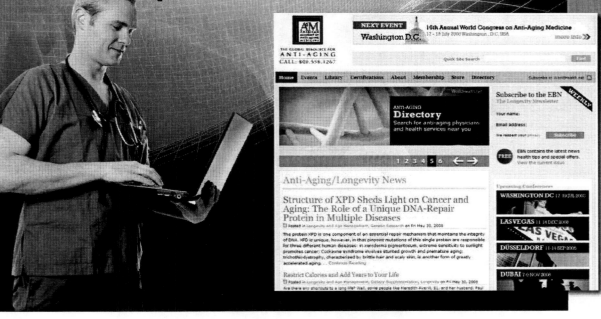

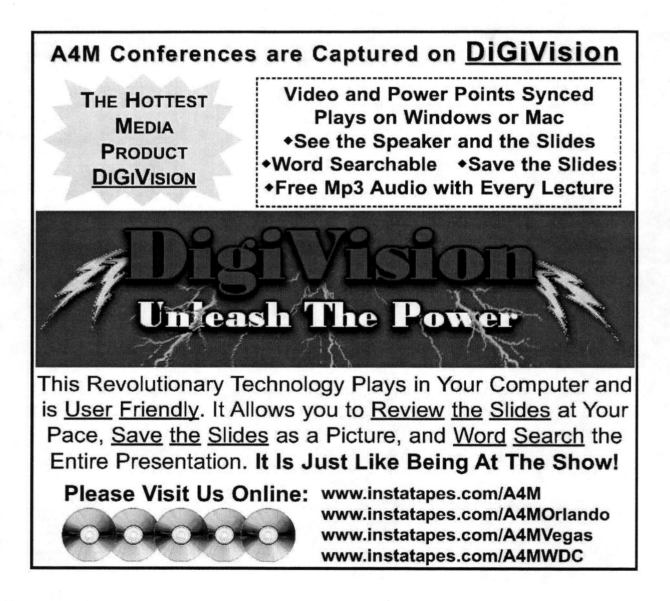